Blockchain for Healthcare Data Management

This fascinating book delves into the transformative role that blockchain technology could play in the security and integrity of patient data within the healthcare sector.

In an era where data breaches and privacy concerns loom large, blockchain has emerged as a potential solution to these challenges, offering a route to streamline healthcare processes, manage data and improve patient outcomes. The book begins by providing a comprehensive overview of its underlying principles, including decentralization, immutability and consensus mechanisms, before exploring, through a range of international case studies, how blockchain has been applied so far within the healthcare sector, from the management of electronic health records and clinical trials to medical billing and supply chain management. The authors also explore the barriers to the wider adoption of blockchain, including financial investment and regulatory issues.

The first book to focus solely on the potential of blockchain within the healthcare sector, it will appeal to international scholars, students and healthcare professionals interested in issues around patient confidentiality, data security and IT management.

Akhil Sharma is currently working as Professor and Principal at the R.J. College of Pharmacy, Raipur, Aligarh, U.P., India.

Shaweta Sharma is currently employed as Professor at Galgotias University, Greater Noida, U.P., India.

Neeraj Kumar Fuloria is currently working as Senior Associate Professor at AIMST University, Malaysia.

Shivkanya Fuloria is currently working as Senior Associate Professor at AIMST University, Malaysia.

Blockchain for Healthcare Data Management

A New Approach to Security and Privacy

Edited by
Shaweta Sharma, Akhil Sharma,
Neeraj Kumar Fuloria and Shivkanya Fuloria

Routledge
Taylor & Francis Group
LONDON AND NEW YORK

First published 2026
by Routledge
4 Park Square, Milton Park, Abingdon, Oxon OX14 4RN

and by Routledge
605 Third Avenue, New York, NY 10158

Routledge is an imprint of the Taylor & Francis Group, an informa business

British Library Cataloguing-in-Publication Data
A catalogue record for this book is available from the British Library

ISBN: 978-1-032-86629-1 (hbk)
ISBN: 978-1-041-00857-6 (pbk)
ISBN: 978-1-003-52991-0 (ebk)

DOI: 10.4324/9781003529910

Typeset in Times New Roman
by codeMantra

Contents

Figures

Tables

Contributors

Neeraj Kumar Fuloria is currently working as Senior Associate Professor, AIMST University, Malaysia. He has over 22 years of experience spanning academics, research and industry. His publication records include three MOOCs, three books, 11 book chapters, 15 patents and 187 research papers. He has successfully obtained nine national and international research grants. His research supervision experience includes mentoring two PhD students (completed), with six ongoing, and guiding six postgraduate students (completed), with two ongoing. He has participated in 126 conferences, trainings, webinars and seminars. Additionally, he has been honoured with six awards for his contributions to the field.

Shivkanya Fuloria is currently working as Senior Associate Professor at AIMST University, Malaysia. She has over 20 years of experience spanning academics, research and industry. She holds qualifications in B. Pharm., M.Pharm., Ph.D. in Pharmacy and a PDCTM. Her publication records include three MOOCs, five books, 11 book chapters, 14 patents and 166 papers. She has supervised one Ph.D., five M.Pharm., two M.Sc. and 27 B.Pharm. students. She has participated in 87 conferences, trainings, webinars and seminars. Additionally, she has been honoured with six awards for his contributions to the field.

Akanksha Sharma is working as Assistant Professor at the R.J. College of Pharmacy, Raipur, Aligarh, U.P., India. She has completed B.Pharm. from the Kashi Institute of Pharmacy, Varanasi in 2018. She has completed M.Pharm. (Pharmaceutics) from Galgotias University in 2020. She has published many research and review papers, mostly in Scopus indexed journals. She is a good motivator and provides guidance to students for being a good pharmacy professional, researcher and to be more human.

Akhil Sharma is currently working as Professor and Principal at the R.J. College of Pharmacy, Raipur, Aligarh, U.P., India. He has completed his Ph.D. in 2016 from Teerthanker Mahaveer University, Moradabad, U.P., India. He has been serving the profession of Pharmacy for more than 15 years. He has published articles in many peer-reviewed national and international journals.

Shaweta Sharma is currently employed as Professor at Galgotias University, Greater Noida, U.P., India. She has completed her Ph.D. in 2017 from Teerthanker Mahaveer University, Moradabad, U.P., India. She has been contributing to academics for more than 15 years. She has published articles in many peer-reviewed national and international journals.

Sunita is working as Assistant Professor at the R.J. College of Pharmacy, Raipur, Aligarh, U.P., India. She has completed B.Pharm. from the I.T.S. College of Pharmacy, Ghaziabad in 2017. She has completed M.Pharm. in Pharmaceutics from the Metro College of Health Sciences and Research, Greater Noida, in 2024. She has published many research and review papers, mostly in Scopus indexed journals. She is a good motivator and provides guidance to students for being a good pharmacy professional, researcher and to be more human.

Shilpa Thukral is currently employed as the Head of the Department at Dnyan Ganga Education Trust's College of Pharmacy, Thane, India. She has completed M.Pharm. in Pharmaceutical Chemistry from Rajiv Academy, Mathura, U.P., India. She has been contributing to academics for more than 15 years. She has published articles in many peer-reviewed national and international reputed journals.

Ashish Verma is working as Assistant Professor at Mangalmay Pharmacy College, Greater Noida, U.P., India. He has completed M.Pharm. in Pharmacology from Monad University. He has two years of teaching and two years of industry experience. He has published several research articles and review articles in national and international reputed journals. He has also published several book chapters with reputed publishers.

Acknowledgement

Authors are highly thankful to their Universities/Colleges for providing library facilities for the literature survey.

1 Introduction to Blockchain Technology in Healthcare

Ashish Verma, Shaweta Sharma, Akanksha Sharma, Sunita, Shivkanya Fuloria and Akhil Sharma

Introduction to Blockchain Architecture

The data is stored on a decentralized node network known as the blockchain. It is an excellent technology that protects sensitive data inside the system. This technology is used to exchange critical data and keep it secure and confidential. It is a perfect tool to keep all the documents together in one secure place. Using a single patient database, crypto reduces the time it takes to search for applicants who meet certain trial criteria. The blockchain can be referred to as a distributed peer-to-peer (P2P) network of personal computers, which is known by the term node and helps to maintain, store, and record historical or transaction data. This makes for a more trustworthy partnership as all those in the network hold the information and maintain an ongoing record of empirical information. It would enable the integration of different networks to organize insights into the value of individual treatment. Hence, blockchain can be truly identified for immutability and security.[1]

There are three high-level concepts in blockchain: block, node, and miner. Blockchain stores none of its data in a central location. Rather, the blockchain is copied and spread across a network of computers.[2] When a new block is added to the blockchain, every computer on the web updates its blockchain. A blockchain system operates over the Internet on a P2P network of computers, all running the protocol with a copy of the transaction ledger, allowing value transmission without an intermediary through machine consensus.[3]

Components of Blockchain

Blockchains leverage high-level cryptographic concepts like hashing, asymmetric key cryptography, and digital signatures, often combined with record-keeping principles. Hashing methods, transactions, public key cryptography (PKC), address & wallet, blocks, and consensus mechanisms are some of the detailed components. Figure 1.1 is depicting the different components of blockchain technology.[4]

DOI: 10.4324/9781003529910-1

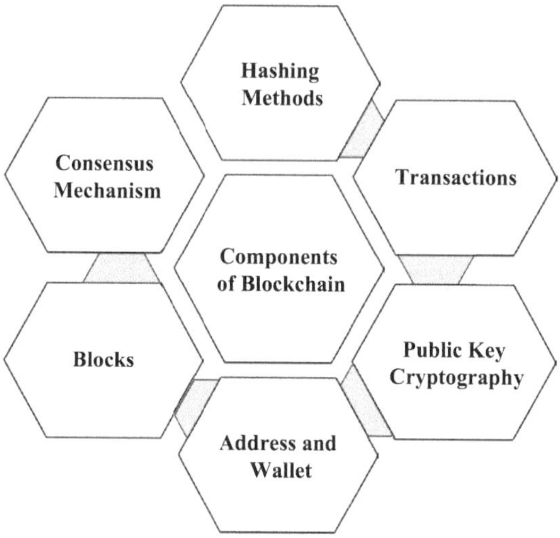

Figure 1.1 Components of blockchain.

Hashing Methods

Hashing functions (a cryptographic mechanism) are the most crucial element of a blockchain. Hashing is a cryptographic method that converts input data of arbitrary length into an output of fixed size that will always be unique. The input can be any text, file, or image; the output is a fixed-size alpha-numeric string. In blockchain, Hashing ensures that the data exchanged among the users is not altered. This can be achieved by calculating the hash of input data. This means that even a small change in input leads to very drastic changes in output(hash). This is because of the security property of the hashing technique in blockchain. (i) Pre-image resistant: Hashing algorithms are typically one-way. It is not possible to determine the input from an output. (ii) Second preimage resistant: Based on the given input, it is impossible to compute the second input that generates the same output. (iii) Collision resistant: Two inputs that produce the same hash output are difficult to find.[2]

Transactions

In blockchain, a transaction is either an interaction of two entities. The transfer of Bitcoin or any other cryptocurrency from one user to another is termed a transaction, whereas, in a business scenario, the transfer of ownership or activities involved in digital assets is considered a transaction. Each block includes 0 or more transactions. Transaction input, output, sender's address, public key, and digital signatures are the data typically found in a transaction. Transactions are mainly used for the transfer of digital objects and data transfer.

In a basic scenario, an individual may permanently publish public data on the blockchain. Or use it to transfer and process the data and store this result in a blockchain, like in a smart contracts system. Beyond mere transmission, the validity and authenticity of the data are crucial. Most importantly, the transaction validity and authenticity of exchanging data are important. This means that validity ensures that the transaction follows blockchain implementation specification protocols, and authenticity indicates that the sender of a transaction possesses the digital assets transmitted. The transaction is digitally signed by the sender using his private key and verifiable by anyone with the sender's public key.[5]

Public Key Cryptography

Asymmetric key cryptography (public key cryptography) is used in blockchain for many functions. In asymmetric key, two keys are used, which are public and private key related mathematically. There are two keys as part of this: a public key that is visible to anyone and a private key that is kept secret. However, the public key is known, and it will be impossible to derive a private key. It can encrypt data with a public key while decrypting with the corresponding private key. This process can be vice-versa.

This cryptographic method offers users authenticity and integrity of the data but also transparency. For this reason, asymmetric key cryptography is slow to compute encryption and decryption. The symmetric key encryption methodology that uses a single key for encryption and decryption is tried and tested, but this signifies trust between users in sharing the keys. To simplify the process, data is encrypted using the symmetric key technique, and then the same symmetric key is encrypted using the asymmetric key technique. Thus, the speed of the asymmetric key algorithm is significantly increased.[6]

Address and Wallet

Addresses typically contain a portion of alphanumeric characters used as transaction points for a sender and receiver. The user's public key is generated using a hash function. There are several ways to derive the addresses depending on different blockchain implementations. Blockchain network users need to keep their private keys secure. Software is used to store them now instead of just manually storing them. Wallets are referred to as the software used to store the private keys. In addition, the wallets can keep the user addresses and public keys besides private keys. Wallets are used to compute how many crypto assets belong to a given trusted person.[7]

Blocks

Software, such as web services, mobile applications, etc., will submit the transactions made by the user to the network. After a transaction submission, the software will send it to one or more nodes. It does not mean the transaction is added to the blockchain. These transactions will be queued on the publishing node and added to the blockchain when the node pulls a block. A block consists of a block header containing the metadata about the block and a block body containing all valid transactions.[8]

Consensus Mechanism

To directly indicate a user to whom blocks publish eventually behind the technology, and that is crucial nowadays in blockchain. When a network node publishes a block, it will discover cryptocurrency. As a result, multiple nodes can compete to publish nodes. Consensus mechanisms can be used to solve this problem. This enables a batch of users who do not rely on each other to collaborate.

Various consensus models are being utilized, such as Proof of Work, Proof of Stake, Proof of Authority, Proof of Elapsed Time, etc. A consensus mechanism is a way of making decisions by which the network users agree and support a decision to benefit their network. In the consensus model, block adding in blockchain requires a miner (node) to solve a cryptographic puzzle. The puzzle-solving process is a large computation and cannot be easily solved. After solving the puzzle, it will be sent to the network for confirmation. The block will be appended to the chain once the verification process is complete.[9]

Types of Blockchain

Bitcoin is the initial application of blockchains created by Satoshi Nakamoto. Originally proposed in 2008, Bitcoin was designed to allow two parties to transact without needing a trusted third party. Instead of relying on trust, the system relies on cryptographic proofs. There are two types of blockchains: permissionless blockchains and permissioned blockchains.

Permissionless Blockchains

Public blockchains are a kind of P2P decentralized network that enables everyone to join the network and write transactions without a trusted third party. Public blockchains are permissionless due to their unattainable access for certain nodes. The network utilizes blockchains to validate, store, and preserve information regarding the transactions taking place over it. These transactions are recorded on the public ledger in blocks. Special nodes called miners verify each transaction exchanged between the different nodes and add it to the blockchain. All transactions are stored in a public blockchain, and its contents are visible to virtually everyone, including adversaries. While the records are on the public ledger, off-chain is where the data is exchanged between parties.[10]

Consensus is required and can only be attained when the miner nodes solve a complex mathematical problem called proof of work; at this point, the block gets appended to the chain. Public blockchains, therefore, require a reward mechanism to encourage users to run nodes in the public network and mine blocks of transactions for the given rewards in terms of CPU time, electricity, etc. Ethereum blockchain is one of the most popular and is used as a public blockchain nowadays.[11] In the Ethereum blockchain, Ether (Ethereum currency) is spawned and issued to the first node that successfully mines the block. A block is verified and gets a permanent place in the chain. When you want to modify or change a block, the hash value of that block has to be recomputed, and all blocks after it, so it is very hard for attackers to forge. In addition, attackers will never be able to change a blockchain since the chain is decentralized and saved in many nodes.

Several research projects have recently been undertaken to use public blockchains in these areas. MedRec most recently followed this. The MedRec model uses the Ethereum platform to build a smart contract-based decentralized medical record-sharing system. This is essential for exchanging medical records among medical stakeholders, patients, and any other third party processing medical or health records. The MedRec system supports two mining modes: Providers can append patients' records at any time but control the data suggested by MedRec. The first is logistic based on the model of Ether as a rewarding mechanism, and the second model uses aggregated and anonymized data as a reward to encourage researchers who would like data to be able to access it, but only if they are the first node who mine the block.[12]

Permissioned Blockchains

Though many attributes of blockchains provide an appropriate basis for decentralized applications like smart healthcare systems, it is impossible to directly store and transmit sensitive data, such as healthcare records, in blockchains without taking the required precautions. Public blockchains are not only about confidentiality but more likely about publicly available data storage that cannot be manipulated without leaving traces.

In addition, sending and storing bulky data on blockchains can create scalability challenges for large-scale and widely adopted applications of blockchains, such as healthcare systems. In response to this, the industry has developed, for commercial applications, a narrower version of the original technology called permissioned blockchains. It is believed that by adding other features to the basic blockchains model, permissioned blockchains offer enhanced confidentiality, privacy, and scalability.[13]

Permissioned blockchains can be further divided into private blockchains and consortium blockchains. While both run on a private network, there has been some focus between the private and consortium blockchains. Both blockchains are permissioned, meaning that access to data and the ability to submit transactions directly to the blockchains are restricted to a predefined set of entities.

Private Blockchains

A private blockchain is a blockchain where write permissions are kept centralized to one organization/entity, but read permissions can be made public or restricted to an arbitrary extent. Private blockchains use a decentralized topology to ensure that only selected participants can see the blockchain's activity, introduce control over which transactions are allowed, and let mining be done safely without proof of work and other related costs.

Due to access limitations overwrite and read rights, private blockchains provide high privacy. The second benefit of private blockchains over public blockchains is the ease at which a company can change/modify the rules in use and reverse transactions. In addition, the validators are public knowledge, so there is no way to add fake blocks to the chain. Moreover, it is possible to solve the scalability issues since people can manually intervene in case faults occur inside very well-connected nodes, and participants within the chain can control block size maximum. Additionally, only verified participants confirm transactions, resulting in lower processing power and, thus, more cost-effective transactions.[14]

Private blockchains are defined as distributed ledgers consisting of blocks with the consensus of the transaction between whoever has permission to enter them. Authorization of any node will make a transaction or block. Without cryptographic hashing, the judge will validate and propagate the transaction.

In private blockchains, trust is not decentralized; the judge adds new records and has a centralized distributed ledger. However, other nodes may have public or somewhat limited read permissions. Each time a transaction occurs, all the nodes involved will notify the judge to record and update the state of this specific transaction onto the ledger. Trust among nodes is an attribute of private blockchains. Therefore, private blockchains are close to a normal distributed database.[15]

Consortium Blockchains

Consortium blockchains are those where the consensus process is controlled by a preselected set of nodes (i.e., entities.) When consensus happens via an agreement to validate the transaction by a group from the prechosen set of nodes, the block gets included in the chain. For instance, if there are five known/trusted nodes in the chain, they must sign the block to be appended to the chain before it is processed/added to the chain, and then a minimum of three entities should be signed.[16]

The read access on a consortium blockchain may be available to everyone (public), or it can be made closed and accessible only by the participants. Also, unlike private blockchains, consortium blockchains are only partially decentralized. The consortium blockchain model is more attractive to companies because, unlike private blockchains, it is decentralized. In healthcare, A consortium blockchain would be deployed using a distributed database across several access points, allowing health organizations to use the dictating ledger to share patients' Electronic Medical Records (EMR) information.[17]

Therefore, on a consortium blockchain, "there is no risk of a breach in PHI security as only people who typically had access to this information were able to obtain it." For instance, the receptionist will be able to see only the identification details of all patients, while a caregiver will view medical records only of his patients. Some previous implementations of building consortium blockchains for healthcare include MedChain, ModelChain, and BlockInsure.[18]

Overview of Blockchain Technology in the Healthcare Sector

Challenges posed by modernization in the current century have necessitated rapid development of technologies over the last decade. In modern-day lives, technologies like the Internet of Things (IoT), Augmented reality, machine learning, and blockchain find their way into daily lives. Blockchain is where information can be shared among the domains that do not trust each other, and we humans have learned to manage a decentralized database. Blockchain will join in the decision-making process in a collaborative and coordinated way. Blockchain technology significantly disrupted business, changing the industry at all levels. It makes new supply chains, healthcare, agriculture, banking, and so on through a trustful atmosphere with security and transparency.

Health informatics is the branch of medical informatics that focuses on the clinical domain and technology translation in healthcare delivery. Healthcare informatics is evolving due to shifts in both technology and healthcare. Health informatics offers the capabilities to furnish health professionals and healthcare organizations with non-divisible knowledge bases, which gives patients a better quality of care services using current technologies. Obtaining and documenting medical and patient data, communicating with healthcare providers, selecting relevant diagnostic means, interpreting lab results, and collecting clinical study information are collectively called Information Processing and Communications within the healthcare sector.

Many countries have widely adopted electronic health records (EHR) and hospital information systems (HISs). At present, HISs are primarily cloud-based, housed by a single data vendor, and have numerous pitfalls, including inadequate security. Consequently, there have been countless instances of breaches and questions around the validity and sharing of data, leading to patients being vulnerable to economic threats and potential social stigma. Attackers find centralized data or information attractive for cyber-attacks, and this results in problems because a persistent view of the patient data needs to be created in the network. Based on these issues, there is a great need for a better database management system that is tamperproof and hackproof as opposed to the current one that has been used for so many decades. It should also have improved data security and the capacity to interface with other IT systems, like finance and admission. In addition to its multi-purpose use in banking and finance, blockchain technology largely satisfied each of these criteria when introduced in 2008.[19]

Blockchain gives marketers a visual of the products used in medicine. Blockchain technologies will clean the health and pharmaceuticals from fake drugs, as all of these medicines will be traceable. It aids in rooting out the reason for fraud. Blockchain can provide this warranty for each patient record to be secured; after developing medical history, blockchain can store it too, and thus, this cannot change. All commodity hardware is used for this decentralized network in the hospital. With these devices, researchers save energy resources that could easily be computed estimates for therapies, medicines, and remedies for a variety of diseases and disorders.

Blockchain is a distributed ledger network where records are added but never deleted or changed, minus an overall consensus. The number of records on each data block with the value of a blockchain hash depends on a cryptographic hash to link blocks of informative data added to the chain. By its distributed blockchain ledger architecture, data cannot be processed in any centralized place; all network users can see and account for it. This decentralized system and no one attack helps the system become more robust and safer. It ensures complete control of the health record and patient care by reducing the exercise of medical practice twice and supervision, saving time and resources for both practitioner and patients. Patient will track where their information flows, and they will make it happen by using health records on the blockchain.[20]

Scholars can use this technology to analyze a large amount of unprocessed information for one group of people. It is beneficial for the development of precision medicine to be made available appropriately for longitudinal studies. Real-time healthcare data can be acquired from the IoT and wearable devices for dynamic parameters, including blood pressure, blood sugar level, etc., and updated on the blockchain. This ensures doctors can help track high-risk patients and provide resources to connect with their careers and families in an emergency. The decentralized nature of a blockchain enables it to be hacked safely, as no single copy of the records is compromised at once.

Blockchain is a distributed database with an imperishable, incremental collection of data records confirmed by participating nodes. This information is documented in a public ledger that details every transaction processed. In parallel, blockchain is also a distributed ledger of cryptographically chained blocks, meaning stacks of transactions exchanging value are aggregated one after another. The principle of decentralization, security, anonymity, and the virtue of the absence of a mediator to control agreement and inalterability are attributes that blockchain also has. Information and data are carried in blocks, and a continuous series of these processing blocks leads us to believe they are transparent and tamperproof.

Blockchain is a decentralized database that nobody owns and is simultaneously owned by everybody, as the contents are available to all parties involved. For example, with Bitcoin, since users process all transactions via a particular pseudonym, the information contained in the blockchain is completely anonymous. This revolutionary system has indeed overcome some of the limitations faced by the existing system. Nevertheless, further exploration in terms of implementation and practicality is much needed and will be discussed in the following sections.[11]

Need for Blockchain in Healthcare

When it comes to healthcare, the need for development increases to even crazier velocities. Today, better-established health facilities must be backed up with the latest technologies. Blockchain would be the key to that change happening in healthcare. Likewise, the health system landscape is transitioning from a patient-centric model to services being rolled out, emphasizing access and appropriate healthcare resources at all times. Healthcare organizations can learn from the blockchain to maintain adequate patient care and quality health facilities. This technology analyzes the scattered data quickly, ultimately eliminating the redundant and time-consuming process of health information exchange, which has also contributed to high health industry costs. Not only will the citizens be able to participate by using blockchain technology through health study programs. More effective research and shared data on public well-being will also improve the treatment of varied communities. The whole healthcare system and organizations are managed through a centralized database.

The biggest challenges to date are data protection, sharing, and interoperability in population health management. Blockchain has addressed this specific issue satisfactorily. Properly implementing this technology improves security, data exchange, interoperability, integrity, and real-time updates & access. Data protection is also a major issue, especially in personalized medicine and wearables. Patients and health workers need safe and simple ways of storing, sending, and retrieving records over networks with no safety risks; hence, the use of blockchain technology to address such issues.[21]

Numerous Features of Blockchain Technology to Promote Global Healthcare Culture

In healthcare, blockchain has a wide range of applications and functions. The ledger technology helps healthcare researchers uncover genetic code by facilitating the secure transfer of patient medical records, managing the drug supply chain, and facilitating the safe transfer of patient medical records. Blockchain has several applications and functions in the healthcare sector. The ledger technology allows healthcare researchers to unravel genetic code by making medical records portable, controlling the drug supply chain, and allowing a secure transfer of patient medical records. Technically obtained and impressive features developed from blockchain technology are applied for healthcare data protection, such as genomics management, electronic data management, medical records, interoperability, digitalized tracking, and issues outbreak. The primary driving factor for the acceptance of blockchain technology in healthcare-related applications is its complete digital attributes.

Blockchain creates transparency in the prescription cycle from manufacturing to pharmacy shelves. Congestion, freight direction, and speed can all be tracked using IoT with the help of blockchain. It provides an opportunity for the timely planning of procurements to avoid disruption and shortage in clinics, pharmacies, and other medical venues for one specific medicine being received. Such digital frameworks, if designed on the pillar of blockchain, would minimize the chances of unfiltered alterations to logistics data. This enhances trust and avoids the illegal manipulation of records, payments, or medications themselves by the multitude of individuals wanting to buy drugs.[22]

This technology can treat patients efficiently while at a competitive rate, saving money. It removes all hindrances in multi-level authentication. It is a perfect security application because blockchain can keep an immutable, decentralized, and transparent patient data record. In addition, although the blockchain is transparent, it is simultaneously private, keeping any person's identifying information behind complex and secure algorithms that can help maintain the privacy of medical records. With its decentralized nature, the technology allows patients, healthcare providers, and doctors to access the same information quickly and securely.

Legislation such as that observed by blockchain technology eases the shift toward patient-led interoperability through patients granting access to their medical data. This allows a patient more control over certain types of personal information and enhances confidentiality. Quality management and enforcing quality practices are hard to measure and implement. Blockchain applications can solve any of these technical issues across the industry. Blockchain dynamics will help regulatory bodies in tracking legal drugs against counterfeits. This ensures that the approved parties can exchange electronic transactions that include information about the patient. Patients who switch medical practitioners may only sign out one consent to exchange their entire history.[23]

Blockchain technology has landed in the healthcare industry, and its acceptance rate is increasing. Moreover, initially, individuals in the health ecosystem embrace the technologies positively. Over the next few years, a holistic vision of blockchain was needed to rebuild the healthcare market by addressing issues currently challenging the existing structure. So, it provides all the information to the physicians, patients, and pharmacists at a specific time. Day and night research, study, and experimentation in all possible ways by medical firms are going on a top-down level, means within the organizations as well as for the health records. Learn More It has proven to be an indispensable tool in healthcare, as it tracks pharmaceuticals, refines payment methods, and decentralizes patient medical history records. Along with required technologies like machine learning and artificial intelligence, the medical industry is mostly based on blockchain. It highlights a few genuine usages of how blockchain will change the healthcare industry. It employs blockchain monitoring technology to optimize the medical supply chain.

Blockchain can potentially create a more sophisticated data storage environment that can capture an entire health history of diagnosis, test reports, prior regimes, and even sensor-based measurements for somebody. A doctor can easily access all available information to make accurate diagnoses and suggestions. Storing all the data in one blockchain system makes it impossible for that data to be lost or shifted. It can use blockchain to steer clear of an organization's internal networks. An encrypted blockchain database with varying degrees of control can effectively defend organizations against risks from outside forces and attacks by many separate individual players forming a cohesive group. Such rescue attacks and related challenges like the corruption of a computer or failure of the hardware will be eliminated if a healthcare organization has properly implemented a blockchain network.[24]

Blockchain Technology in the Development of Healthcare Services

Blockchain technology can implement healthcare pristine cultural perspectives and overall development. Various associated industrial/medical care supporters or providers helping carry out the investigation and studies for accomplishing the applications of blockchain in the health industry and its major domains.

Under blockchain, new patient data cards will be developed by medical practitioners in various hospitals. Information that is newly added is generally a repetition, causing a waste of time, which can be a dangerous health malfunction. The location in the supply chain provides its own privileges or accessibility options for everyone. Also, if the medication detail is contained in a block, then that block will have a hash connected to that block.

Additionally, the data transparency in the blockchain framework will aid in tracing the original root path and eliminate the trade of counterfeit medication. When the patient goes to a new clinic, they open a new medical card on them and put it in a certain facility. These particulars are usually net and therefore incomplete by the general public; they include captured records of attention providers accessible at the amenities involved. Problems in the blockchain can easily piece together the data processing. Such technology will generate open and similar blockchain medical records worldwide.[25]

Clinical trials in healthcare are underway to determine whether such therapies can act as a treatment or partial cure for a specific disease. Scientists can record data on test results, number of people, patient files, and a variety of other different variables. Authentication of data generated in clinical trials is critical for assuring scientists, pharmaceuticals, and policymakers that results are high quality. Blockchain technology could offer higher transparency and accountability in clinical trials. Because it is only through an understanding of patient problems that the processing of medical history works, which gives tremendous record-keeping power to the healthcare blockchain as clinicians and patients access the blocks. The use of blockchain in the supply chain is very trendy, and it also makes sense for medicines in the healthcare sector.

Blockchain makes it easier to consider what health professionals should be practicing and providing. This blockchain prowess works in healthcare to manage approval efficiently and faster processing and acquisition. The lineup is used to prevent waste, and it's easier to stand in a line, unlock productivity, and make the workflow cleaner with blockchain. It will promote fully personalized medicine, clinical guidance, and blockchain is one of the most widespread technologies ever encountered by humanity, enabling health-related practical research through its applications. The latest among such blockchains is mainly focused on the fact that this platform can help reshape the face of healthcare better according to their belief. This will be an ever-reliable and constant digital register in the healthcare industry. They will bolster several challenges in blockchain healthcare technologies, including clinical trials, patient records management, and prescription tracing.[26]

Blockchains have proven applications in healthcare for making the right decisions in the health ecosystem. The distributed blockchain platform provides the health market with options to follow fraud, cut down on overhead expenses, work reliable production jobs, eliminate duplication of effort, and enact transparency in the health ecosystem. It is also utilized to store assets immutably, confidently, and decentralized. Clinical trials and approval organizations for the subject are the areas where blockchain can boost the reliability, suitability, and accountability of medical professionals and researchers. The benefit for patients is that their medical histories are protected more confidently and that their diagnostic accuracy improves the chances of further care.

Patients will now have more of a say in processing their health records. They will be permitted to have access to data and exchange it as partners with the blockchain community, thus providing additional security and privacy. The promise of blockchain has far-reaching implications for stakeholders across healthcare. This technology is likely to interact with disparate networks to provide insight and assess the importance of treatment based on this information.

In the long term, an electronic medical records blockchain network nationwide will drive efficiencies and advance better patient health outcomes. Blockchain is a common ledger of transactions linked together in blocks and stored in an e-book. In this medical field, medical details such as patient life, logs of the medical equipment, or temperature of medical products can be recorded while shipping.[27]

Applications of Blockchain Technology in Healthcare

Blockchain, being a decentralized and distributed technology, has vast implications in the healthcare domain. Blockchain technology is primarily applied to the banking and finance market, but now it is intended for providing safer information sharing between providers, payers, and patients within healthcare systems. Researchers have begun investigating possible uses for blockchain technology in healthcare sectors, owing to blockchain's immense potential and real-world applicability within the healthcare system. The application of blockchain technology in the healthcare sector is shown in Figure 1.2 and discussed below.

Blockchains in Electronic Health Records

Digitization of medical health records: the need over the past three decades has been led by medical practitioners, hospitals, and healthcare devices since more the facility and ease of access, sharing also forms the backbone of better tackled timely decisions. Currently, most applications for blockchain technologies in healthcare are focused on electronic medical records.

EHRs are never built for lifetime records across institutions, and patients scatter their data among many different institutions as life circumstances pull them from one provider to another; they lose convenient access to all prior data. With its need for an innovative resolution for the secure management of EHRs that encourages patients to participate in their present and previous health data, blockchain technology has been raised by numerous investigators to facilitate the maintenance of EHRs.[28]

MedRec is a prototype incorporating unique blockchain advantages to provide security in authentication, privacy, integrity, and data sharing. Built on a decentralized records management system, the project says that it allows for a complete, immutable history for each patient while enabling easy access to a respective health record across different providers and treatment organizations.

Unlike MedRec, it does not store medical records, and there is no adjustment time. It places a hash of the record on a blockchain and notifies the patient, who is ultimately in control of how that record can flow. The stamp certifies an unchanged

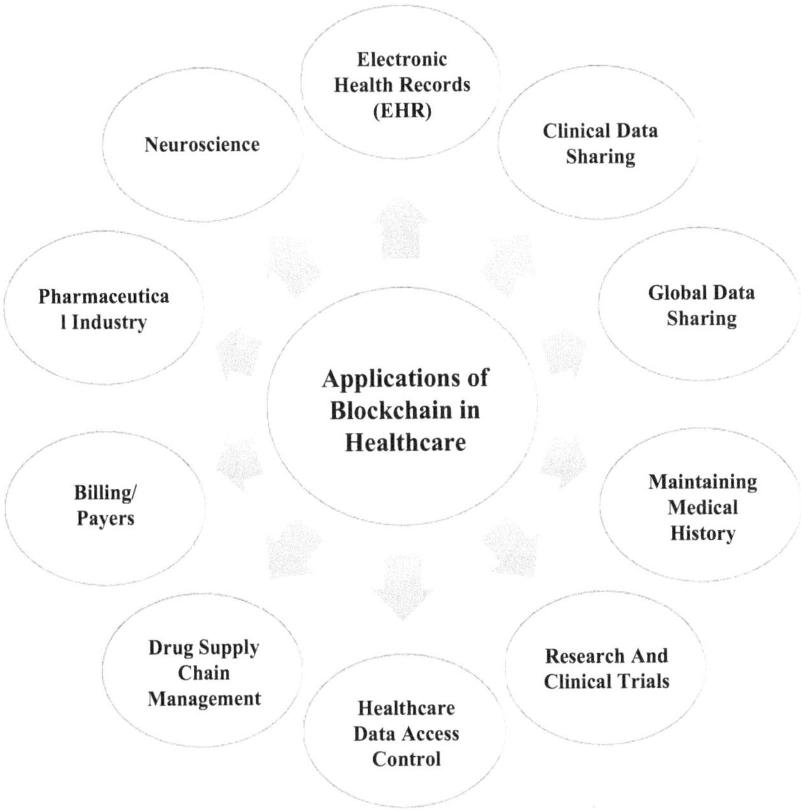

Figure 1.2 Applications of blockchain in Healthcare.

copy of the document was obtained. It also transfers the control power from the institution to point and charge as an owner. This both empowers and gives more weight to the patient. For those patients who would not like to manage their data, the organization associations are supposed to act as patient advocates for this endeavor.

However, several crucial limitations exist during the EHR implementation process related to medical data sharing, including loss of control of data, provenance, auditing, and secured data trailing on medical data. Considering such restrictions, the new MeDShare is a trusted and reliable blockchain-based scheme for medical data dissemination between untrusted private sectors. For example, MeDShare can be applied to sharing medical data and storing EHRs between cloud service providers, hospitals, and healthcare research organizations, ensuring where the data came from, and who accesses it with audit control based on user identity as well as entity type while allowing potential less threat of privacy leakage or violation detection.[29]

EHRs usually have very sensitive and valuable patient-related data, which is very common and often must be shared amongst clinicians, radiologists, healthcare service providers, pharmacists, and research technicians (for proper diagnosis and treatment of the patient). This extremely sensitive patient information is stored, transmitted, and distributed among various entities while the patient is being treated. The sensitivity of these records being exposed can lead to immediate endangerment of a patient's health as well as difficulty in keeping track of all up-to-date information regarding the patient's history. For patients who are struggling with chronic diseases (e.g., cancer and HIV) the incidence of these hazards may be even further exacerbated due to an extensive period of pre-and-post treatment, follow-ups, and rehabilitative procedures.

As a maybe global growth in use case on blockchain battery treatment is but to take shape, it could be because of patients' extremely strong assurance in the technology as it allows patients them unchanging and permanently preserves medical documents because any attempt at access or alteration can be instantly marked all over the blockchain. Not only is this important for patient integrity, but it also detects any criminal activities, such as massive fraud or alteration of records. In addition, sharing and reviewing approved medicinal service records will be vastly simpler. When a patient visit occurs, it is immediately visible to all of that patient's providers. With the appropriate patient-caring algorithms, narcotics bugs, hypersensitivities, and drug solutions may be arranged overall blockchain records very rapidly without having to go through tedious pharmaceutical compromise forms. Different potential applications of blockchain tech will accordingly advance more mind-blowing access to care, medical record management, instant clinical information validation, expanded protection, and improved efficient care arrangement.[30]

Blockchains in Clinical Data Sharing

An important and main scope of the blockchain in healthcare is sharing medical data among several stakeholders within the system. EHR and EMR contain sensitive and critical medical data of the patient, which is to be stored, shared, processed, and accessed securely. So, to better the healthcare services and improve their quality, it is essential for medical info to be frequently stored and shared among all concerned parties like patients, doctors, hospitals or healthcare service providers, drug stores or pharmacies, as well as insurance companies and researchers. Mediators between these kinds of critical data sharing thus need to be equipped with solid transparency and accountability mechanisms during data transactions. Hence, in such cases, blockchain provides more transparency as a distributed ledger for all parties involved in the network. Blockchain offers verification and management mechanisms of data in a trustable manner while being aware of the transactions between parties.[31]

Blockchains in Global Data Sharing

In addition, in some cases, patients go abroad as tourists or for other reasons. Also, there are times when they might need to see a doctor to treat any illness. So, the doctors/hospitals in different countries should have all the patient healthcare information to provide greater health services. Using blockchain-based methods, this medical data can effortlessly be passed to demanding parties in foreign countries, and the patient can be permitted to manage all details. For instance, The medical history of the respective patient in case the respective patient has an allergy to some medicines or knowledge about his recent treatment should be well known to provide better medicolegal treatment outside the country. For that, the service provider should comfortably access the medical history.[32]

Blockchains in Maintaining Medical History

The patient's medical history can also be efficiently recorded and stored using blockchain technology. For instance, at times, patients go to unconnected hospitals, which means the entire chronology of the clinical history may not be accessible or easily managed (because of scatter and inaccessibility of prior documents). For such problems, blockchain can be helpful because whenever a hospital has a visit, it maintains all its records history. Also, as some disconnected data of medical/laboratory reports are unavailable, the patients again have to undergo the same test. Repeating the same laboratory test increases the cost, but repeating some tests is also dangerous (due to high radiation).[33]

Blockchains in Research and Clinical Trials

Clinical trials are the second most important and meaningful process in the healthcare sector, and proper supervision is needed at all trial stages, for instance the mechanism and monitoring of trials and management of the required data from these trials. This trial will be a significant resource drain as numerous parties must coordinate with one another. The trust measured in these trial phases was also huge among the many entities involved. As a result, blockchain can be an important way to go in such research tests where each intermediate step can be easily tracked, and the information can be used and analyzed with minimal wasted time.[34]

Blockchains in Healthcare Data Access Control

Recent innovations can weaken user control/grip on their data. When it comes to healthcare data, for example, most users remain oblivious about who accesses their medical data, what other entities they use them for, and if they are actually authorized to get over those records. For instance, in the case of EHR/EMR, many healthcare service providers are linked, and in that scenario, patients do not know who is accessing their medical data or which parties are to its storage or sharing. This would enable patients to read their medical data and share it with other healthcare professionals in a more secure and safer vehicle while assuring that only verified persons can read, write, or modify the data by utilizing blockchain technology.[35]

Blockchains in Drug Supply Chain Management

Managing medical drug supply is vital in the wide range of fields of modern medicine. Still, this sector is ridden with different complexities and losses due to counterfeiters and pilfering. Moreover, blockchain can retain the traceability of these supply chain activities and improve the integrity of the entire process. Using the blockchain will also allow authorized individuals to authenticate the drugs and their supply chain. Hence, tracking drug supply chain management in the different phases can be essential with the help of blockchain to allow access to only those users who use proper credentials.[36]

Blockchains in Billing/Payers

Conventional patient billing systems are regarded as the most cumbersome and open to medical billing fraud. Moreover, the process in most of these cases must be more time-consuming and resource-draining in collecting all relevant invoices. Blockchain-based payment solutions will likely simplify billing because traditional billing approaches take days to claim the bills. Moreover, if the insurance company is a part of the payment process, it takes even longer to file a claim on the bills. In such cases where payment is the bread and butter for an insurance company, Blockchain would come in extremely handy. Moreover, this can also speed up the processing of insurance claims and reduce additional requirements regarding resources to provide service for time and cost.[37]

Blockchains in Pharmaceutical Industry

Pharmaceuticals is a rapidly growing and indispensable industry at the forefront of healthcare delivery. Apart from enabling the launch of new and novel medications in the market, the pharmaceutical industry also plays an integral role in ensuring that medical products and drugs sold to end consumers are safe and legitimate. Moreover, even the pharmaceutical industry helps evaluate and process safe medicines, which ultimately help faster patient recovery. Usually, drug companies continuously struggle with instance-wise tracking their product to identify those quickly. As a result, it poses extreme threats of counterfeiters penetrating through the production or even injecting fake medications into the system. Thus, the inevitable production and distribution of counterfeit drugs has resulted in one of the vital yet global health hazards, specifically in developing countries. Effectively identifying the best-fit technologies for monitoring and assuring production processes of potential COVID-19 drugs, it could be possible to use blockchain during the research & development and production phases of these drugs.[38]

Hyperledger, a research foundation on blockchain technology-based projects, has launched the first project on blockchain, using it primarily as a tool to inspect and battle counterfeit medicines. However, having a worldwide digital technologies system that aids in monitoring, evaluating, and delivering the entire process of developing and supplying pharmaceutical drugs is highly needed for reliable and authentic delivery to patients, particularly in developing countries. A long-term solution to protect against counterfeit medications can be introduced using a digital drug control system (DDCS). Pharmaceutical giants Sanofi, Pfizer, and Amgen initiated a collaborative pilot project to inspect and assess new medicines using blockchain-based DDCS. Using an approach such as blockchain would enable the tracking and tracing of not only drug production and existing location in real-time but also allow for enhanced traceability of counterfeit drugs, security of drug supply system, and ensuring the quality of medicines supplied to consumers or end-users.[39]

Blockchains in Neuroscience

News and analysis focused on blockchain applications is booming, with neuroscience no exception. Modern neural technologies aim to create a new paradigm that will not rely on mechanical interaction with the surrounding infrastructure, meaning having one control device and data using mental commands. These neural devices can read brain activity patterns and convert them into commands to control external devices. They also identify the current cognitive state of a person from their brain activity data. Neural interface devices, equipped with multiple sensors, chips, and communication devices responsible for reading and interpreting brain signals, are designed to solve this sophisticated task. They sense the electrical activity from the brain, and later, this signal is analyzed and sent to a device under control. Everything occurs in that one gadget, which the individual wears on their head. Blockchain philosophy will store those brain signals in the neural interface using complex algorithms and big data. One of the companies that confirmed that they'll be using blockchain tech is Neurogress. Registered in Geneva and formed in 2017, the firm is focused on building neural-control systems, enabling users to control robotic arms, drones, smart appliances, and AR/VR (augmented reality/virtual reality) devices with their thoughts.[40]

The focus of Neurogress's control system is that it uses machine learning to improve its reading-brain accuracy. This goal entails retaining 90% of brain data to train the AI utilized by the system. In other words, they are demanding the "big data of user neural activity," with a whitepaper from the company referencing how "exabytes (1 exabyte = 1 billion of gigabytes) of memory" will be required for storage capacity alone, as exhibited in the Human Brain Project. Consequently, it should come as no surprise that Neurogress intends to utilize blockchain, which, in the view of third-party developers of this technology, "solves the problem of security and privacy of data storage." This data is then recorded in the decentralized blockchain, so it becomes "resistant to hacking attacks" and thus more private. Simultaneously, applying blockchain technology makes the Neurogress system "open and transparent for potential users of services on the Neurogress platform." Due to information transparency and easy traceability of abnormal activity, the system will ensure the security and confidentiality of personal data.[41]

Security and Privacy Challenges of Blockchain Technology in Healthcare Sectors

The fact that performing a transaction without trusted third parties exposes security and privacy vulnerabilities is the problem that blockchains solve. While smart contracts between health providers to grant others access to certain data or patient records are constructed on blockchains, the question arises regarding who else has access to this data and if they even have authorization. The nature of the implementation of blockchains is another major issue as it does not provide privacy or security for data, at least for the Protected Health Information (PHIs) and EMR to be viable.[42]

One more security threat that can happen is a measurement known as the Sybil attack. If we talk about this attack is a network-based attack in which a single attacker or group of attackers disguise themselves as multiple nodes on a network. This attack can also disconnect the attacked node from the chain network and prevent it from partaking in any chain activities. Inference of private data can also be another issue that arises. For instance, if the hash values of patients' private keys were written directly onto the block and a specific doctor knows a certain patient's private key, they can be used to derive information about when and how many times that patient visited the hospital. It could put the privacy of patients at risk.

In addition, Blockchain relies only on a collection of cryptographic algorithms for integrity. If quantum computers ever become able to produce private keys, there is the possibility that this would threaten the entire network's security and integrity. This is so because instead of binary bits, quantum computers use qubits. Hence, it has faster processing speeds, allowing an attacker to trick blocks by recomputing the hash value of those blocks in polynomial time.[43]

Future Prospects of Blockchain Technology in Healthcare Sectors

Blockchain will have a significant technical impact on humanity's world, and the value and potential of blockchain healthcare have yet to scratch the surface. Blockchain healthcare will revolutionize technology, transform sectors and upend human society's present order, legal recognition, and value systems. With the progressive maturation of blockchain technology, the following development trends are expected to materialize.

Zero-Knowledge Proof

By definition, the blockchain is one of the most transparent things. ZenLedger uses zero-knowledge proof technology, so while anyone can read the entire ledger, any node in the Bitcoin system can download all the stored data that may not relate to an organization or individual. To run that smart contract, they use the data but do not disclose the actual content of the data.[44]

Artificial Intelligence

It can be used for artificial intelligence to create a decentralized marketplace and collaboration platform for different AI components, including data, algorithms, and computing power. It could potentially herald an entirely new era of artificial intelligence and artistry. The decision-reliability, clarity, and transparency of all processes to which blockchain in healthcare is applied will be enhanced. Since every information on the blockchain is public, artificial intelligence will be the basis for anti-counterfeiting and privacy protection.[45]

Internet of Things

In the future, the role of healthcare blockchain technology could be supportive as it may bring another level of trust and security to IoT data while enabling more efficiency, scalability, and standardization. The advent of blockchain-enabled the IoT devices in healthcare will allow patients to determine who sees the data such devices collect, thus increasing security against hackers and providing a reliable log of who has accessed the recorded data. Based on that conditions are monitored by an IoT sensor, the smart contracts that underpin a blockchain-based solution may automate payments in supply chains.[46]

Conclusion

Blockchain technology is poised to bring revolutionary changes in healthcare as enormous volumes of sensitive patient data can now be stored securely, privately, and transparently. It has the potential to provide greater trust, security, and interoperability in healthcare systems by exploring blockchain architecture's key components, such as hashing functions, PKC, transactions, and consensus. Blockchain has many attractive features, most importantly as a permissionless and optionally also findable in numerous networks (private and consortium). It is deployable over various use cases, such as EHR or drug-supply chains. This makes it imperative to build further integrative, efficient, and patient-centered healthcare systems with the help of available data, which can only be provided worldwide based on appropriate privacy and security regulations. Healthcare blockchain applications hit many of the top issues that the industry is facing. Blockchain can create a secure healthcare ecosystem with a trusted medical history where shared clinical data in treating individual cases and global research collaboration can occur seamlessly without duplicating efforts. However, as with new technology, blockchain faces security and regulatory compliance challenges. Blockchain in healthcare will likely have enhanced use cases bundled with other advanced technologies, including but not limited to Zero-Knowledge Proofs, Artificial Intelligence, and the IoT, which could strengthen its proposition by providing improved privacy, automation, and real-time monitoring. In conclusion, though blockchain holds great promise for healthcare, widespread adoption will require addressing important challenges, including scalability, standardization, and regulatory hurdles. Still, blockchain offers tremendous potential for a better, more secure, transparent approach to future healthcare built on trust between patients and enterprises.

References

1 Haleem, Abid, Mohd Javaid, Ravi Pratap Singh, Rajiv Suman, and Shanay Rab. "Blockchain technology applications in healthcare: An overview." *International Journal of Intelligent Networks* 2 (2021): 130–139.

2 Sarmah, Simanta Shekhar. "Understanding blockchain technology." *Computer Science and Engineering* 8, no. 2 (2018): 23–29.

3 Aggarwal, Shubhani, Neeraj Kumar and Pethuru Raj. "Core components of blockchain." In Zoe Kruze, Leticia Lima, James Selvam, Alan Studholme (eds), *Advances in Computers*, vol. 121, pp. 193–209. Elsevier, 2021.

4 Wang, Maoning, Meijiao Duan, and Jianming Zhu. "Research on the security criteria of hash functions in the blockchain." In *Proceedings of the 2nd ACM Workshop on Blockchains, Cryptocurrencies, and Contracts*, pp. 47–55. 2018.

5 Jourdan, Marc, Sebastien Blandin, Laura Wynter, and Pralhad Deshpande. "Characterizing entities in the Bitcoin blockchain." In *2018 IEEE International Conference on Data Mining Workshops (ICDMW)*, pp. 55–62. IEEE, 2018.

6 Sathya, A. R., and Barnali Gupta Banik. "A comprehensive study of blockchain services: future of cryptography." *International Journal of Advanced Computer Science and Applications* 11, no. 10 (2020): 279–288.

7 Jayaprakash, Varsha, and Amit Kumar Tyagi. "Security optimization of resource-constrained Internet of Healthcare Things (IOHT) devices using asymmetric cryptography for blockchain network." In *International Conference on Network Security and Blockchain Technology*, pp. 225–236. Singapore: Springer Nature Singapore, 2021.

8 Sandeep Kumar Panda, Ajay Kumar Jena, Santosh Kumar Swain, Suresh Chandra Satapathy. "Blockchain technology: Introduction, applications, challenges." In *Blockchain Technology: Applications and Challenges*, pp. 1–11. Cham: Springer International Publishing, 2021.

9 Lashkari, Bahareh, and Petr Musilek. "A comprehensive review of blockchain consensus mechanisms." *IEEE Access* 9 (2021): 43620–43652.

10 Hasselgren, Anton, Katina Kralevska, Danilo Gligoroski, Sindre A. Pedersen, and Arild Faxvaag. "Blockchain in healthcare and health sciences—A scoping review." *International Journal of Medical Informatics* 134 (2020): 104040.

12 Alhadhrami, Zainab, Salma Alghfeli, Mariam Alghfeli, Juhar Ahmed Abedlla, and Khaled Shuaib. "Introducing blockchains for healthcare." In *2017 International Conference on Electrical and Computing Technologies and Applications (ICECTA)*, pp. 1–4. IEEE, 2017.

13 Hu, Yining, Ahsan Manzoor, Parinya Ekparinya, Madhusanka Liyanage, Kanchana Thilakarathna, Guillaume Jourjon, and Aruna Seneviratne. "A delay-tolerant payment scheme based on the Ethereum blockchain." *IEEE Access* 7 (2019): 33159–33172.

14 Yaqoob, Ibrar, Khaled Salah, Raja Jayaraman, and Yousof Al-Hammadi. "Blockchain for healthcare data management: Opportunities, challenges, and future recommendations." *Neural Computing and Applications* 34, (2022): 1–16.

15 Zheng, Zibin, Shaoan Xie, Hong-Ning Dai, Xiangping Chen, and Huaimin Wang. "Blockchain challenges and opportunities: A survey." *International Journal of Web and Grid Services* 14, no. 4 (2018): 352–375.

16 Dias, Joao Pedro, Luís Reis, Hugo Sereno Ferreira, and Ângelo Martins. "Blockchain for access control in e-health scenarios." *arXiv preprint arXiv:1805.12267* (2018).

17 Chen, Yaoliang, Shi Chen, Jiao Liang, Lance Warren Feagan, Weili Han, Sheng Huang, and X. Sean Wang. "Decentralized data access control over consortium blockchains." *Information Systems* 94 (2020): 101590.

18 Elgamal, Esraa, Walaa Medhat, Mohamed Abd Elfatah, and Nashwa Abdelbaki. "Blockchain in healthcare for achieving patients' privacy." In *2023 20th Learning and Technology Conference (L&T)*, pp. 59–64. IEEE, 2023.

19 Javaid, Mohd, Abid Haleem, Ravi Pratap Singh, Rajiv Suman, and Shahbaz Khan. "A review of Blockchain Technology applications for financial services." *BenchCouncil Transactions on Benchmarks, Standards and Evaluations* 2, no. 3 (2022): 100073.

20 Ballamudi, Koteswara Rao. "Blockchain as a type of distributed ledger technology." *Asian Journal of Humanity, Art and Literature* 3, no. 2 (2016): 127–136.

11 Elangovan, Deepa, Chiau Soon Long, Faizah Safina Bakrin, Ching Siang Tan, Khang Wen Goh, Siang Fei Yeoh, Mei Jun Loy, Zahid Hussain, Kah Seng Lee, Azam Che Idris, Long Chiau Ming. "The use of blockchain technology in the health care sector: systematic review." *JMIR Medical Informatics* 10, no. 1 (2022): e17278.

21 Chakrabarty, Shambhu Prasad, and Souvik Mukherjee. "Transforming healthcare sector in India through blockchain technology: Challenges and opportunities from legal perspectives." *Transformations Through Blockchain Technology: The New Digital Revolution* (2022): 231–248.

22 Jamil, Faisal, Lei Hang, KyuHyung Kim, and DoHyeun Kim. "A novel medical blockchain model for drug supply chain integrity management in a smart hospital." *Electronics* 8, no. 5 (2019): 505.

23 Kumar, Adarsh, Rajalakshmi Krishnamurthi, Anand Nayyar, Kriti Sharma, Vinay Grover, and Eklas Hossain. "A novel smart healthcare design, simulation, and implementation using healthcare 4.0 processes." *IEEE Access* 8 (2020): 118433–118471.

24 Pandey, Prateek, and Ratnesh Litoriya. "Implementing healthcare services on a large scale: Challenges and remedies based on blockchain technology." *Health Policy and Technology* 9, no. 1 (2020): 69–78.

25 Cerchione, Roberto, Piera Centobelli, Emanuela Riccio, Stefano Abbate, and Eugenio Oropallo. "Blockchain's coming to hospital to digitalize healthcare services: Designing a distributed electronic health record ecosystem." *Technovation* 120 (2023): 102480.

26 Singh, Suruchi, Satish Kumar Sharma, Pavas Mehrotra, Pankaj Bhatt, and Monika Kaurav. "Blockchain technology for efficient data management in healthcare system: Opportunity, challenges and future perspectives." *Materials Today: Proceedings* 62 (2022): 5042–5046.

27 Onik, Md Mehedi Hassan, Satyabrata Aich, Jinhong Yang, Chul-Soo Kim, and Hee-Cheol Kim. "Blockchain in healthcare: Challenges and solutions." In *Big Data Analytics for Intelligent Healthcare Management*, pp. 197–226. Palm Bay, FL: Apple Academic Press Inc., 2019.

28 Quinn, Martha, Jane Forman, Molly Harrod, Suzanne Winter, Karen E. Fowler, Sarah L. Krein, Ashwin Gupta, Sanjay Saint, Hardeep Singh, and Vineet Chopra. "Electronic health records, communication, and data sharing: Challenges and opportunities for improving the diagnostic process." *Diagnosis* 6, no. 3 (2019): 241–248.

29 Alzahrani, Ahmed Ghurmullah M., Ahmed Alenezi, A. Mershed, Hany Atlam, Fathy Mousa, and Gary Wills. "A framework for data sharing between healthcare providers using blockchain." In *IoTBDS 2020 - Proceedings of the 5th International Conference on Internet of Things, Big Data and Security*. SciTePress, vol. 1 (2020): 349–358.

30 Kaswan, Kuldeep Singh, Jagjit Singh Dhatterwal, and Santar Pal Singh. "Blockchain technology for health care." In *Healthcare and Knowledge Management for Society 5.0*, pp. 1–20. Boca Raton, FL: CRC Press, 2021.

31 Kanagi, Karamo, Cooper Cheng-Yuan Ku, Li-Kai Lin, and Wen-Huai Hsieh. "Efficient clinical data sharing framework based on blockchain technology." *Methods of Information in Medicine* 59, no. 06 (2020): 193–204.

32 Biswas, Sujit, Kashif Sharif, Fan Li, Anupam Kumar Bairagi, Zohaib Latif, and Saraju P. Mohanty. "Globechain: An interoperable blockchain for global sharing of healthcare data—A COVID-19 perspective." *IEEE Consumer Electronics Magazine* 10, no. 5 (2021): 64–69.

33 Tith, Dara, Joong-Sun Lee, Hiroyuki Suzuki, W. M. A. B. Wijesundara, Naoko Taira, Takashi Obi, and Nagaaki Ohyama. "Application of blockchain to maintaining patient

records in electronic health record for enhanced privacy, scalability, and availability." *Healthcare Informatics Research* 26, no. 1 (2020): 3–12.
34 Omar, Ilhaam A., Raja Jayaraman, Khaled Salah, Ibrar Yaqoob, and Samer Ellahham. "Applications of blockchain technology in clinical trials: Review and open challenges." *Arabian Journal for Science and Engineering* 46, no. 4 (2021): 3001–3015.
35 Ramani, Vidhya, Tanesh Kumar, An Bracken, Madhusanka Liyanage, and Mika Ylianttila. "Secure and efficient data accessibility in blockchain-based healthcare systems." In *2018 IEEE Global Communications Conference (GLOBECOM)*, pp. 206–212. IEEE, 2018.
36 Xu, Xiang, Ning Tian, Haoyu Gao, Hong Lei, Zixuan Liu, and Zhiwei Liu. "A survey on application of blockchain technology in drug supply chain management." In *2023 IEEE 8th International Conference on Big Data Analytics (ICBDA)*, pp. 62–71. IEEE, 2023.
37 Rahman, Md Shafiur, Md Amirul Islam, Md Ashraf Uddin, and Giovanni Stea. "A survey of blockchain-based IoT eHealthcare: Applications, research issues, and challenges." *Internet of Things* 19 (2022): 100551.
38 Uddin, Mueen. "Blockchain Medledger: Hyperledger fabric enabled drug traceability system for counterfeit drugs in pharmaceutical industry." *International Journal of Pharmaceutics* 597 (2021): 120235.
39 Lokesh, M., Suhail Ahmed, and Saifulla Khan. "Block chain based supply chain management for counterfeit drugs in pharmaceutical industry." *International Journal of Scientific Research in Computer Science and Engineering Information Technology* 7, no. 1 (2021): 100–108.
40 Porkodi, S., and D. Kesavaraja. "Blockchain in healthcare sector." In Sandeep Kumar Panda, Ahmed A. Elngar, Valentina Emilia Balas, Mohammed Kayed (eds), *Bitcoin and Blockchain*, pp. 163–182. CRC Press, 2020.
41 Karpagam, G. R. "A survey about fusion of blockchain technology in various application realms." In *ICCAP 2021: Proceedings of the First International Conference on Combinatorial and Optimization, ICCAP 2021, December 7–8, 2021, Chennai, India*, p. 430. European Alliance for Innovation, 2021.
42 Zhang, Rui, Rui Xue, and Ling Liu. "Security and privacy for healthcare blockchains." *IEEE Transactions on Services Computing* 15, no. 6 (2021): 3668–3686.
43 Dey, Nivedita, Mrityunjay Ghosh, and Amlan Chakrabarti. "Quantum solutions to possible challenges of blockchain technology." In Adarsh Kumar, Sukhpal Singh Gill, Ajith Abraham (eds), *Quantum and Blockchain for Modern Computing Systems: Vision and Advancements: Quantum and Blockchain Technologies: Current Trends and Challenges*, pp. 249–282. Cham: Springer International Publishing, 2022.
44 Feng, Tao, Pu Yang, Chunyan Liu, Junli Fang, and Rong Ma. "Blockchain data privacy protection and sharing scheme based on zero-knowledge proof." *Wireless Communications and Mobile Computing* 2022, no. 1 (2022): 1040662.
45 Tagde, Priti, Sandeep Tagde, Tanima Bhattacharya, Pooja Tagde, Hitesh Chopra, Rokeya Akter, Deepak Kaushik, and Md Habibur Rahman. "Blockchain and artificial intelligence technology in e-Health." *Environmental Science and Pollution Research* 28 (2021): 52810–52831.
46 Singh, Saurabh, Shailendra Rathore, Osama Alfarraj, Amr Tolba, and Byungun Yoon. "A framework for privacy-preservation of IoT healthcare data using Federated Learning and blockchain technology." *Future Generation Computer Systems* 129 (2022): 380–388.

2 The Evolution of Patient Data Security

Sunita, Akhil Sharma, Ashish Verma, Akanksha Sharma, Neeraj Kumar Fuloria and Shaweta Sharma

Introduction

Blockchain technology is an evolution of a database framework for sharing information transparently within a business network. A blockchain database uses a chain of blocks to store data. It is chronologically consistent because you cannot delete or alter the chain without every node agreeing on it. Consequently, blockchain can help you build a/changeable or immutable ledger to keep track of orders, payments, accounts and other transactions. The system is able to prevent unauthorised entries of transactions, and it also builds the consistency of these managed records for a shared view among all parties.[1]

Blockchain for Healthcare Data Security

Blockchain is poised to revolutionise the security of healthcare data and meet rising data breach threats while maintaining patient privacy. As the healthcare industry faces a surge in data breaches, with more than 41 million records reported as compromised only during the first half of 2023, there is an increasingly high demand for stronger security controls to protect patient information. Blockchain for Healthcare Data Security are depicted in Figure 2.1.[2]

Enhancing Data Security

The decentralised, immutable nature of blockchain technology can transform the way healthcare data is managed. Blockchain removes single points of failure by decentralising data, decreasing the chances of loss and unauthorised access. Blockchain uses cryptographic algorithms that provide absolute mathematical certainty that data will not be breached and that patient records cannot be altered without detection. An irreversible log of each transaction or record change is maintained, thus providing a transparent audit trail that increases the level of accountability and trust within this physician–patient interaction.[3]

DOI: 10.4324/9781003529910-2

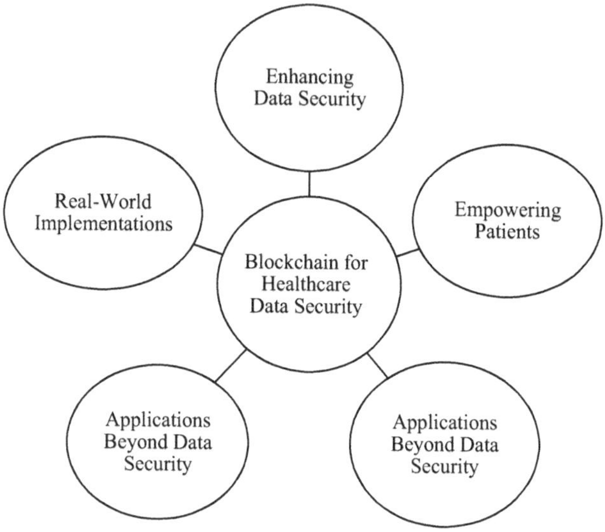

Figure 2.1 Blockchain for Healthcare Data Security.

Empowering Patients

The most important benefit of blockchain in the healthcare industry is that it allows patients to take control of their health data. Using blockchain, patients would be able to manage who can see their medical records, and all access activity would be tracked transparently. Such autonomy can protect privacy and also cultivate an individual feeling of ownership of their health data. With more and more patients concerned about data security (95% are worried about their data being stolen or leaked), the natural trust that comes with blockchain can help ease some of these patient fears.[4]

Applications beyond Data Security

The potential of blockchain extends to securing patient data, but it also serves a major role in improving healthcare supply chain management. Blockchain reduces fraud and guarantees the legitimacy of medical products by ensuring transparency and traceability from pharmaceutical production to the actual delivery. In clinical trials, it can improve transparency by reducing the manipulation of clinical data, thus contributing to both patient safety and confidence in healthcare systems.[5]

Real-World Implementations

A number of healthcare organisations are already utilising blockchain for applications, including patient consent management and secure health record tracking. These implementations demonstrate the ability of the technology to redefine how patient data is managed while adhering to privacy standards. As an example, medical chains are developing blockchain-based electronic medical records (EMRs) that track every change to a patient's record and provide patients with the ability to explicitly consent or deny sharing their data with providers or researchers.[6]

Need for Enhanced Patient Data Security

The need for enhanced patient data security in healthcare has become increasingly critical due to the rising number of data breaches and the sensitive nature of health information. Several key factors underscore this urgency:

Patient Confidentiality

Healthcare data has extremely sensitive information, such as medical histories, diagnoses, and personal identifiers. This information needs to be protected for patient confidentiality and trust. These breaches can be caused by identity theft, fraud, and other malicious activities that pose a serious threat to the patient's well-being and negatively impact their confidence in healthcare systems.[7]

Compliance with Regulations

Healthcare organisations have a number of legal and ethical obligations when it comes to patient data protection. Regulatory mechanisms like the Health Insurance Portability and Accountability Act (HIPAA) in the U.S. have established stringent requirements for ensuring the safety of patient data. Failure to comply could lead to significant fines, criminal penalties, or loss of reputation.[8]

Prevention of Data Breaches

A data breach in the healthcare domain can induce dire repercussions, such as financial losses, damage to reputation and inconvenience to patient safety. Protected health information (PHI) has its fair share of value on the dark web, which makes healthcare systems a primary target for cybercriminals. For instance, a single medical record can receive far more money than other forms of personal data. This is where robust security measures come into play to mitigate these risks.[9]

Continuity of Care

Accessing accurate and secure patient information is a fundamental step to providing quality care. In order to make the best decisions, communicators need robust and timely data. Breaches in security or access problems hamper continuity of care and compromise patient safety if this data is lost.[10]

Impact on Research and Development

Healthcare data is essential in medical research and development. However, anonymised datasets are crucial for the citation of trends and the preparation of new therapies. Maintaining the integrity of this data gives researchers access to critical information (without violating patient privacy).[11]

Rising Cybersecurity Threats

Cybercriminals have been targeting the healthcare sector due to its vulnerabilities and the privacy of patients. Disruptive cybersecurity threats like malware, ransomware and phishing attacks which very serious potential dangers to healthcare agencies. Applying thorough cybersecurity encryption, access controls, and regular audits is essential for protecting sensitive data.[12]

Operational Efficiency

Secure healthcare data systems allow for information to be exchanged among providers, enabling improved coordination and collaboration. This also helps ensure faster decision-making where healthcare providers are able to access and evaluate clinical information in real time, which significantly reduces redundancies surrounding tests and procedures, thereby improving the efficiency of delivery.[13]

Challenges in Traditional Patient Data Security

Blockchain is a newly developed technology that brings benefits and opportunities to other sectors, such as cryptocurrency, digital currency, and financial services. However, this technology comes with challenges that should be addressed. This section discusses a few of these major challenges. Challenges in Traditional Patient Data Security are shown in Figure 2.2.

Data Breaches

Healthcare data breaches can be defined as "illegitimate access or disclosure of the PHI that compromises the privacy and security of it".[14]

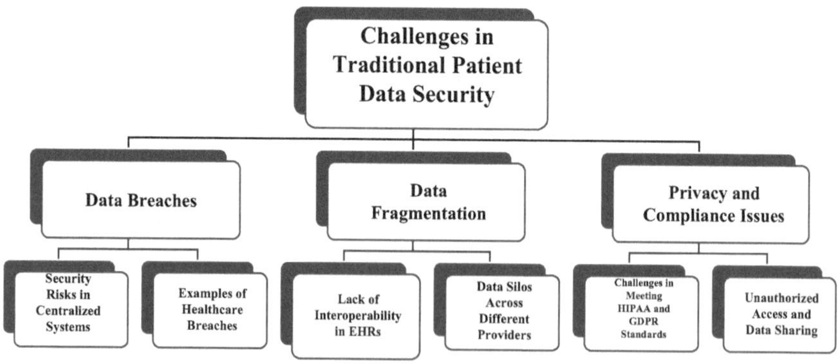

Figure 2.2 Challenges in Traditional Patient Data Security.

Security Risks in Centralised Systems

Centralised systems have a single point of control, which has a huge security risk because they are inherently vulnerable. The primary risk is the single point of failure, where the central server or authority on which everything relies can be attacked or technically fail, resulting in a massive service outage. There are trust issues as well because users have to rely on the central authority to store their data securely. Organisations could end up facing legal proceedings as a result of the breach, which will quickly lead to a crisis of trust between users and the services that deign to protect their sensitive information but fail at any given moment. Centralised systems also have scalability limitations; as user demand increases along with the resources consumed, this can lead to bottlenecks and performance degradation. The increased attack surface is also a major issue, as compromising a single point could give attackers access to significant data. It is necessary to look back at the recent outbreaks of major cloud outages and cryptocurrency exchange hacks. Moreover, centralised systems increase censorship and control since governments or other entities can restrict data access and limit the freedom of users. Such vulnerabilities expose the dangers of centralised architectures in different domains.[15]

Examples of Healthcare Breaches

The healthcare sector has seen many data breaches that highlight the issues with centralised systems that implement data storage. For example, the Anthem Inc. breach from 2015, which is one of the largest healthcare breaches, revealed key personal information for nearly 78 million people, such as names, birth dates, social security numbers and other sensitive data stored in Anthem's centrally located databases. Likewise, with the Premera Blue Cross breach of 2014, hackers used vulnerabilities in Premera's security protocols associated with its centralised data storage systems to access protected personal and financial information for approximately 11 million members. One of the most major breaches happened in 2014, when hackers penetrated Community Health Systems' centralised network, downloading data from 4.5 million patients, like their names, addresses, birth dates and social security numbers. The incidents are a reminder of the threat posed by centralised data systems in the healthcare industry.[16]

Data Fragmentation

Data fragmentation in healthcare is a result of a lack of interoperability in electronic health records (EHRs) and data silos across different providers.

Lack of Interoperability in EHRs

Interoperability is the key to effective communication and data exchange among EHRs, but it remains a daunting task for the healthcare industry. The foremost problem is patient identification because of the lack of a national patient identifier to match patient records between different systems. As a result, records for the same patient may not be linked (in as much as 50% of cases), increasing costs and reducing patient safety. A second challenge is the presence of disparate standards and protocols; many EHR vendors use proprietary communication protocols, making seamless data exchange difficult. Even if systems can technically share the relevant data, differing formats and requirements for what constitutes a complete data set make effective communication difficult. The high costs of integration also hinder a small healthcare provider from upgrading, which can lead them to avoid seeking interoperability solutions. Lastly, regulatory challenges complicate efforts, as regulations like the Medicare and Medicaid Promoting Interoperability Programs are difficult to meet due to the complexities of existing EHR systems, further hindering progress in achieving widespread interoperability.[17]

Data Silos across Different Providers

In the healthcare domain, data silos refer to a situation when some information is isolated within departments or organisations for various reasons, such as governance and or regulations, which limits both effective sharing and collaboration of that shared knowledge, which leads to multiple challenges. Fragmented patient information is one of the biggest challenges; without interoperability, providers using two different EHR systems have difficulty accessing full health records. This can lead to treatment delays or avoidable medical errors. The absence of integration results in a higher administrative burden as healthcare professionals waste valuable time looking up relevant patient data from multiple systems, taking their focus away from patient care and inflating operational costs. A compromised infrastructure leads to limited care coordination, which becomes a major problem in the setting of chronic care where multi-disciplinary delivery is unavoidable. If providers do not have seamless access to all relevant health information, they may miss out on critical insights necessary for total treatment plans. Ultimately, data silos hurt public health, hindering tracking of disease trends or outbreaks or effectively assessing population health to adjust to emerging public health crises.[18]

Privacy and Compliance Issues

Challenges in Meeting HIPAA and GDPR Standards

Strict security controls are mandated under the HIPAA and General Data Protection Regulation (GDPR) to protect sensitive health data. The crucial elements of this practice are data encryption and storage; organisations must ensure that patient information remains encrypted when stored locally or in the cloud, as well as during transmission, to meet regulatory standards. Furthermore, consent management is an important aspect that HIPAA and GDPR cover because both regulations require patients to provide explicit consent before PHI can be collected, processed, or shared. In the case of healthcare in a global arena, maintaining a record of this consent is especially burdensome across platforms and jurisdictions. Data minimisation and purpose limitation, also a principle of the GDPR, states that personal data shall not be collected or processed unless necessary and must only be used for specific purposes. These can be significant in ensuring compliance in clinical research, healthcare analytics, or shared medical platform settings due to the power of the volume of data in analytics. Similarly, well-known cross-border data transfer challenges exist as GDPR prohibits the transfer of personal data outside the European Economic Area unless equivalent data protection standards are satisfied. Cloud-based services and international research involving healthcare organisations must comply with HIPAA as well as GDPR when sending data across borders. Finally, GDRP gives everyone the right to access, rectification, and erasure, which means that people can have access to their data and can correct or erase wrong information about them easily. However, as these requests become more frequent, implementing mechanisms to handle these needs effectively can become operationally complicated, particularly for large, interconnected health systems.[19]

Unauthorised Access and Data Sharing

In healthcare organisations, patient data can be targeted from both internal and external sides. Organisations must ensure the required security systems are in place to comply with regulations like HIPAA and GDPR. Most of the internal threats occur when an employee accesses personal health information (PHI), with or without their intentions, which leads to the breach of HIPAA compliance. To mitigate these risks, organisations should implement regular audits, role-based access controls and rigorous employee education programs. Conversely, external threats like phishing, ransomware, and hacking can compromise patient data security in the long run. To combat these weaknesses, strong cybersecurity protocols, continuous system monitoring, and frequent updates are required.[20]

Misuse of data is another prevalent risk, especially when entities mistakenly reveal information about third-party vendors/subcontractors without precautions upon attaining the consent of patients that violate HIPAA and GDPR. It is also equally important to ensure third-party service providers are regulated in terms of data protection. The increased adoption of cloud-based platforms in healthcare creates additional vulnerabilities, with misconfigured cloud services or security settings exposing sensitive patient data. Lastly, weak data governance may also violate privacy law because organisations fail to have policies or procedures for determining the pathways by which this PHI will be accessed and shared. Setting clear boundaries and governance structure is paramount to remain compliant and safeguard patient information.[21]

Blockchain Technology: A New Paradigm

Core Features of Blockchain

Decentralisation

Blockchain works on a decentralised network in the absence of any central authority that will control the system. In a decentralised system, each participant (or node) holds equal power and has a complete copy of the database, which ensures that no one can dominate or influence the data. This makes it more secure and less vulnerable to data breaches.[22]

Immutability

Data recorded on a blockchain cannot be changed. It also means that this cannot be altered or erased without the agreement of most of the nodes in the network. This is implemented with the help of cryptographic principles and is extremely tamper-resistant.[23]

Transparency and Traceability

Blockchain transparency means that all transactions are visible to the public and can be audited by anyone. This openness creates confidence among users and also guarantees that each transaction can be effortlessly tracked back, which is particularly valuable for applications such as supply chain management.[24]

Blockchain vs. Traditional Systems

Comparisons in Data Security and Management

The centralised nature of the traditional database is another weak point since they are managed by one single entity, which is prone to hacking and data manipulation. Unlike blockchain, where all participants collectively maintain data integrity through decentralisation, it is much harder to alter or destroy information through cyber-attacks.[25]

Enhanced Privacy and Security through Encryption

Blockchain uses contemporary cryptographic approaches to protect the data it contains. Each block includes the unique cryptographic hash of the previous one, making it very hard to break into or tamper with. Although classical databases implement security-like access controls, due to the centralised architecture, they are more vulnerable to breaches.[26]

Smart Contracts for Automated Data Access

Self-Executing Contracts for Secure Data Exchange

Smart contracts are essentially self-executing agreements that are written in code and follow specific rules. Their execution is triggered under particular conditions, which removes intermediates and minimises transaction fees. It automates processes and assists with data exchange, which improves efficiency.[27]

Managing Consent and Data Permissions

smart contracts are also capable of handling consent and data permissions. To maintain privacy, they are making sure only authorised parties have access to the data, and only those who are entitled can change it, enabling secure transactions over the blockchain network.[28]

Blockchain in Healthcare Data Security

Decentralised Electronic Health Records

Creating Secure, Interoperable EHR Systems

Decentralised, secure and tamper-proof EHRs can be built on blockchain. The secure storing of patient records will ensure that every healthcare system works at its full potential while maintaining the integrity of data with real-time access and updates through its distributed ledger technology. This supports interoperability between the many hospitals, clinics and healthcare providers, enabling a swift and secure transfer of data.[29]

Empowering Patients with Control over Their Data

Through blockchain, patients will be in full control of their medical data and thus be able to grant or deny access to providers. Patients can control access to their data via smart contracts, protecting privacy and enabling compliance with regulations such as GDPR and HIPAA.[4]

Secure Data Sharing among Providers

Trustless Data Exchange between Hospitals, Clinics, and Labs

Blockchain provides a trustless environment in which healthcare entities can share data securely, such as hospitals, clinics, and laboratories. Blockchain helps avoid sharing data with unauthorised parties, which increases security and the efficiency of medical data flows by removing intermediaries.[30]

Reducing Redundancy and Ensuring Data Accuracy

Blockchain removes duplication by storing one authenticated document representing an individual patient record. This also helps eliminate duplicate tests or procedures and ensures that all of the healthcare providers have access to the most current information, thereby decreasing errors and increasing the quality of care.[31]

Medical Supply Chain Management

Blockchain for Tracking Pharmaceuticals and Devices

Blockchain offers pharmaceutical and medical device traceability from manufacturer to patient in a secure manner across the healthcare supply chain. It can track each step that a product makes, preventing any counterfeit drug or device from entering the supply chain. Blockchain guarantees supply chain integrity by creating an immutable record of transactions.[32]

Ensuring the Integrity and Authenticity of Medical Products

Blockchain can be used to verify the provenance of pharmaceuticals and medical devices, providing healthcare providers with assurance that the products they are using are real. It eliminates the chance of fraudulent practices and guarantees that medical goods adhere to legal guidelines.[33]

Clinical Trials and Research

Ensuring Transparency and Security in Clinical Data

Blockchain offers a secure and transparent way to manage clinical trial data. It ensures that every piece of information relating to the clinical trial, such as protocol, patient data and results, are securely stored and can be readily verified, which reduces the risk of tampering or data manipulation.[34]

Reducing Fraud in Research Data and Consent Management

Blockchain helps provide transparency and immutability to the entire record and thus be able to affect the integrity of the research with respect to all other data related to that clinical trial. This means obtaining informed consent from the participants in a secure and verifiable way as a preventive measure for ethical violations and fraud.[35]

Blockchain and Compliance with Healthcare Regulations

HIPAA and GDPR Compliance

How Blockchain Ensures Data Privacy and Security

Blockchain technology ensures encrypted and decentralised storage, making management of sensitive patient data secure while complying with HIPAA and GDPR. Blockchain stores data in an immutable and distributed manner, hence protecting against illegitimate access, tampering or loss of data accidentally. That involves getting access to sensitive data through permission keys or smart contracts, where privacy is ensured by blockchain using cryptographic hashing.[36]

Permissioned vs. Public Blockchains for Regulatory Compliance

Permissioned blockchains, where only authorised participants can access or modify the data, are ideal for healthcare due to their ability to ensure compliance with HIPAA and GDPR. Such blockchains afford stricter access control through role-based permissions for healthcare providers. Although some public blockchains like Ethereum allow anyone to interact with them, this is not a good fit for healthcare since the lack of access control would hinder privacy. Thus, they can satisfy regulatory compliance by limiting access while guaranteeing transparency and helping patients maintain their privacy on permissioned blockchains.[37]

Audit Trails and Data Traceability

Using Blockchain for Tamper-Proof Records and Audits

The immutable nature of blockchain itself creates a clear, tamper-proof audit trail with data transactions being securely recorded that cannot be altered. For example, audit logs of data access, modification or sharing are essential for regulatory compliance in the field of healthcare and other industries where sensitive data is handled. Apart from this, each access request regarding patient data (who accessed it and its purpose) is recorded on a blockchain; hence, tracking of data flow becomes evident and proves to be beneficial during audits.[38]

Simplifying Regulatory Reporting

Blockchain simplifies regulatory reporting through automated audit report generation required by HIPAA, GDPR or other healthcare standards. Because all transactions and interactions with health data are automatically recorded in a blockchain, the necessary comprehensive reports can be easily extracted from this information by healthcare providers for regulators, minimising administrative burden while ensuring accuracy. With blockchain, healthcare entities can respond much faster to regulatory contacts and data breaches, as both are very transparent and traceable.[39]

Emerging Blockchain Applications in Healthcare

Telemedicine and Remote Monitoring

Securing Patient Data in Telehealth Platforms Using Blockchain

In telemedicine, blockchain technology can guarantee the security and privacy of patient data by building a decentralised information system used for the transmission of encrypted data regarding health statuses. Telehealth platforms can also use blockchain to protect video consultations, health records, and diagnostic reports so that only relevant healthcare professionals have access to this information. This alleviates worries about data breaches, particularly when transferring highly confidential medical records across (potentially) insecure channels.[40]

Blockchain-Based Authentication for Wearables and IoT Devices

Wearable health devices and Internet of Things (IoT) sensors integrated with blockchain can generate safe, accessible data from these devices. Using decentralised authentication protocols, blockchain can ensure that only trusted devices will collect health data and transmit it to healthcare systems. This preserves the security and privacy of data collected from wearables but enhances the reliability of remote monitoring for chronic diseases, fitness tracking, and other health management systems.[41]

AI and Blockchain Synergy

Combining AI with Blockchain for Predictive Healthcare

Combining AI and blockchain will transform predictive healthcare through large dataset sharing for AI-modelled use cases. In this way, the data that is used for AI algorithms remains uncompromised and private due to blockchain. At the same time, AI technology can give insights from these diagnosis records by predicting disease trajectory, suggesting personalised treatment, or optimising resource allocation in healthcare systems. Blockchain guarantees the reliability of data, which improves the performance and accuracy of AI models in healthcare applications.[42]

Enhancing Security in AI-Driven Healthcare Systems

Healthcare systems powered by AI have access to sensitive patient information, and blockchain can bring a transparent and immutable environment for data storage. They enable tracking of the provenance of training datasets, assuring that AI models are based on correct and compliant data. Moreover, blockchain can also protect AI models from adversarial attacks through secure verification procedures, ensuring that healthcare predictions and diagnostics are made with reliable inputs.[43]

Patient Empowerment and Self-Sovereign Identity

Giving Patients Control over Their Digital Health Identity

SSI is a new blockchain application which allows patients to own and govern their digital health identity. Patients can own their health data and even decide to whom they share them, thanks to blockchain, making centralised databases in healthcare a thing of the past. Patients would have their medical records, their prescriptions, and the history of the treatment option stored securely on the blockchain. They can share this information with healthcare providers, researchers or insurers when needed, which will put them in control of their healthcare.[44]

Blockchain for Managing Patient Consent

Patient consent for sharing health data can also leverage blockchain by maintaining a record of how data is shared and obtaining consent transparently while following the HIPAA and GDPR. Using blockchain smart contracts, patients are able to grant and revoke consent at any moment, providing a secure, constant, auditable record of exactly when and how researchers can access their data. It ensures patients' rights are preserved and provides an extensive but intuitive consent process for healthcare providers, researchers, and insurance companies seeking to use data in a clinical trial, treatment or analytics.[38]

Challenges and Barriers to Adoption

Scalability Issues

Blockchain Transaction Speed vs. Healthcare Data Demands

Scalability is one of the biggest obstacles in front of blockchain adoption, especially for industries like healthcare that demand high transaction throughput. For example, Bitcoin processes around seven transactions per second (TPS), whereas systems such as Visa can easily process roughly 1,700 TPS. This discrepancy indicates the inability of current blockchain technology to support data-driven applications in the health sector.

Solutions: Layer 2 Scaling, Off-Chain Storage

Layer 2 solutions and off-chain storage are the two major approaches to solving this scale issue in healthcare around blockchain technology. Layer 2 solutions work as secondary protocols that are built on the main blockchain, offloading transactions away from the primary network. This includes state channels and sidechains that increase the transaction throughput of these improvements without sacrificing underlying chain security. Similarly, off-chain storage helps improve transaction speeds and lower costs by allowing some data to be stored outside the blockchain, reducing the burden of on-chain storage while still maintaining access to necessary information. These approaches are essential for meeting the high data demands of the healthcare sector.[45]

Cost and Integration

Financial and Technical Challenges of Implementing Blockchain

Blockchain Technology has high monetary and technical barriers to implementation. Cost implications pertaining to infrastructure, maintenance, and workforce training necessary for organisations will need to be considered so that blockchain systems can be managed properly. Such financial obstacles might prevent prospective adopters from switching over to blockchain solutions.

Integration with Existing Healthcare Systems

The merging of the blockchain with legacy systems in healthcare presents additional challenges. The blockchain technologies being developed are unlikely to easily interface with the legacy systems that many healthcare organisations continue to use. Such integration complexity can result in high costs and a long implementation delivery cycle.[46]

Data Privacy vs. Transparenc y Dilemma

Balancing Blockchain's Transparency with Patient Confidentiality

The most well-known characteristic of blockchain, which is it being transparent, dominates the main reason for using this technology in healthcare as patient secrecy. Transparency is crucial for trust and accountability, but it also opens the door to other issues with revealing sensitive patient information. It is essential to strike a balance between the two in order for blockchain adoption to succeed in healthcare.

Cryptographic Solutions like Zero-Knowledge Proofs

In order to ensure the demand for privacy, at a minimum, how transparent the system behaves, some cryptographic solutions are provided, like zero-knowledge proofs (ZKPs). With ZKPs, one party proves to the other that something holds without revealing any more information than just this information being true. This approach can assist in maintaining patient privacy and providing required confirmation on the data.[47]

Future of Blockchain in Healthcare

Interoperability, the use of AI tools to mine data from decentralised sources and quantum-resistant technology are all areas where blockchain's potential in healthcare looks promising. Soon, we will have a global health and care blockchain ecosystem with secure transmission of data from HCPs to research facilities and patients within and across borders. To achieve this, standards for cross-blockchain data sharing that provide uniform protocols for secure and efficient data transfer are needed.

AI and blockchain are two technologies that will only complement each other to use healthcare systems, strengthen their potential for real-time threat detection, and secure data analytics. While AI can scrutinise innumerable healthcare data to discover security breaches, blockchain offers a tamper-proof proposition that acts as a cementing foundation for ensuring data integrity. This harmony enables a predictive healthcare and personalised medicine system to thrive without contravening data privacy rights.

Beyond these advancements, there must also be considerations as to the age of quantum computing, which could potentially serve as a huge risk to blockchain due to threats to foundational cryptographic techniques. Protecting healthcare data against future quantum attacks will require quantum-resistant blockchain solutions. However, blockchain systems need enhanced encryption techniques, particularly post-quantum cryptography, to be future-proof and provide long-lasting security. Dealing with such emerging challenges and opportunities, blockchain can transform healthcare, ensuring secure, interoperable, and intelligent systems for new-generation healthcare delivery.[47]

Conclusion

In conclusion, has a lot of potential to change the nature of healthcare data security with a distributed ledger system that is transparent and accurate to improve the management of highly sensitive medical information. Blockchain has the potential to solve a host of challenges we face today with patient data privacy and regulatory compliance through its capacity for secure, interoperable sharing across healthcare networks. It provides patients with control of their digital health records, allowing them to manage consent securely and decreasing exposure to unauthorised access or manipulation difficulties. In the future, blockchain will enable a more patient-centric model as the healthcare ecosystem moves to decentralised models of care in which patients can share their health data with providers wherever and whenever they choose. Blockchain will further be enhanced with the integration of advanced technologies such as AI and quantum-resistance cryptography, which will support real-time threat detection while preparing the system for future security threats. Blockchain will be an integral part of the next generation of data management systems that are designed to be secure, scalable and patient-centric as the healthcare industry continues to evolve. Due to its ability to protect privacy, provide data integrity and allow seamless interoperability across disparate healthcare systems, it will be an essential pillar of the continued evolution of patient data security.

References

1 Dong, Shi, Khushnood Abbas, Meixi Li, and Joarder Kamruzzaman. "Blockchain technology and application: An overview." *PeerJ Computer Science* 9 (2023): e1705.

2 Attaran, Mohsen. "Blockchain technology in healthcare: Challenges and opportunities." *International Journal of Healthcare Management* 15, no. 1 (2022): 70–83.

3 Christo, Mary Subaja, V. Elizabeth Jesi, Uma Priyadarsini, V. Anbarasu, Hridya Venugopal, and Marimuthu Karuppiah. "Ensuring improved security in medical data using ECC and blockchain technology with edge devices." *Security and Communication Networks* 2021, no. 1 (2021): 6966206.

4 Anik, Fahim Islam, Nazmus Sakib, Hossain Shahriar, Yixin Xie, Helal An Nahiyan, and Sheikh Iqbal Ahamed. "Unraveling a blockchain-based framework towards patient empowerment: A scoping review envisioning future smart health technologies." *Smart Health* 29 (2023): 100401.

5 Hussien, Hassan Mansur, Sharifah Md Yasin, S. N. I. Udzir, Aws Alaa Zaidan, and Bilal Bahaa Zaidan. "A systematic review for enabling a blockchain technology in healthcare application: taxonomy, substantial analysis, motivations, challenges, recommendations and future direction." *Journal of Medical Systems* 43 (2019): 1–35.

6 Liu, Fang, and Demosthenes Panagiotakos. "Real-world data: A brief review of the methods, applications, challenges and opportunities." *BMC Medical Research Methodology* 22, no. 1 (2022): 287.

7 Beltran-Aroca, Cristina M., Eloy Girela-Lopez, Eliseo Collazo-Chao, Manuel Montero-Pérez-Barquero, and Maria C. Muñoz-Villanueva. "Confidentiality breaches in clinical practice: What happens in hospitals?" *BMC Medical Ethics* 17 (2016): 1–12.

8 Chowdhury, Omar, Andreas Gampe, Jianwei Niu, Jeffery von Ronne, Jared Bennett, Anupam Datta, Limin Jia, and William H. Winsborough. "Privacy promises that can be kept: A policy analysis method with application to the HIPAA privacy rule." In *Proceedings of the 18th ACM Symposium on Access Control Models and Technologies,* pp. 3–14. 2013.

9 Alanazi, Abdullah T. "Clinicians' perspectives on healthcare cybersecurity and cyber threats." *Cureus*, 15, no. 10 (2023): 1–9.

10 Seh, Adil Hussain, Mohammad Zarour, Mamdouh Alenezi, Amal Krishna Sarkar, Alka Agrawal, Rajeev Kumar, and Raees Ahmad Khan. "Healthcare data breaches: Insights and implications." *Healthcare* 8, no. 2 (2020): 133.
11 Ahmed, Awais, Rui Xi, Mengshu Hou, Syed Attique Shah, and Sufian Hameed. "Harnessing big data analytics for healthcare: A comprehensive review of frameworks, implications, applications, and impacts." 11, *IEEE Access* (2023): 112891–112928.
12 Burke, Wendy, Andrew Stranieri, Taiwo Oseni, and Iqbal Gondal. "The need for cybersecurity self-evaluation in healthcare." *BMC Medical Informatics and Decision Making* 24, no. 1 (2024): 133.
13 Torab-Miandoab, Amir, Taha Samad-Soltani, Ahmadreza Jodati, and Peyman Rezaei-Hachesu. "Interoperability of heterogeneous health information systems: a systematic literature review." *BMC Medical Informatics and Decision Making* 23, no. 1 (2023): 18.
14 Abouelmehdi, Karim, Abderrahim Beni-Hessane, and Hayat Khaloufi. "Big healthcare data: Preserving security and privacy." *Journal of Big Data* 5, no. 1 (2018): 1–18.
15 Hathaliya, Jigna J., and Sudeep Tanwar. "An exhaustive survey on security and privacy issues in Healthcare 4.0." *Computer Communications* 153 (2020): 311–335.
16 Chernyshev, Maxim, Sherali Zeadally, and Zubair Baig. "Healthcare data breaches: Implications for digital forensic readiness." *Journal of Medical Systems* 43 (2019): 1–12.
17 Samal, Lipika, Patricia C. Dykes, Jeffrey O. Greenberg, Omar Hasan, Arjun K. Venkatesh, Lynn A. Volk, and David W. Bates. "Care coordination gaps due to lack of interoperability in the United States: A qualitative study and literature review." *BMC Health Services Research* 16 (2016): 1–8.
18 Ranchal, Rohit, Paul Bastide, Xu Wang, Aris Gkoulalas-Divanis, Maneesh Mehra, Senthil Bakthavachalam, Hui Lei, and Ajay Mohindra. "Disrupting healthcare silos: Addressing data volume, velocity and variety with a cloud-native healthcare data ingestion service." *IEEE Journal of Biomedical and Health Informatics* 24, no. 11 (2020): 3182–3188.
19 Chen, Jim Q., and Allen Benusa. "HIPAA security compliance challenges: The case for small healthcare providers." *International Journal of Healthcare Management* 10, no. 2 (2017): 135–146.
20 Mazurek, Michelle L., J. P. Arsenault, Joanna Bresee, Nitin Gupta, Iulia Ion, Christina Johns, Daniel Lee et al. "Access control for home data sharing: Attitudes, needs and practices." In *Proceedings of the SIGCHI Conference on Human Factors in Computing Systems*, pp. 645–654, 2010.
21 Ness, Roberta B., and Joint Policy Committee. "Influence of the HIPAA privacy rule on health research." *JAMA* 298, no. 18 (2007): 2164–2170.
22 Cimiterra, Martin, and Jackie Krafft. "Blockchain as a new digital paradigm." *Elgar Encyclopedia on the Economics of Knowledge and Innovation* (2022): 22–30.
23 Tripathi, Gautami, Mohd Abdul Ahad, and Gabriella Casalino. "A comprehensive review of blockchain technology: Underlying principles and historical background with future challenges." *Decision Analytics Journal* 9 (2023): 100344.
24 Sunny, Justin, Naveen Undralla, and V. Madhusudanan Pillai. "Supply chain transparency through blockchain-based traceability: An overview with demonstration." *Computers & Industrial Engineering* 150 (2020): 106895.
25 Bodkhe, Umesh, Sudeep Tanwar, Karan Parekh, Pimal Khanpara, Sudhanshu Tyagi, Neeraj Kumar, and Mamoun Alazab. "Blockchain for industry 4.0: A comprehensive review." *IEEE Access* 8 (2020): 79764–79800.

26 Alzoubi, Mahd M. "Investigating the synergy of Blockchain and AI: Enhancing security, efficiency, and transparency." *Journal of Cyber Security Technology* (2024): 1–29.

27 Pradhan, Nihar Ranjan, and Akhilendra Pratap Singh. "Smart contracts for the automated control system in blockchain-based smart cities." *Journal of Ambient Intelligence and Smart Environments* 13, no. 3 (2021): 253–267.

28 Merlec, Mpyana Mwamba, Youn Kyu Lee, Seng-Phil Hong, and Hoh Peter In. "A smart contract-based dynamic consent management system for personal data usage under GDPR." *Sensors* 21, no. 23 (2021): 7994.

29 Shuaib, Khaled, Juhar Abdella, Farag Sallabi, and Mohamed Adel Serhani. "Secure decentralised electronic health records sharing system based on blockchains." *Journal of King Saud University-Computer and Information Sciences* 34, no. 8 (2022): 5045–5058.

30 Taloba, Ahmed I., Alanazi Rayan, Ahmed Elhadad, Amr Abozeid, Osama R. Shahin, and Rasha M. Abd El-Aziz. "A framework for secure healthcare data management using blockchain technology." *International Journal of Advanced Computer Science and Applications* 12, no. 12 (2021): 639–646.

31 Cernian, Alexandra, Bogdan Tiganoaia, Ioan Sacala, Adrian Pavel, and Alin Iftemi. "PatientDataChain: A blockchain-based approach to integrate personal health records." *Sensors* 20, no. 22 (2020): 6538.

32 Nanda, Saroj Kumar, Sandeep Kumar Panda, and Madhabananda Dash. "Medical supply chain integrated with blockchain and IoT to track the logistics of medical products." *Multimedia Tools and Applications* 82, no. 21 (2023): 32917–32939.

33 Jamil, Faisal, Lei Hang, KyuHyung Kim, and DoHyeun Kim. "A novel medical blockchain model for drug supply chain integrity management in a smart hospital." *Electronics* 8, no. 5 (2019): 505.

34 Minssen, Timo, Neethu Rajam, and Marcel Bogers. "Clinical trial data transparency and GDPR compliance: Implications for data sharing and open innovation." *Science and Public Policy* 47, no. 5 (2020): 616–626.

35 Kennedy, James E. "Addressing researcher fraud: retrospective, real-time, and preventive strategies–including legal points and data management that prevents fraud." *Frontiers in Research Metrics and Analytics* 9 (2024): 1397649.

36 Ettaloui, Nehal, Sara Arezki, and Taoufiq Gadi. "An Overview of the blockchain-based electronic health record and compliance with GDPR and HIPAA." In Javier González Argote, Yousef Farhaoui, *The International Conference on Artificial Intelligence and Smart Environment,* pp. 405–412. Cham: Springer Nature Switzerland, 2023.

37 Velmovitsky, Pedro Elkind, Pedro Augusto Da Silva E. Souza Miranda, Hélène Vaillancourt, Tania Donovska, Jennifer Teague, and Plinio Pelegrini Morita. "A blockchain-based consent platform for active assisted living: Modelling study and conceptual framework." *Journal of Medical Internet Research* 22, no. 12 (2020): e20832.

38 Lei, Moyixi, Shuangyin Liu, Na Luo, Xinting Yang, and Chuanheng Sun. "Trusted-auditing chain: A security blockchain prototype used in agriculture traceability." *Heliyon* 8, no. 11 (2022).

39 Ghadi, Yazeed Yasin, Tehseen Mazhar, Tariq Shahzad, Muhammad Amir khan, Alaa Abd-Alrazaq, Arfan Ahmed, and Habib Hamam. "The role of blockchain is to secure the internet of medical things." *Scientific Reports* 14, no. 1 (2024): 18422.

40 Ahmad, Raja Wasim, Khaled Salah, Raja Jayaraman, Ibrar Yaqoob, Samer Ellahham, and Mohammed Omar. "The role of blockchain technology in telehealth and telemedicine." *International Journal of Medical Informatics* 148 (2021): 104399.

41 Sharma, Aashima, Sanmeet Kaur, and Maninder Singh. "A comprehensive review on blockchain and Internet of Things in healthcare." *Transactions on Emerging Telecommunications Technologies* 32, no. 10 (2021): e4333.
42 Kasula, Balaram Yadav. "Synergizing AI, IoT, and Blockchain: Empowering next-generation smart systems in healthcare." *International Journal of Sustainable Development in Computing Science* 5, no. 2 (2023): 60–64.
43 Charles, W., N. Marler, L. Long, and S. Manion. "Blockchain compliance by design: Regulatory considerations for blockchain in clinical research." *Frontiers in Blockchain* 2, Article 18 (2019): 1–18.
44 Siqueira, Alexandre, Arlindo Flavio Da Conceição, and Vladimir Rocha. "Blockchains and self-sovereign identities applied to healthcare solutions: A systematic review." *arXiv preprint arXiv:2104.12298* (2021).
45 Tortola, Domenico, Andrea Lisi, Paolo Mori, and Laura Ricci. "Tethering Layer 2 solutions to the blockchain: A survey on proving schemes." *Computer Communications* 225 (2024): 289–310.
46 AbuHalimeh, Ahmed, and Omar Ali. "Comprehensive review for healthcare data quality challenges in blockchain technology." *Frontiers in Big Data* 6 (2023): 1173620.
47 Loreti, Pierpaolo, Lorenzo Bracciale, Emanuele Raso, Giuseppe Bianchi, Eleonora Riva Sanseverino, and Pierluigi Gallo. "Privacy and transparency in blockchain-based smart grid operations." 11, *IEEE Access* (2023): 120666–120679.

3 Challenges in Traditional Healthcare Data Management

Sunita, Ashish Verma, Akanksha Sharma, Shaweta Sharma, Shilpa Thukral and Akhil Sharma

Introduction

Healthcare data management (HDM), also known as clinical data management or health information management, refers to the process of managing healthcare data stored in digital formats. HDM contains multiple data types, such as electronic medical records (EMRs), electronic health records (EHRs) accessed through a digital database and various scanned handwritten clinical notes. Digital transformation helped the healthcare sector to transfer and maintain patient records in an electronic format. Generally, these records consist of patient demographics (age, residence address, and sex), medication-associated records (laboratory results, drug prescriptions, physician referrals/visits, and treatment history), and administrative information (insurance claims/billing/reimbursement processes). HDM now involves integrating and analysing that data to improve care delivery and generate insights for better medical outcomes – all while safeguarding data privacy and security.[1,2]

Importance of Addressing Challenges

Overcoming issues in legacy healthcare data provides relief and clarity directly associated with patient care, operational efficiency, and regulatory compliance. The adoption of digital healthcare systems has brought about these massive and complicated data sets, which is, in itself, a big challenge due to the complexities relating to fragmentation and integration among them. Incomplete patient records are a by-product of fragmented data sources that obstruct diagnosis and treatment decisions, compromising patient safety and care quality.

Proper data management is essential to adhere to regulations like HIPAA that require strict measures around data privacy and security. Failing to comply can lead to heavy fines and damage to the organisation's reputation. Furthermore, as healthcare organisations work to implement a more holistic model of patient care, establishing stronger interoperability makes it easier for providers to collaborate on patient care, which can enhance health outcomes and lead to more individualised treatment plans. If healthcare organisations proactively tackle these issues, healthcare organisations can leverage their data more effectively, improve

DOI: 10.4324/9781003529910-3

decision-making processes, and ultimately provide higher-quality care while maintaining operational efficiency in a rapidly evolving digital landscape.[3,4]

Significance of Health Data Management

Handling this health data is crucial not only because it is expected to organise medical data but also because it integrates them and allows analysis. It allows for better patient care and greater efficiency. Encryption protects privacy in healthcare and cybersecurity, while HDM drives insights that improve health outcomes.

This includes a number of healthcare organisations that assemble claims data, EMR abstracts, enrolment data, and medical programs. Top-performing organisations take advantage of EMR feeds and data on disease management programs. Few organisations leverage non-health data assets that draw on enriched clinical or informal health data such as remote monitoring, wearables, patient lifestyle information, and patient experience surveys. When this level of capabilities in HDM is surpassed, more institutions are likely to amass a greater breadth of health information and data, mix it to generate new insights, and improve patient care outcomes.[5]

Top Challenges in Healthcare Data Management

HDM challenges involve working with stakeholders, including healthcare providers and patients. Aligning data processes and technologies to meet the requirements of all participants in the healthcare value chain can sometimes be daunting due to differing regulatory standards, data interoperability challenges, varying levels of technological adoption, and concerns over data privacy and security. Top Challenges in Healthcare Data Management are depicted in (Figure 3.1):

Data Fragmented

Healthcare data has various formats, including digital data in spreadsheets or databases, visual content, files like PDF and docx, scanned documents, and more complex data such as DICOM for MRI scans. Data duplication and collection preservation of the data in different formats are major issues that burden hospitals, public health organisations, payers, pharmacies, and patients.[6]

For patient health data to be actionable, it needs to be based on a singular source of truth. Various IT tools and software solutions can now eliminate duplicates by automating the data collection process of standardisation from diverse formats as well as EHR systems. Remember that a person still needs to connect those data systems to make them accessible, exchangeable, and interoperable.[7]

Data Storage Capability

Healthcare data just continues to increase regularly. Patients go through many tests and therapies in their lifetime, and a new treatment or drug is always available

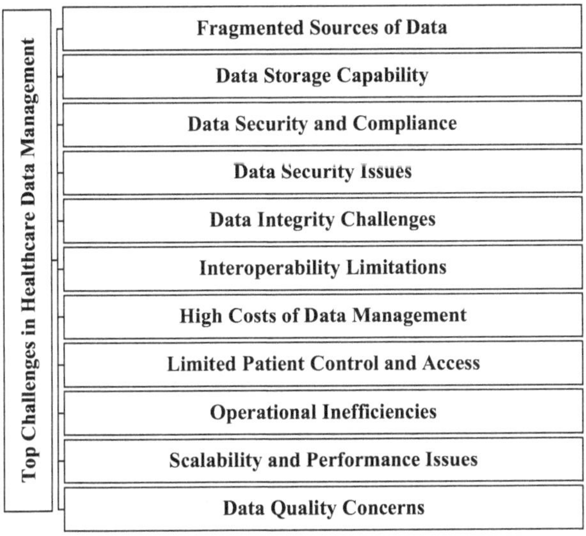

Figure 3.1 Top Challenges in Healthcare Data Management.

in the market. Shockingly, the healthcare industry generates 30% of the world's data. Managing such vast amounts of information presents significant challenges, including high costs and security risks. As a result, many healthcare organisations are moving towards advanced cloud storage options to ensure scalability, robustness, and security.[8]

Data Security and Compliance

The secrecy and integrity of the data shall be preserved so that it will never fall into the wrong hands or get corrupted. The key step needed to move forward towards a more value-based care model that rewards quality and transparency around billing rather than a misaligned fee-for-service process is secure data sharing. It also helps safeguard sensitive patient data from unauthorised access that could lead to malicious use, such as ransomware attacks.[9]

Furthermore, data protection should be HIPAA compliant (government access, encryption, security standards of stored and transmitted data). It should also be resilient to cyber threats so that when healthcare data is consumed and used by the system, it can maintain its trustworthiness and privacy.[10]

The critical issue of data security in health care arises from the sensitivity of patient information and the increasing sophistication of cyber threats. Ransomware alerts healthcare providers of data loss and being locked out from systems until a ransom is paid, which rivals the cost of patient care for managing data breaches and other cybersecurity threats. Data breaches are usually the most expensive for healthcare organisations, each exceeding $10 million. These vulnerabilities are compounded by weak encryption and authentication mechanisms. The lack of protective measures makes the system vulnerable to unauthorised access and exploitation of sensitive data. The reliance on outdated software and hardware compounds these issues, as many healthcare facilities struggle to keep up with necessary updates due to budget constraints.[11]

Additionally, insider threats present an additional barrier. Mishandling data or being the victim of phishing scams are common pitfalls that inadvertently undermine security. In addition, malicious intent from insiders may lead to deliberate data breaches, which can have a very detrimental effect on the trust in patients and the integrity of organisations. Dealing with these intersectional issues is crucial to protecting patient data and, more broadly, the integrity of the healthcare system.[12]

Data Integrity Challenges

Some of the most important data integrity challenges in healthcare focus on ensuring that patient data remains accurate and reliable, which is essential for making clinical decisions to address health issues while also ensuring patient safety. One significant issue is the risk of data tampering, where unauthorised modifications can lead to a lack of trustworthy records. This takes away the amount of faith healthcare providers and patients have in using the data for diagnosing or treatment plans. Moreover, errors in data entry or record discrepancies often lead to incomplete and inaccurate data, which can result in misdiagnosis, improper treatment, and even harm to patients. Furthermore, poor audit trails complicate the situation by making it difficult to track changes made to data over time. Such a lack of transparency can create a reduced level of duty among the providers since it is hard to tell who changed what and for which purpose. When combined, these challenges illustrate a pressing need for sound data management that safeguards healthcare data because lapses in this area can have drastic consequences for patient care and organisational credibility.[13,14]

Interoperability Limitations

The lack of interoperability in health care creates immense business challenges and prevents the combination of information across disparate systems. Legacy systems are another reason for system compatibility issues, as older technologies can rarely exchange information with modern solutions resulting in data silos and inefficiencies. Such incompatibility creates a challenge in data sharing, as organisations are faced with the steep cost of trying to bridge the technology divide. A second major issue is the unkind plethora of non-standardised data formats, as well as varying coding systems such as ICD and CPT. Without common standards, data exchange between systems often requires significant mapping work, which is time-consuming and error-prone. The absence of standardisation creates ambiguity and makes the aggregation of health data difficult, leading to a negative impact on patient care. Moreover, numerous healthcare organisations exchange data manually, and this procedure is slow and vulnerable to human errors. Such manual transfers can slow up access to a patient's vital data and increase the chances of miscommunication between healthcare suppliers. Thus, these interoperability constraints not only hinder operational efficiency but also jeopardise patient care quality, highlighting the urgent need for more efficient integration strategies within the healthcare context.[15,16]

High Costs of Data Management

Rising data management costs in the healthcare domain are one of the most critical factors contributing to jeopardising financial sustainability and inefficiency, as evidenced by various studies. Another area that stands out with significant expenditure as healthcare organisations deal with massive amounts of information produced every day from EHR, imaging, and other clinical solutions is storage and backup costs. Therefore, the demand for high-capacity data storage solutions and constant updating to keep the data untarnished adds largely to total operational expenditure. Likewise, high-priced manner upgrades are necessary for legacy infrastructure: lots of times, the existing things get historic and are out-of-date. Most health organisations are highly challenged to integrate legacy systems with new technologies, resulting in higher costs associated with both hardware and software upgrades as well. Modernising is vital for better data management functionality and interoperability with other health information systems. Healthcare providers need to implement technologies and processes that support compliance with regulations around patient data privacy and security, such as HIPAA. Compliance often necessitates continual training, audits, and systems upgrades, all of which are related to the cost base associated with data. Cumulatively, these factors highlight the imperative for healthcare organisations to lay out a roadmap towards reducing these costs while simultaneously preserving their delivery of high-quality patient care and data integrity.[17,18]

Limited Patient Control and Access

Limited patient control and access to healthcare data is a pressing issue that significantly impacts patient autonomy and engagement in their care. One major concern is restricted data ownership, where patients often cannot easily access their medical records. This lack of access not only hinders patients from being fully informed about their health but also limits their ability to participate actively in treatment decisions. Furthermore, data portability issues create further barriers, as transferring medical records from one provider to another can be fraught with difficulties. Patients may encounter challenges such as incompatible systems or the unavailability of standardised formats, making it cumbersome to move their health information seamlessly between different healthcare providers. Moreover, transparency gaps exacerbate the situation by creating a lack of visibility into how patient data is being used. Patients often remain unaware of who accesses their information and for what purposes, which can lead to mistrust in the healthcare system. This lack of transparency not only affects patient confidence but also raises ethical concerns regarding data privacy and consent. Addressing these limitations is crucial for empowering patients, enhancing their engagement in healthcare processes, and ensuring that they have control over their health information.[19,20]

Operational Inefficiencies

Operational inefficiencies in HDM can significantly hinder the effectiveness and quality of patient care. One of the primary contributors to these inefficiencies is the reliance on manual processes, particularly time-consuming data entry tasks. Healthcare professionals often spend excessive amounts of time inputting information into various systems, which not only detracts from their ability to focus on patient care but also increases the likelihood of human errors that can compromise data accuracy. Also, slow data retrieval poses a major challenge, as accessing real-time data is crucial for informed decision-making in clinical settings. Delays in retrieving patient information can result in missed opportunities for timely interventions, negatively impacting patient outcomes. This sluggishness is often exacerbated by fragmented systems that do not communicate effectively with one another, leading to further delays in accessing critical health information. Moreover, the duplication of efforts through redundant record-keeping creates unnecessary administrative burdens. When multiple departments or systems maintain separate records for the same patient, it not only wastes resources but also increases the risk of inconsistencies and errors in the data. Such redundancy can lead to confusion among healthcare providers and ultimately detracts from the overall efficiency of healthcare delivery. Addressing these operational inefficiencies is essential for streamlining processes, enhancing productivity, and improving the quality of care provided to patients.[21,22]

Scalability and Performance Issues

Scalability and performance issues in HDM are critical challenges that organisations must address to handle the increasing demands of patient data effectively. The exponential growth of healthcare data has created a pressing need for systems that can manage larger volumes without sacrificing performance. As patient records, imaging, and other data sources expand, healthcare information systems must have sufficient storage capacity and efficient retrieval mechanisms to ensure real-time access to critical information.[23]

However, many healthcare organisations face performance bottlenecks, particularly in centralised systems where slow response times can hinder clinical workflows. Delays in accessing patient information can impede timely decision-making, ultimately affecting patient care outcomes. The reliance on legacy systems often exacerbates these issues, as outdated technology may not support the rapid processing of large datasets or accommodate the growing number of users needing access to information.

Furthermore, limited flexibility for expansion presents additional challenges. Many existing systems struggle to scale effectively, making it difficult to adapt to new technologies or increased workloads. This rigidity can lead to inefficiencies

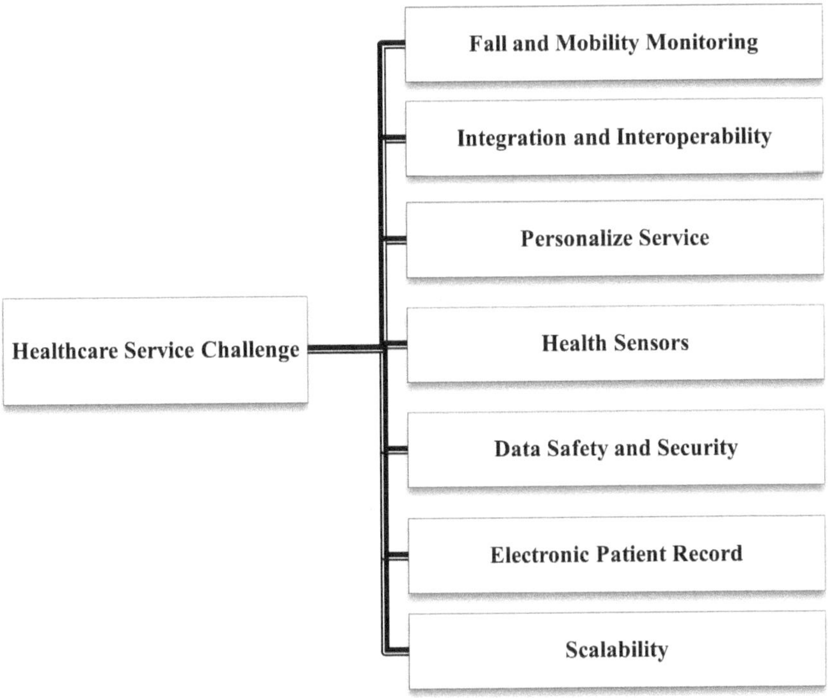

Figure 3.2 Scalability and Performance Issues.

and increased operational costs as organisations attempt to integrate new solutions with outdated infrastructure. To overcome these scalability and performance issues, healthcare organisations should consider adopting cloud-based solutions, modular architectures, and automation technologies that enhance system flexibility and responsiveness while ensuring robust performance (Figure 3.2) is summarizing the issues arises during Scalability and Performance .[24]

Data Quality Concerns

Data quality concerns in healthcare are critical for ensuring accurate patient care and effective decision-making. One significant issue is inconsistent data collection, which often arises from variability in data entry standards across different healthcare providers and systems. This inconsistency can lead to discrepancies in patient records, making it challenging for clinicians to rely on the information available for treatment decisions. Additionally, the presence of duplicate or redundant records exacerbates data quality issues, with studies indicating that healthcare organisations can experience duplication rates as high as 10–30%. Duplicate records occur when multiple entries exist for the same patient, often due to errors during data entry or registration processes. This redundancy not only complicates patient care but can also lead to medical errors and increased costs associated with unnecessary tests or treatments. Moreover, misclassification or mistakes in data labelling further compromise data integrity. Incorrectly labelled information can result from typographical errors, outdated information, or misunderstandings during data entry. Such inaccuracies can severely impact clinical workflows and patient safety, as healthcare providers may act on incomplete or erroneous data. Addressing these data quality concerns is essential for improving patient outcomes, enhancing operational efficiency, and ensuring compliance with regulatory standards in the healthcare sector.[25,26]

Effective Healthcare Data Management

HDM is known for its complexity. Some best practices healthcare organisations can adopt to help strategically streamline data management.[14]

Collect the Right Data

Healthcare data is sourced from various databases within an integrated care system. Whether from hospital EHRs or population health platforms, proper processes and tools are vital for managing the data effectively.[27]

Healthcare organisations must define the potential sources for extracting valuable data. Identifying the correct data to collect helps in the later stages of setting priorities for each data type and integrating the right tools to retrieve the data needed.[28]

Identify Key Data Elements

Start with your healthcare organisation's goals and align the essential data elements, such as patient health outcomes, treatment efficacy, and operational performance metrics.[29]

Ensure Data Quality at the Source

Implement processes to ensure the data collected is accurate, complete, and entered correctly at the point of care. This might involve training staff on the importance of data accuracy and correctly inputting data.[30]

Leverage Technology

EHRs and other digital tools can be used to automate data collection where possible. This reduces the likelihood of human error and ensures a more comprehensive data collection.[31]

Interpret Data

Hospital data systems extract data from various sources to make medication decisions. This process relies on data interpretation.

Use Advanced Analytics Tools

Deploy analytics tools that can handle large volumes of data and provide insights through predictive analytics, machine learning algorithms, and data visualisation techniques.[32]

Cross-Disciplinary Teams

Form teams comprising healthcare professionals, data scientists, and IT experts to interpret the data, and if those resources aren't in-house, consider a technology vendor for support! This multidisciplinary approach ensures that insights are clinically relevant and actionable.

Continuous Learning and Adaptation

Make data interpretation an ongoing process. As new data comes in and the healthcare landscape evolves, continuously refine your analysis methods to adapt to these changes.[33,34]

Manage Data Storage Growth

Embrace Scalable Solutions

Opt for cloud-based storage solutions that offer scalability. As your data storage needs grow, cloud services can easily accommodate this increase without significant upfront investments in physical infrastructure.[35]

Regular Data Audits and Cleanup

Conduct regular audits of your data storage to identify redundant, obsolete, or trivial (ROT) information. Removing ROT data helps manage storage costs and improves system performance.[36]

Implement Data Lifecycle Management

Establish policies for data retention, archiving, and deletion based on regulatory requirements and the data's ongoing value to the organisation. This not only helps in managing storage growth but also ensures compliance with data protection regulations (Figure 3.3) is showing the Data Lifecycle management.[37]

Decode Data Access Requirements

Extracted data often comes in various formats and is subject to different accessibility regulations. Healthcare organisations must understand all the data access requirements to ensure a clear data management plan. Also, healthcare organisations can enable Healthcare Information Exchange, which allows different devices, applications, and systems to collaborate, access, and exchange medical data. Aim

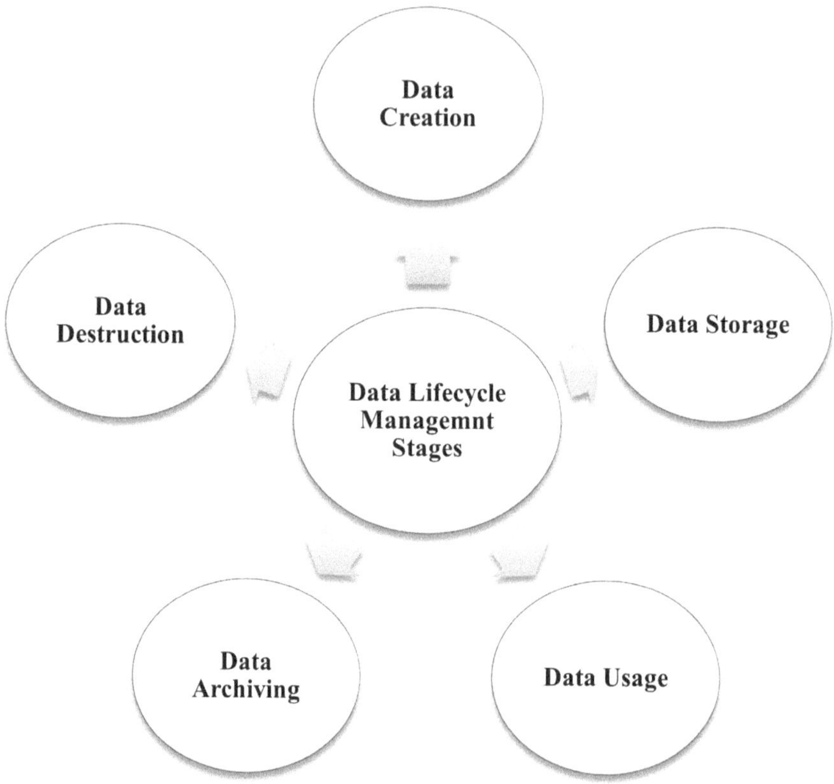

Figure 3.3 Data Lifecycle Management.

for a continued goal of simplifying the process of accessing and retrieving healthcare data.[38]

Implement Data Management Software

Several health information systems overlook a crucial practice – investing in data management solutions. HDM often comes with challenges, particularly during setup. Providers may need specialised tools such as system connectors or APIs to implement and operate data management practices effectively. Strategic investments in collaboration with data management experts or technology providers should be used to enhance your data management system processes.[39]

Solutions to Meet Healthcare Data Management Challenges

HDM is known for its complexity. It comprises various processes like storage, data entry, AI, processing, accessibility, security, and predictive modelling. Some of the advantages of technology in healthcare include helping in implementing solutions and medical enterprises, as well as facilitating, informing, and streamlining processes. It includes:

Technologies for Data Entry

Healthcare enterprises use technologies for data entries to aggregate and collect data from various systems and resources in different formats. This helps in storing the data in a central repository. Providers are using IoT to monitor patients remotely through smart and wearable devices. Providers can collect and monitor data from their homes. Providers are using customer-relationship management tools and platforms to understand patient needs and improve their holistic experience. OCR technologies enable providers to digitise the texts and minimise manual errors.[40]

Access to Technologies and Data Storage

Providers use data storage and have access to technologies like automated tasks, HIPAA compliance, improved access, and security. In place of using traditional on-premise geolocations, they are now towards safer and cloud-based solutions.

Cloud data storage offers flexible information storage capacity and low maintenance costs. It also allows providers, stakeholders, and organisations to have easy access to adopting hybrid and remote work policies and mobile apps. Providers are allowed to increase or reduce this HDM software space as needed instead of investing in on-premise platforms or servers. Cloud-based technologies and other hosting solutions have a lower risk of health data breaches than on-premise servers as this data is stored in various locations and is more secure.[41]

Data Security, Fraud Technology Detection, and Security

Processing data in real time is crucial to providers and healthcare organisations. HDM allows them to adopt newer technologies and healthcare database management systems as a lot of data needs to be collected, which can be too much for traditional systems. This data is stored in various resources and formats.

AI and ML are allowing providing to diagnose patients more accurately and forecast medical concerns and their progress. This helps in working in real-time, improving the overall efficacy of providers, doctors, and nurses, and assists in providing better health results for patients. To ensure data management in healthcare, providers also need to ensure optimum data security. Implementing security technologies helps control access and integrate encryption during storage or transmission.

Providers can now also use fraud detection and prevention systems to monitor any suspicious activities that can be inspected more closely. Data-driven fraud prevention is now aided by artificial intelligence as it offers higher fraud prevention and detection power that is more cost-efficient for organisations.[42]

Optimum Scalability for Data Architectures

HDM enables providers to generate an exponential amount of data every second to mine it for valuable patient insights. With digital innovation and new technologies making headway towards availability, data output will grow further.

Healthcare professionals are adopting cloud storage and computing to predict inevitable future growth. On-premise storage methods are now limited as healthcare organisations and enterprises are investing more in provider data management solutions. Cloud-based solutions will provide optimum output for data architectures and scale up the business when new hardware is invested in.[43]

Predictive Modelling and Data Intelligence

Healthcare professionals incorporate and employ a wide range of analytical tools and methods to understand the data that has been collected. It helps in deriving the right value. Through assistance from data intelligence, providers will improve treatment outcomes, recognise threats early, and personalise their treatment when it comes to taking preventive and cautious actions.

With predictive modelling technologies using AI, providers can utilise patient records and other health information and data to detect any chronic conditions or high-risk medical events proactively, hence preventing them from happening. The predictive modelling lowers internal healthcare process expenditures and tailors treatment plans according to the patient's medical requirements.[44]

Conclusion

In conclusion, traditional HDM faces significant challenges that hinder the efficient and secure handling of patient information. Issues such as data fragmentation, lack of interoperability, security vulnerabilities, and inconsistent data standards present considerable barriers to optimising patient outcomes and operational efficiencies. The reliance on legacy systems and manual processes further exacerbates these problems, leading to potential data inaccuracies, increased administrative burden, and limited real-time access to critical health data.

As healthcare continues to evolve towards more patient-centred and data-driven approaches, it is imperative to address these challenges. Solutions must prioritise interoperability, standardisation of data formats, and enhanced cybersecurity measures to protect patient privacy. Additionally, the adoption of innovative technologies, such as blockchain, artificial intelligence, and cloud computing, can offer transformative potential in overcoming current limitations. These technologies promise to streamline data integration, enhance security, and facilitate seamless data exchange across healthcare ecosystems.

Ultimately, resolving these challenges requires a concerted effort from stakeholders across the healthcare spectrum, including policymakers, healthcare providers, and technology developers. Collaborative efforts to modernise infrastructure, establish robust data governance frameworks and implement forward-looking policies will be crucial to unlocking the full potential of healthcare data. By doing so, the healthcare industry can pave the way for more secure, efficient, and interoperable data management systems that better support patient care and advance medical research.

References

1 Bazel, Mahmood A., Fathey Mohammed, and Mazida Ahmed. "Blockchain technology in healthcare big data management: Benefits, applications and challenges." In *2021 1st International Conference on Emerging Smart Technologies and Applications (eSmarTA)*, pp. 1–8. IEEE, 2021.
2 Yaqoob, Ibrar, Khaled Salah, Raja Jayaraman, and Yousof Al-Hammadi. "Blockchain for healthcare data management: Opportunities, challenges, and future recommendations." *Neural Computing and Applications* 34 (2022): 1–16.
3 Pastorino, Roberta, Corrado De Vito, Giuseppe Migliara, Katrin Glocker, Ilona Binenbaum, Walter Ricciardi, and Stefania Boccia. "Benefits and challenges of Big Data in healthcare: An overview of the European initiatives." *European Journal of Public Health* 29, no. Supplement_3 (2019): 23–27.
4 Martin, Erika G., and Grace M. Begany. "Opening government health data to the public: Benefits, challenges, and lessons learned from early innovators." *Journal of the American Medical Informatics Association* 24, no. 2 (2017): 345–351.
5 Cylus, Jonathan, Irene Papanicolas, Peter C. Smith, and World Health Organization. *Health System Efficiency: How to Make Measurement Matter for Policy and Management*. World Health Organization. Regional Office for Europe, 2016. Health Policy Series No. 46 www.healthobservatory.eu.
6 Cribb, Alan. "Shaping the future." In *Healthcare in Transition*, pp. 153–184. Policy Press, 2017.
7 Ciriani, Valentina, Sabrina De Capitani Di Vimercati, Sara Foresti, Sushil Jajodia, Stefano Paraboschi, and Pierangela Samarati. "Combining fragmentation and encryption to protect privacy in data storage." *ACM Transactions on Information and System Security (TISSEC)* 13, no. 3 (2010): 1–33.
8 Binnig, G., Michel Despont, Ute Drechsler, Walter Haeberle, M. Lutwyche, Peter Vettiger, H. J. Mamin, B. W. Chui, and Th W. Kenny. "Ultrahigh-density atomic force microscopy data storage with erase capability." *Applied Physics Letters* 74, no. 9 (1999): 1329–1331.
9 Nass, Sharyl J., Laura A. Levit, and Lawrence O. Gostin. "The value and importance of health information privacy." In *Beyond the HIPAA Privacy Rule: Enhancing Privacy, Improving Health Through Research*. Washington, DC: National Academies Press (US), 2009.
10 Coronado, Anthony J., and Timothy L. Wong. "Healthcare cybersecurity risk management: Keys to an effective plan." *Biomedical Instrumentation & Technology* 48, no. s1 (2014): 26–30.
11 Coventry, Lynne, and Dawn Branley. "Cybersecurity in healthcare: A narrative review of trends, threats and ways forward." *Maturitas* 113 (2018): 48–52.
12 He, Ying, Aliyu Aliyu, Mark Evans, and Cunjin Luo. "Health care cybersecurity challenges and solutions under the climate of COVID-19: Scoping review." *Journal of Medical Internet Research* 23, no. 4 (2021): e21747.

13 Hassan, Ammar. "Ensuring data integrity in clinical trials: A comprehensive overview." (2023): 1–32.

14 Vimalachandran, Pasupathy, Hua Wang, Yanchun Zhang, Ben Heyward, and Frank Whittaker. "Ensuring data integrity in electronic health records: A quality health care implication." In *2016 International Conference on Orange Technologies (ICOT)*, pp. 20–27. IEEE, 2016.

15 Mahmud, Redowan, Fernando Luiz Koch, and Rajkumar Buyya. "Cloud-fog interoperability in IoT-enabled healthcare solutions." In *Proceedings of the 19th International Conference on Distributed Computing and Networking*, pp. 1–10. 2018.

16 Adenuga, Olugbenga A., Ray M. Kekwaletswe, and Alfred Coleman. "eHealth integration and interoperability issues: Towards a solution through enterprise architecture." *Health Information Science and Systems* 3 (2015): 1–8.

17 Charlson, Mary, Robert E. Charlson, William Briggs, and James Hollenberg. "Can disease management target patients most likely to generate high costs? The impact of comorbidity." *Journal of General Internal Medicine* 22 (2007): 464–469.

18 Pothukuchi, A. Shastri, Lakshmi Vasuda Kota, and Vinay Mallikarjunaradhya. "A critical analysis of the challenges and opportunities to optimize storage costs for big data in the cloud." *Asian Journal of Multidisciplinary Research & Review* 25, no. 1 (2021): 132–144.

19 Entwistle, Vikki A., Stacy M. Carter, Alan Cribb, and Kirsten McCaffery. "Supporting patient autonomy: The importance of clinician-patient relationships." *Journal of General Internal Medicine* 25 (2010): 741–745.

20 Heidelberg, M., A. Kelman, J. Hopkins, and M. E. Allen. "The evolution of data ethics in clinical research and drug development." *Ethics, Medicine and Public Health* 14 (2020): 100517.

21 Syed, Rehan, Rebekah Eden, Tendai Makasi, Ignatius Chukwudi, Azumah Mamudu, Mostafa Kamalpour, Dakshi Kapugama Geeganage Sareh Sadeghianasl, Sander J J Leemans ,Kanika Goel ,Robert Andrews ,Moe Thandar Wynn ,Arthur Ter Hofstede ,Trina Myers "Digital health data quality issues: Systematic review." Journal of Medical Internet Research 25 (2023): e42615.

22 Langell, John T. "Evidence-based medicine: A data-driven approach to lean healthcare operations." *International Journal of Healthcare Management* 14, no. 1 (2021): 226–229.

23 Mazlan, Ahmad Akmaluddin, Salwani Mohd Daud, Suriani Mohd Sam, Hafiza Abas, Siti Zaleha Abdul Rasid, and Muhammad Fathi Yusof. "Scalability challenges in healthcare blockchain system—A systematic review." *IEEE Access* 8 (2020): 23663–23673.

24 Brataas, Gunnar, Erlend Stav, Sebastian Lehrig, Steffen Becker, Goran Kopčak, and Darko Huljenic. "CloudScale: Scalability management for cloud systems." In *Proceedings of the 4th ACM/SPEC International Conference on Performance Engineering*, pp. 335–338. 2013.

25 Bernardi, Filipe Andrade, Domingos Alves, Nathalia Crepaldi, Diego Bettiol Yamada, Vinicius Costa Lima, and Rui Rijo. "Data quality in health research: Integrative literature review." *Journal of Medical Internet Research* 25 (2023): e41446.

26 Johnson, Steven G., Stuart Speedie, Gyorgy Simon, Vipin Kumar, and Bonnie L. Westra. "Quantifying the effect of data quality on the validity of an eMeasure." *Applied Clinical Informatics* 8, no. 04 (2017): 1012–1021.

27 Kumar, Yogesh, Kanika Sood, Surabhi Kaul, and Richa Vasuja. "Big data analytics and its benefits in healthcare." *Big Data Analytics in Healthcare* (2020): 3–21.

28 Ahmadi, Maryam. "Identification of the necessary data elements to report AIDS: A systematic review." *Electronic Physician* 9, no. 12 (2017): 5920–5931.

29 Management Group Liefer Laura A. 51 Wetterstrand Kris A. 51 Good Peter J. 51 Feingold Elise A. 51 Guyer Mark S. 51 Collins Francis S. 52, Baylor College of Medicine Human Genome Sequencing Center*, Washington University Genome Sequencing Center*, Broad Institute*, Children's Hospital Oakland Research Institute*, and Mark Gerstein. "Identification and analysis of functional elements in 1% of the human genome by the ENCODE pilot project." *Nature* 447, no. 7146 (2007): 799–816.

30 Baigent, Colin, Frank E. Harrell, Marc Buyse, Jonathan R. Emberson, and Douglas G. Altman. "Ensuring trial validity by data quality assurance and diversification of monitoring methods." *Clinical Trials* 5, no. 1 (2008): 49–55.

31 Pérez-Stable, Eliseo J., Beda Jean-Francois, and Courtney Ferrell Aklin. "Leveraging advances in technology to promote health equity." *Medical Care* 57 (2019): S101–S103.

32 Aroraa, Gaurav, Chitra Lele, and Munish Jindal. *Data Analytics: Principles, Tools, and Practices: A Complete Guide for Advanced Data Analytics Using the Latest Trends, Tools, and Technologies (English Edition)*. Noida, Uttar Pradesh: BPB Publications, 2022.

33 Smith, Andrea, and Melissa Severn. "An overview of continuous learning artificial intelligence-enabled medical devices." *Canadian Journal of Health Technologies* 2, no. 5 (2022): 1–15.

34 Johnson, Ebunoluwa, Omorinsola Bibire Seyi-Lande, Gbenga Sheriff Adeleke, Chinazor Prisca Amajuoyi, and Bayode Dona Simpson. "Developing scalable data solutions for small and medium enterprises: Challenges and best practices." *International Journal of Management & Entrepreneurship Research* 6, no. 6 (2024): 1910–1935.

35 Patel, Kaushikkumar. "Mastering cloud scalability: Strategies, challenges, and future directions: Navigating complexities of scaling in digital era." In *Emerging Trends in Cloud Computing Analytics, Scalability, and Service Models*, pp. 155–169. Hershey, Pennsylvania, New York, New York Beijing, China. Dina Darwish: IGI Global, 2024.

36 Mahanti, Rupa. *Data Quality: Dimensions, Measurement, Strategy, Management, and Governance*. North America, Mexico: Quality Press, 2019.

37 Zhang, Yingfeng, Shan Ren, Yang Liu, Tomohiko Sakao, and Donald Huisingh. "A framework for Big Data-driven product lifecycle management." *Journal of Cleaner Production* 159 (2017): 229–240.

38 Stanciu, Alexandru. "Data management plan for healthcare: Following FAIR principles and addressing cybersecurity aspects. A systematic review using InstructGPT." *medRxiv* (2023): 2023-04.

39 Hulsen, Tim. "Challenges and solutions for big data in personalised healthcare." In Ahmed A. Moustafa (ed), *Big Data in Psychiatry# x0026; Neurology*, pp. 69–94. Washington, DC: Academic Press, 2021.

40 Tse, Daniel, Chung-kin Chow, Ting-pong Ly, Chung-yan Tong, and Kwok-wah Tam. "The challenges of big data governance in healthcare." In *2018 17th IEEE International Conference on Trust, Security and Privacy in Computing and Communications/12th IEEE International Conference on Big Data Science and Engineering (TrustCom/BigDataSE)*, pp. 1632–1636. IEEE, 2018.

41 Sachdeva, Sonali, Saurabh Bhatia, Ahmed Al Harrasi, Yasir Abbas Shah, Khalid Anwer, Anil K. Philip, Syed Faisal Abbas Shah, Ajmal Khan, and Sobia Ahsan Halim. "Unraveling the role of cloud computing in health care system and biomedical sciences." *Heliyon* 10: (2024), 1–15.

42 Liu, Brent J., Zheng Zhou, and H. K. Huang. "A HIPAA-compliant architecture for securing clinical images." *Journal of Digital Imaging* 19 (2006): 172–180.
43 Hilal, Waleed, S. Andrew Gadsden, and John Yawney. "Financial fraud: A review of anomaly detection techniques and recent advances." *Expert Systems with Applications* 193 (2022): 116429.
44 Liu, Vincent X., David W. Bates, Jenna Wiens, and Nigam H. Shah. "The number needed to benefit: Estimating the value of predictive analytics in healthcare." *Journal of the American Medical Informatics Association* 26, no. 12 (2019): 1655–1659.

4 Smart Contracts Transforming Healthcare Transactions

Akanksha Sharma, Ashish Verma, Sunita, Akhil Sharma, Shivkanya Fuloria and Shaweta Sharma

Introduction

Previously known as a written contract, which requires agreement in written form, a smart contract is an application that uses blockchain technology to provide two parties with a written agreement in digital form. However, this makes the agreement less effective because it can lead to errors and fraud on the part of one party, making it less secure and more likely to be lost or damaged. These days, practically every industrial activity uses smart contracts. The smart contract is another example of a smart contract. It was initially identified in 1994 by Nick Szabo and was intended to enable attorneys to enter into a particular contract between parties. Even though Satoshi Nakamoto initially discovered the blockchain in 2008, it is a peer-to-peer, decentralized, and transparent method of exchanging information that allows all parties to interact directly without the need for a middleman by creating digital currency, or bitcoin.[1,2]

The blockchain cannot host a huge amount of data, but if it replicates the entity and engages all users to obtain every data to be permanently saved on the blockchain could solve this issue. A cryptographic system safeguards such data and confidentiality of data is targeted by cryptography. The process serves as a way for Smart Contracts to enter into a contract with the transaction, written on a blockchain network that acts as data storage security for Smart Contracts themselves.

An Ethereum system, a popular computer programming system, is where this blockchain technology is implemented. Since blockchain is not able to store huge amounts of data, developers must create decentralized applications (dApps) in order to create Smart Contracts. These dApps must involve all parties and have no priority entities; all data will be stored on blockchain permanently, protected by cryptographic and encryption systems whose goal is to store data confidentiality so that the stored data won't vanish or be altered by anybody.[1–3]

The implementation of smart contracts within blockchain facilitates the identification of ownership, thereby preventing unauthorized tracking or data manipulation. Additionally, smart contracts offer flexibility, enabling efficient operation without the necessity of third-party intermediaries, such as lawyers and notaries, thus reducing costs and saving time by eliminating lengthy queues for document

DOI: 10.4324/9781003529910-4

agreements between the involved parties, which can be executed via electronic signatures.[2]

During the digital transformation of the healthcare industry, one emerging technology that has recently gained attention is blockchain technology. It has been implemented to transform the conventional approach that medical systems and enterprises have adopted in the healthcare sector for decades. Information and Communication Technologies and blockchain are pivotal technologies for the decentralization and digitalization of healthcare institutions, thereby creating a contemporary and entirely digital healthcare environment accessible to both patients and service providers.[2]

These healthcare data management applications create many utilities in the field of patient record control and access, payments and claims management, medical IoT security management, researcher data verification, and medical research grants transparency exchange for financial auditing. Such applications make use of fast, up-to-the-minute modifications to a secure, decentralized blockchain ledger to interpret, observe and also adjust healthcare details. This also helps medical healthcare institutions to halt any unauthorized person from gaining entry to essential information.[4]

Healthcare management comprises various processes including managing funds, employees, patients, lawyers, logistics, inventories, etc. Hence handling repetitive tasks associated with the actual treatment of patients in medical workflows can be mapped out as a series of conditional steps. They are intended to improve effectiveness, productivity, and compliance in hospitals and other healthcare service providers and also establish stronger internal controls so that risk exposure, work cycles, and overhead can be minimized.[2,5]

Potential Benefits in the Healthcare Industry

For medical researchers, healthcare providers, and individuals alike, blockchain technology offers a wealth of advantages. A central repository of all health data stored over a real-time tracking of personalized data and permissions being set on the level and scale of an individual would benefit both research and personalized medicine equally. Big data in health is essential for enabling new understandings of illness, accelerating biomedical research, tracking medication development in real time, and creating individualized treatment regimens based on environmental, lifestyle, and genetic factors. Because patients from various socioeconomic and cultural backgrounds and geographical locations contribute to a shared data system using blockchain, the data set's breadth would be wide. Blockchain delivers the best data for long-term research since it gathers a person's health information throughout the course of their lifetime.[6]

Healthcare blockchain extends the accessibility of health data to encompass previously marginalized communities that have been underserved by the medical community or historically excluded from scientific engagement. As a common data environment, the blockchain facilitates interest from "hard-to-reach"[2] audiences and makes results produced by the general public more reflective. A healthcare blockchain could also promote a new type of app as health providers which would bypass current medical research and create individualized treatment pathways. Instead of an informed discussion based on the intuition-derived best option, the patient and healthcare provider would have access to the same information to facilitate a conversation around research-based treatment options.[2]

Concepts of Healthcare Transaction Using Blockchain

A distributed ledger known as a blockchain is kept up to date by several peers on a peer-to-peer network. Such technology functions without the need for a central governing body or administration of data storage. Data is accessed by various nodes and encryption and replication are used to preserve data quality. Blockchain was first introduced by Nakamoto in a white paper. As a result, the idea of transferring money online between parties directly rather than via a financial institution was born. The main goal was to develop a non-trusting system that utilizes peer-to-peer distributed ledger technology to overcome the double-spending problem by demonstrating computational consistency across chronological sequences of transactions.[1] The name blockchain indicates a chain of blocks in which every block contains some data about the past, present, and future of itself. Each block is very important in linking one to the previous one and the next one also comes into the system to be attached to the chain. Each block mainly records and verifies the transaction messages between blocks. Essentially it makes it so a block in the chain cannot be deleted or edited without changing every block afterwards.[7]

In other words, a blockchain network is a distributed database that has historical data from all previous trades and operates according to an algorithm selected in advance which indicates how these transactions should be carried out and approved as well as how the entire network should operate between its participants. Furthermore, this framework is generally known as a disseminated registry since information in each company gets put away by means of each hub working in one of the separate systems.

Blocks of transactions are combined together by hashing the previous block's record. Thus the basic feature of the bitcoin network security as a property of immutability is enforced. As the blockchain expands, any previous block will become increasingly impervious to interference: Because the hash values in the following block headers will vary entirely depending on how the hash function operates, an attacker would be quickly neutralized because the local register would no longer match any of those keys even with slight modifications.[8]

Security Vulnerabilities of Blockchain Technology

Complexity of smart contracts and blockchain technology can cause the vulnerabilities of blockchain-based applications. These are critical issues that a malicious attacker can exploit and do serious harm to the system. Some common blockchain vulnerabilities are discussed below:

Gas Transaction Fee Attacks

Some blockchain platforms like Ethereum transact via some fee system called gas fee. Attackers can then overload a targeted smart contract with an unreasonable amount of gas fees in order to delay or even make the transaction fail.[9]

Transaction Replay Attacks

Some smart contracts allow undoing or redoing transactions before processing a transaction. This feature can be abused by attackers to consume resources by performing the same action.

Front-Running Attacks

Front-running attacks happen through attackers when they observe the unconfirmed actions of a user and try to make use of that chance by performing an analytical move on behalf of him, achieving benefit by taking an action in the same nature directly or indirectly.[10]

Blockchain Protocol Weaknesses

The protocols used by such blockchain-based applications may not be so robust. These vulnerabilities can be exploited by malicious attackers to manipulate consensus mechanisms or break the integrity of data.[11]

Phishing and Social Engineering Attacks

The protocols used by such blockchain-based applications may not be so robust. These vulnerabilities can be exploited by malicious attackers to manipulate consensus mechanisms or break the integrity of data.[12]

Centralized dApps Issues

Certain components of some blockchain applications may be hosted on centralized servers. It can lead to security and data integrity concerns as components stored in a centralized location can be exposed to cyber-attacks.

Overview of Smart Contract Platforms

Smart contracts are a type of computer program used to define an agreement or ruleset between members of a blockchain network. Smart contracts can be used to guarantee that the terms of a contract are fulfilled, while at the same time making it expensive to breach the contract. Smart contract can be executed automatically, as part of a transaction on the blockchain network, and does not require a third party to perform. In other words, whenever a participant node receives a transaction, the smart contract corresponding to that transaction will be executed to verify that the transaction is valid and whether or not the conditions stipulated in the contract are met. If the transaction is confirmed to be valid, the outcome is written into the blockchain. They cryptographically guarantee business logic, offer blockchain read access to the public, and make sure that an operation over an asset is performed in a verifiable transaction-free manner with no chance of conflict or dispute, while suppressing any charges or involvement from intermediaries.[13]

There is a variety of smart contract applications across domains. They can be used for banking transactions, to register anything that one owns, or to manage access control of specific assets. In each case, the smart contract has all conditions and terms agreed by every stakeholder in their particular process. Smart contract platforms are a fundamental element of crypto and blockchain technology, enabling developers to build DApps and run transactions in a trustless, open-source as well as secure environment. The following is a description of three popular smart contract systems:

Ethereum

Ethereum is the most popular and one of the most used smart contract platforms as it offers Turing-complete programming language to allow users the ability to create DApps and complex smart contracts. It is the backbone of the decentralized finance (DeFi) ecosystem, containing lending protocols, many decentralized exchanges, and other financial software. The proof-of-work (PoW) consensus method used by Ethereum 1.0 is energy-intensive, however, by transitioning the upgrade uses less energy as it has adopted a proof-of-stake consensus mechanism that allows for greater scalability.[14]

Cardano

Cardano is a third-generation blockchain and aspires to give us an eco-friendly alternative to Ethereum. It employs peer-reviewed codebase with a proof-of-stake consensus mechanism for security and scalability. Cardano built a new smart contract language called Plutus, and it is far more secure and user-friendly than Solidity–the current language used for developing applications on Ethereum.[15]

Polkadot

Multi-chain networks like Polkadot provide interoperability between different blockchain networks. The core is implemented in a sharded manner to enhance its scalability and performance, while the smart contract language has been made simple enough for even nondevelopers. Developers can build dedicated parachains that integrate with one another and connect to outside networks on Polkadot.

Smart contract platforms are a key part of the blockchain ecosystem as they allow for various applications and use cases to take place across many industries, like real estate and finance, to healthcare and supply chain management. By providing a secure, efficient, and trustless way to conduct transactions and agreements, they encourage innovation and change the way people interact socially.[16]

Importance of Smart Contract Platforms

Platforms for smart contracts offer a safe and efficient way to execute transactions and agreements between two or more parties in a decentralized, trustless environment, making it an integral part of blockchain technology. The following are some of the main justifications for the significance of smart contract platforms in blockchain technology are shown in Figure 4.1.

Automation

Smart contract platforms automate agreement execution, eliminating intermediaries' need, decreasing the risk of errors, and increase effectiveness of the transaction process.

Transparency

Smart contracts are transparent, as they are visible on blockchain, guaranteeing a record of the transaction that cannot be changed and allowing all parties involved to access the same information.

Security

Smart contracts are performed on a decentralized blockchain network, they cannot be manipulated or hacked and are basically secure. A smart contract is not auditable or modifiable after it is deployed on blockchain network, ensuring a very high level of integrity and trust.

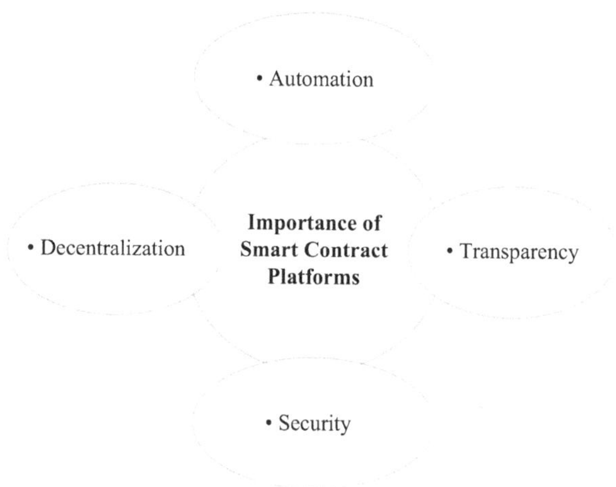

Figure 4.1 Importance of Smart Contract Platforms.

Versatility

Smart contract platforms allow the creation of contracts ranging from simple transactions to complex multi-party arrangements and including various conditions and requirements.[17,18]

Decentralization

Smart contract platforms work in decentralized, peer-to-peer setup so there is no entity that monitors the transaction process. This assurance ensures increased transparency, safety, and trust in the transaction process.

All digital contract platforms are considered to be an important part of the modern economy blockchain technology, enabling a range of innovative applications across a variety of sectors like real estate, healthcare and finance, supply chain management, and other industries. They offer a useful solution to guarding and automating transactions, while also serving as a vehicle to open up new spaces for party engagement and interaction.[19]

Role of Smart Contract Platforms in Facilitating Blockchain-Based Applications

Smart contracts platforms are used to build many different kinds of blockchain applications. Among the most popular use cases is DeFi. DeFi applications allow users to conduct different financial activities, like lending, borrowing, and trading. And they are built on smart contract platforms. With smart contracts, these applications can execute entirely autonomously and in a decentralized manner without intermediaries or other third parties.

Smart contracts are also being used in supply chain management platforms. Utilizing blockchain technology and smart contracts, each participant in the supply chain can make an immutable record of all actions related to the production and delivery of goods. It helps reduce fraud, increases transparency, and improves supply chain efficiency.

In the healthcare sector, smart contracts are utilized to prepare an efficient and safe way of record keeping. Smart contracts and blockchain technology allow medical records to be stored on a transparent and secure basis, assuring that patients have control over their data once again, but can share it safely with healthcare professionals. Smart contract platforms are a fundamental part of the blockchain ecosystem, facilitating multiple applications and use cases throughout industries.[20,21]

Interoperability between Different Smart Contract Platforms

The need for interoperability between several smart contract platforms gains great importance as the blockchain ecosystem develops. For independent blockchain networks and smart contract platforms to interoperate, communicate, and share info between each other (interoperability), they need more reliable ecosystems that are entirely linked with one another. There are pros and cons for each platform. Still, developers are trying to amalgamate the benefits of different platforms in order to get more out of software and create solutions that can better withstand both mobile wounds and desktop artillery. It enables developers to build complex and interconnected apps that leverage the unique properties of different platforms by creating interoperability across different smart contract platforms. For example, a DeFi program can use one platform for its lending protocols and another for its decentralized exchange to take advantage of both platforms and offer users more services.[22]

The demand for interoperability is most acute in the DeFi space where there is increasing demand for more composable, multi-chain applications. To ensure the flow of resources and data across different platforms, DeFi apps must be extremely interoperable. For example, the Polkadot ecosystem supports interoperability across multiple blockchain protocols and allows developers to build applications that can communicate across several platforms. While the primary focus of Cosmos had been to provide a more scalable and sustainable basis for building interconnected Blockchain ecosystems, it was also interested in enabling interoperability between different networks of blockchain. Blockchain landscape has gone through a major transition with such a stronger focus on the cross-chain expansion of the ecosystem between different smart contract platforms.[23]

Application of Smart Contracts

In the system of blockchain, a smart contract is a segment of a software which runs a series of events using a consensus process. A smart contract may be used in a variety of fields to automate the system and remove third-party transactions.[24] The various smart contract using cases and blockchain-based applications are discussed below and shown in Figure 4.2.

Internet of Things (IoT)

IoT is a promising field of research. IoT devices are resource-constrained devices that have less memory power also low processing power. As the CISCO report mentions, a number of IoT devices linked with various applications has already surpassed the world's population. Some of the many smart homes, smart cities, smart transportation, and applications for monitoring environments based on blockchain technology already exist as research. Therefore, the idea of smart contracts can be further integrated with blockchain technology to increase the autonomy of IoT.[25]

Supply Chain

The supply chain management system comprises various transaction levels. There are some terms and conditions of each level. The supply chain system involves multiple systems. Numerous supply chain system sectors, including shipping, transportation, and food manufacturing. In each of these situations, a digital ledger database adds information, trust, and most importantly, no third parties. Everything in an open system of the supply chain sector in a distributed manner with enhanced reliability and trustfulness due to the blockchain system.[24,26]

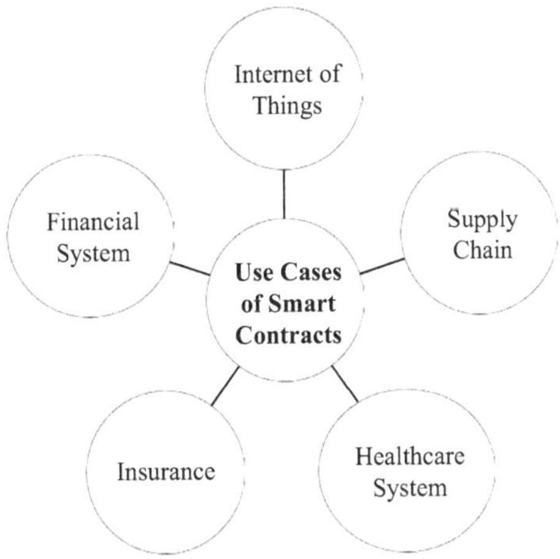

Figure 4.2 Applications of Smart Contracts.

When a smart contract is integrated with a blockchain system, the system's operation becomes secure and independent. A few smart conditions must be created as programs and added to the blockchain system so that these smart contracts will run whenever a transaction takes place. The blockchain nodes carry out the validation and verification. Smart contract events are initiated if the network node agrees to certain requirements. Lastly, the blockchain system records the transaction. Smart contracts are increasing transparency in our supply chains and aiding the flow of goods while rebuilding trust in trade.[24,27]

Healthcare System

As anticipated, the advancement of technology has led to an increase in the level of living for people. By making use of these newly invented gadgets and helping technologies, humans can keep track of his or her well-being while sitting at home. Many devices are developed to understand certain characteristics of the body. This is a low-end device and can be collected nearby and processed locally which gives you quick information. The use of blockchain technology reduces patients' privacy and maintains that data in a digital ledger format. In that kind of system, it is possible to use a smart contract to make the system less dependent on manual processes and more automated. A smart contract enables humans to establish terms and conditions that take effect when data is gathered. After that, it will run these smart contracts and cause the appropriate things to happen.[24,28]

Insurance

The current insurance model processes claims over a long period of time. There is enormous ambiguity happens among various stakeholders in processing. A smart contract-based system can streamline procedures, and blockchain technology can be used to build an ecosystem that is transparent and safe without the involvement of third parties. It fires corresponding events whenever a smart contract is successfully executed.

Financial System

The Bitcoin cryptocurrency system invented blockchain technology, which was initially utilized for financial systems only. In a conventional banking system when you want to transfer money from one account into other accounts, it involves a third party. On the other hand, in the blockchain system, the transaction is peer-to-peer and does not utilize a central storage. The smart contract and blockchain-based financial industry are a boon; however, the implementation of this technology involves extensive research in this domain.[29]

Healthcare Smart Contracts Based on Blockchain

The blockchain smart contract system for healthcare was built on Ethereum. Being open-source, it has a thriving community and a substantial public DApp repository, making it one of the largest public blockchain networks today. This platform just adopted the Ethash PoW consensus technique, which is being modified by engineers to become a proof-of-stake (PoS) scalability algorithm in the upcoming years.[1,2]

A consensus technique like Delegated Proof-of-Stake or Practical Byzantine Fault Tolerance would be perfect for distributed application architecture. By matching DFS content against the ledger, DApp could identify discrepancies, such as inserting data without proper authorization and the absence of entities. Every stage has a timeline mark for the audit. A high-level programming language called Solidity, which has key components including functions, events, state variables, and modifiers, is used to write even smart contracts. To deploy contracts on the testnet and pay for transaction fees using the testnet ethers, we have used Remix and Kovan test network.[30–32]

Current medical records stored on different nodes throughout the network are intelligently represented using Ethereum smart contracts. Instructions for managing these attributes are cryptographically authenticated and included in blockchain transactions. Only through valid transactions that cause data modification do the contract's state-transition features implement policies. As long as it can be calculated, such regulations can enforce any restriction relating to a particular medical record. For example, a policy may require that both the patients and the healthcare professionals should send individual consent transactions before a third party gets permission to view data. A blockchain-based smart contract solution can streamline and secure intricate medical procedures by automating consent, ensuring compliance, managing multi-party coordination, and maintaining transparent, tamper-proof records. These include data access permissions between healthcare ecosystem participants and smart contracts designed for various medical workflows.[2,33]

It is possible that a smart contract be built to keep everything in its accountability ledger, from conditions controlling who has what permission levels to when and where data can be accessed with the involvement of various stakeholders carrying out varying activities. It will also bring ease in interaction between doctor and patient. Smart contracts encode data authorization rules. They provide a unique id for each activity carried out, which facilitates the tracing of all operations from the point of origin until the surrender.[2,33]

Relevant Scenarios have been clearly outlined, with all processes and functions thoroughly described and encoded into smart contracts. The operation can be managed directly through the smart contract itself, eliminating the need to have some kind of centralized entity that manages and approves this process which will drastically reduce the administrative cost of working processes. The data hash, which contains all medical record data, is nevertheless stored locally in database storage to preserve efficiency and economic viability.

Every data transaction is digitally signed using the private key of the owner, which could be a patient or a physician. The block content of a peer-to-peer private network represents the shared viewing rights and data ownership of its participants. They can use smart contracts, which are enabled by blockchain technology, to automate and track particular passing states (such as a change in viewing privileges or the generation of a new system record). Relationships between patients and providers are tracked using smart contracts on an Ethereum blockchain. Using a cryptographic hash of the record on-chain, these contracts associate a medical record with viewing rights and data retrieval instructions (essentially, information pointers) to stop external servers from altering the payload and interfering with the record's execution.

A provider adds an associated record for a specific patient, and the patient permits the records in providers. Parties receiving novel information in both cases are automatically notified and have the opportunity to verify the proposed record prior to data being accepted or refused. Participants are kept informed and active in the development of their records as a result.

Prioritizing utilization, this system also has a unique contract that compiles each user's references of patient-provider relationships, making it simpler to obtain an address to verify whether or not a medical history has been updated. Manage identity verification using public key cryptography and employ a DNS-type solution that associates a user's Ethereum address with an established and commonly used form of identification, such as their name or social security number. When permissions are requested, they get directed to the blockchain and then back to the server for database authentication to verify permissions, and all the data exchange which is outside the chain of server between provider and patient database is handled by a syncing algorithm.[2,34]

Implementation of Smart Contract in Healthcare

Various medical workflows with particular medical processes have been created and executed through blockchain smart contract system. Issuing general medicine prescriptions to heal complex diseases and their process like treatment methods for the surgery individuals are a few of these. The solution lowers the administrative burden, which benefits patients, doctors, and healthcare organizations by designing these medical smart contracts. It aids in data retrieval and analysis for healthcare and also manages other complex medical data and procedures.[35]

Medical Prescriptions Handling

The primary objective is to streamline the process of receiving medical prescriptions by removing long waiting periods, eliminating fraud from the system, and reducing the number of errors brought on by misinterpretations by doctors. It uses a smart contract to transmit a prescription to the patient's medical records. After that, the prescription is encrypted on the Ethereum blockchain, and a pharmacy is granted authorization by the patient and the primary care physician to read it using this smart contract.

The drug is then available for the patient to pick up after the pharmacy uses smart contracts to send the medication, dose, and expiration date to the patient's medical records. The medicine satisfaction between hospitals and drug stores under the smart contract functions. After a patient visit, physicians spend less time explaining medicine orders or talking with pharmacies when using a certain digitally assisted clinical decision software.[36]

Sharing Laboratory Test Data

By enabling laboratories, doctors, clinics, and other stakeholders to enter and exchange medical data of patients across several parties, the ultimate objective is to retrieve and distribute information with the use of blockchain smart contracts. Think of a scenario in which a patient goes to a lab to have a blood test. Once the results are processed, the laboratory would enter them through the patient records and then through the Ethereum blockchain, from which notice of the processing result of the test is sent to them so as for them to decide whether or not to allow one lab to encode these data and enter it on Ethereum blockchain. The patient gives permission for this data to be published on the blockchain. Through their Ethereum blockchain, the emergency room would have instant access to patient information in the event of an emergency and the patient refused to cooperate, allowing them to treat the patient appropriately.[2,37]

A patient's medical history will be published on the healthcare blockchain when they are able to store laboratory findings on their laptop and do not need to make arrangements for documents to be faxed to other healthcare providers. Additionally, they ensure that all medical professionals have the data necessary to deliver available care. By faxing or mailing each test result singularly to suppliers, laboratories reduce the regulatory costs of printing. Labs and patients get to the medicinal services blockchain, wherein they can receive instalments from protection organizations that prompt the data to be prepared for a claim or pharmaceutical organizations that choose the information for utilization in contemplates. This will provide emergency clinics and specialists free entry to unified treatment information on their patients, diminishing authoritative burden and costs.[2,38]

Facilitating Efficient Communication between Physicians and Patients

The patient requests a condition from their doctor. This request gets automatically sent to the primary physician via a smart contract mechanism. An explanation of how a physician will deal with responses and requests, providing a recommendation and referring patients to specialists for aftercare as necessary. Any patient data pertaining to treatment history should be included in the EHR. The patient's record is kept in a local database that is subject to rules about who can access it and how much. Smart contracts on the Ethereum blockchain are used to manage these constraints.[2,39]

A patient requests a particular treatment or medication. As a result, it uses the rigorous structure of the agreement to transmit this application to the appropriate expert. The EMR has to report any patient data pertaining to historical treatment. Patient records are saved in nearby databases with clearly stated guidelines on who may access the records and to what extent. An Ethereum blockchain's agreeable contracts are used to handle these guidelines.

Compared to recommendations from a web search, patients who seek health information on a specific subject are given recommendations that are far more suited to their needs. Another version is given to senior physicians so they can profit from their knowledge without overbooking their schedules. By employing them for branding in their specialty, junior doctors can investigate a new patient market. Immediate compensation ensures that patients queue to see junior doctors recommended.[40]

Flow of Data for Reimbursement of Healthcare

The primary goal is to expedite the healthcare system's reimbursement procedure. Instead of keeping their patients on hold while they wait for the payer's reaction, doctors will be able to start therapy right away using this method. The entire procedure will be tracked via automated smart contract execution. Decreasing-and eventually eradicating-the need for humans to review prior authorization requests and respond manually, with error-prone effort, and decreasing appeals that often happen as a result of the incorrect read of handwritten free-form prior authorization forms.[2]

The blockchain smart contracts that include the authorization policies are published by the health insurance business. The blockchain then receives an application from a clinician seeking pre-authorization for a medication, surgery, or specialist visit. Authorization is automatically determined by the payer's medical policy smart contract utilizing the patient's medical records, which are kept on the Ethereum blockchain, and the request data. The provider will then receive the authorization data right away. Additionally, the patient could instantly verify whether the insurance had approved it, as could any labs, pharmacies, specialists, and other parties to whom the patient had granted access.[2]

Payers, who now spend a lot of money manually examining and responding to requests, would save a lot of money by using an automated prior authorization process. This will enable medical professionals to continue treating patients without having to wait for a payer's reaction. That means they will no longer have to worry whether their insurance pays for the treatment the doctor thinks is best for them. Providing doctors and patients with access to prior authorization information in real-time enables them to collaborate on creating a patient-centred treatment plan based on the specific requirements of the patient and adherence to insurance benefits.[2,41]

Clinical Trial Smart Contracts

Offering pharmaceutical and medical device companies a simpler and more affordable alternative to the traditional clinical trial recruitment procedure, which often requires large financial outlays to buy patient contact information from outside data sources and to run intensive pull-marketing campaigns. The goal is to enable users to implement smart contracts linked to clinical trials on an Ethereum network, which would eventually result in safer medications and heightened interest of the public in medical research. Smart contracts will be used to maintain metadata at this phase, such as registration of protocol, preconfigured study information, and enrolment and screening records.[42]

Clinical trials are experiments that a pharmaceutical company conducts on actual candidates, and the company identifies those candidates using metadata found on the Ethereum blockchain. The organization then texts certain patients, inviting them to grant entry to their medical history, which includes relevant lab study outcomes. If patient gave their agreement, a pharmaceutical company's bill could be performed by numerous smart contracts, with the patient receiving a portion of the costs and the laboratories receiving the remaining portion to provide the patient with a positive test result. Manufacturers of pharmaceuticals and medical devices will save a lot of money on data acquisitions and marketing initiatives by directly targeting eligible consumers. In the meantime, patients would be compensated for taking part in studies and have access to new therapy choices. There would be a new method for laboratories engaged in reporting findings to make money off of their data.[43]

Outpatient Surgical Procedure

In a busy clinic, surgery is such a burdensome process. The right EHR Surgical Workflow System can help busy practices by shaping a complicated process into a single stepwise, streamlined workflow. This EHR Surgical Workflow system is designed to operate completely autonomously and, over its different stages, can be integrated with Ethereum blockchain smart contracts. This makes it possible for front desk staff, administrators, and billers to do duties that are essential to the workflow from pre-operative to post-operative management of patients. After that, data is easily added to patients' precise prior surgical records.

The patients' initial evaluation and permission might be recorded using the smart contract's characteristics. The steps in the workflow are a component of the surgical patient journey. These include scheduling surgeries, obtaining medical clearance, obtaining pre-approvals, doing pre-operative testing, and documenting consent. A visit is registered, treatment is reported, and then paid during that process. This will be helpful to go back and look at old surgical cases or cancelled surgeries.[44]

Future Directions in Smart Contract Platforms

The future of smart contracts may be understood by addressing the following aspects, which are depicted in Figure 4.3.

Possibility of Smart Contracts with Multiple Chains

As the blockchain ecosystem grows, the need for communication between different blockchains has become more important. As a result, multi-chain solutions that implement data sharing and communication between multiple blockchain networks have been developed. Multi-chain solutions could enable one of the new use cases for blockchain technology multi-chain smart contracts. An underlying feature of multi-chain smart contracts is that it's designed to run on multiple blockchain networks, which enables the developers to create more complex and advanced decentralized apps.[45]

Using multi-chain solutions, developers can create Ethereum-based smart contracts, which are not limited to the specific underlying blockchain network. Rather than be limited to a single unique decentralized app, the development of other smart contracts can then operate across these smart contracts as well as onto other blockchain networks that allow their smart contracts to work with each other, forming more complex and versatile decentralized apps. A multi-chain smart contract, for example, could be used to facilitate cross-chain trading between multiple tokens. Enabling this would allow people to exchange different cryptos with one another without the use of a standardized central exchange. It may also be utilized in the

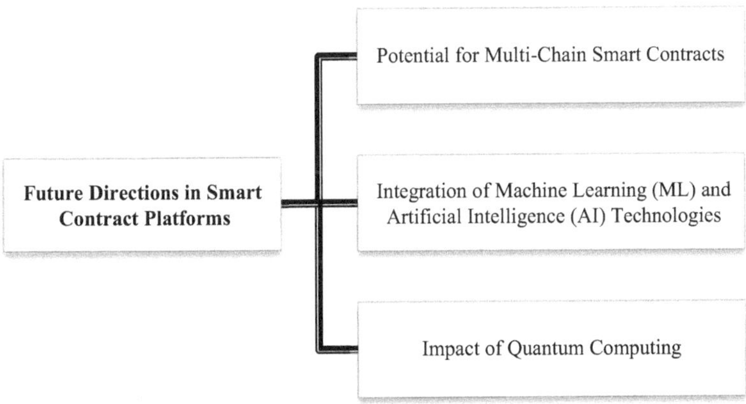

Figure 4.3 Future Directions in Smart Contract Platforms.

creation of cross-chain decentralized autonomous organizations (DAOs), allowing for global decentralized governance and management.[46]

Combining Artificial Intelligence with Machine Learning Technologies

As smart contract systems and primitives continue to mature, an increasing interest in combining artificial intelligence (AI) and machine learning (ML) technologies is observed. This could allow for new smart contract use cases and applications by enabling more complex and intelligent decentralized systems. AI and ML technology can provide enhanced security to smart contract platforms. For example, ML algorithms can be used to detect potential security threats and analyse network data Smart contracts can then automatically cause their behaviour to change in response to a threat.[47]

Smart contract platforms can utilize AI and ML technologies to enhance their usability as well as functionality and security. Using natural language processing and other AI technologies, for example, chatbots and virtual assistants can reach out to consumers in a more human-friendly manner facilitating interaction between smart contracts and the end-consumer. A lot of problems remain unresolved in the early stage of the development of integration between smart contract platforms and AI and ML technologies. Smart contracts that leverage AI and ML algorithms raise questions regarding the accountability and transparency of these systems. AI and ML algorithms, however, can require significant computational resources, which intensify concerns about the scalability of these systems. Overall, the integration of smart contract platforms with AI and ML technologies may enable new use cases and applications for blockchain technology.[48]

Impact of Quantum Computing

Smart contract platforms are an important element of blockchain as they allow the creation and deployment of DApps. Quantum computing is a developing technology that has raised questions about the security and stability of smart contract platforms. Because the technology behind quantum computing is designed to break correlated cryptographic algorithms used to secure blockchain networks, it can exert an important impact on the security of smart contract platforms. That can give access to the security of smart contract platforms, which may allow money theft or malicious code execution.

To overcome this challenge, researchers and developers are exploring the implementation of quantum-resistant cryptographic protocols that are designed to be secure against the attacks of future quantum computers. These protocols involve mathematical techniques that withstand quantum computer attacks. Quantum computing could affect the stability of smart contract systems and raise security issues. But since quantum computers run at a much faster speed than the old-fashioned ones always used, there could be scalability issues for smart contract platforms. This could raise performance issues as the platforms are unable to keep pace with the number of transactions being processed. In response to these challenges, researchers and programmers are exploring methods like quantum-resistant consensus algorithms and approaches to augment the scalability and efficiency of smart contract suites against quantum computing.[49]

Conclusion

Smart contracts are transforming healthcare transactions by enabling more secure, transparent, and efficient processes. These automated contracts driven by blockchain have the potential to transform the management and sharing of private health data, leveraging automation, and reducing the need for administrative burden while also providing assurances of data integrity. Blockchain with smart contracts can help to automate many important healthcare processes, ranging from medical prescriptions to laboratory data exchange to patient-physician communication, but also critical functions in healthcare reimbursements and clinical trials.

While smart contracts have their set of benefits, blockchain is not devoid of challenges. There are security vulnerabilities that can be fatal, like gas transaction fee attacks, transaction replay attacks and front-running attacks. Additionally, protocols can be weak, and issues arise in many other ways as well, for example, phishing or social engineering. In addition, centralized dApps come with trust and governance issues of their own.

Emerging leaders in blockchain-based applications, smart contract platforms like Ethereum, Cardano, and Polkadot have taken centre stage. These frameworks enable decentralized healthcare solutions, notably automating processes, ensuring transparency and security while decentralizing the process. Even with NFTs, interoperability between smart contract platforms is an important factor in the extensibility and uptake of blockchain solutions internationally, including in healthcare.

An optimistic future of smart contracts in the healthcare sector envisions streamlined administrative processes, automated claims management, enhanced data security, and improved transparency in patient care and clinical trials. For example, multi-chain smart contracts promise improved cross-platform capabilities. In addition to this, the synergy of ML together with AI and blockchain could also increase the quality of accuracy and customization in healthcare services. Another potential frontier is quantum computing, which can boost the computational performance of blockchain networks. Despite the challenges ahead, smart contracts have the property to revolutionize healthcare transactions. With these advancements, the technology should continue to spur innovation and enhance some areas within healthcare delivery by increasing patient safety, streamlining operations, and protecting data access.

References

1 Fauziah, Zaleha, Haznah Latifah, Xavier Omar, Alfiah Khoirunisa, and Shofiyul Millah. "Application of blockchain technology in smart contracts: A systematic literature review." *Aptisi Transactions on Technopreneurship (ATT)* 2, no. 2 (2020): 160–166.
2 Khatoon, Asma. "A blockchain-based smart contract system for healthcare management." *Electronics* 9, no. 1 (2020): 94.
3 Bocek, Thomas, and Burkhard Stiller. "Smart contracts–blockchains in the wings." In *Digital Marketplaces Unleashed*, pp. 169–184. Berlin, Heidelberg: Springer, 2017.

4 Onik, Md Mehedi Hassan, Satyabrata Aich, Jinhong Yang, Chul-Soo Kim, and Hee-Cheol Kim. "Blockchain in healthcare: Challenges and solutions." In Nilanjan Dey, Himansu Das, ... Himansu Sekhar Behera (eds), *Big Data Analytics for Intelligent Healthcare Management*, pp. 197–226. New Jersey and Canada: Academic Press, 2019.
5 Liu, Chuanren, Hui Xiong, Spiros Papadimitriou, Yong Ge, and Keli Xiao. "A proactive workflow model for healthcare operation and management." *IEEE Transactions on Knowledge and Data Engineering* 29, no. 3 (2016): 586–598.
6 Abu-Elezz, Israa, Asma Hassan, Anjanarani Nazeemudeen, Mowafa Househ, and Alaa Abd-Alrazaq. "The benefits and threats of blockchain technology in healthcare: A scoping review." *International Journal of Medical Informatics* 142 (2020): 104246.
7 Belchior, Rafael, André Vasconcelos, Sérgio Guerreiro, and Miguel Correia. "A survey on blockchain interoperability: Past, present, and future trends." *ACM Computing Surveys (CSUR)* 54, no. 8 (2021): 1–41.
8 Kumar, Tanesh, Vidhya Ramani, Ijaz Ahmad, An Braeken, Erkki Harjula, and Mika Ylianttila. "Blockchain utilization in healthcare: Key requirements and challenges." In *2018 IEEE 20th International Conference on E-Health Networking, Applications and Services (Healthcom)*, pp. 1–7. IEEE, 2018.
9 Zarir, Abdullah A., Gustavo A. Oliva, Zhen M. Jiang, and Ahmed E. Hassan. "Developing cost-effective blockchain-powered applications: A case study of the gas usage of smart contract transactions in the ethereum blockchain platform." *ACM Transactions on Software Engineering and Methodology (TOSEM)* 30, no. 3 (2021): 1–38.
10 Eskandari, Shayan, Seyedehmahsa Moosavi, and Jeremy Clark. "Sok: Transparent dishonesty: Front-running attacks on blockchain." In *Financial Cryptography and Data Security: FC 2019 International Workshops, VOTING and WTSC, St. Kitts, St. Kitts and Nevis, February 18–22, 2019, Revised Selected Papers 23*, pp. 170–189. Springer International Publishing, 2020.
11 Cheng, Jieren, Luyi Xie, Xiangyan Tang, Naixue Xiong, and Boyi Liu. "A survey of security threats and defence on Blockchain." *Multimedia Tools and Applications* 80 (2021): 30623–30652.
12 Andryukhin, A. A. "Phishing attacks and preventions in blockchain-based projects." In *2019 International Conference on Engineering Technologies and Computer Science (EnT)*, pp. 15–19. IEEE, 2019.
13 Khan, Shafaq Naheed, Faiza Loukil, Chirine Ghedira-Guegan, Elhadj Benkhelifa, and Anoud Bani-Hani. "Blockchain smart contracts: Applications, challenges, and future trends." *Peer-to-Peer Networking and Applications* 14 (2021): 2901–2925.
14 Metcalfe, William. "Ethereum, smart contracts, DApps." *Blockchain and Crypt Currency* 77 (2020): 77–93.
15 Li, Li, Jiahao Wu, and Wei Cui. "A review of blockchain cross-chain technology." *IET Blockchain* 3, no. 3 (2023): 149–158.
16 Wall, Eric, and Gustaf Malm. "Using blockchain technology and smart contracts to create a distributed securities depository." (2016). https://lup.lub.lu.se/luur/download?func=downloadFile&recordOId=8885750&fileOId=8887911
17 Sayeed, Sarwar, Hector Marco-Gisbert, and Tom Caira. "Smart contract: Attacks and protections." *IEEE Access* 8 (2020): 24416–24427.
18 Tyagi, Shobha, Chennakesava Gogireddy, Chandu Varikuppala, and Koteswararao Nalabothu. "Study of smart contracts." In *Proceedings of the International Conference on Innovative Computing & Communication (ICICC)*, pp. 1–8, 2022.
19 Hewa, Tharaka Mawanane, Yining Hu, Madhusanka Liyanage, Salil S. Kanhare, and Mika Ylianttila. "Survey on blockchain-based smart contracts: Technical aspects and future research." *IEEE Access* 9 (2021): 87643–87662.

20 Omar, Ilhaam A., Raja Jayaraman, Mazin S. Debe, Khaled Salah, Ibrar Yaqoob, and Mohammed Omar. "Automating procurement contracts in the healthcare supply chain using blockchain smart contracts." *IEEE Access* 9 (2021): 37397–37409.
21 Linn, Laure A., and Martha B. Koo. "Blockchain for health data and its potential use in health it and health care related research." In *ONC/NIST Use of Blockchain for Healthcare and Research Workshop*. Gaithersburg: ONC/NIST, pp. 1–10, 2016.
22 Alamsyah, Andry, Gede Natha Wijaya Kusuma, and Dian Puteri Ramadhani. "A review on decentralized finance ecosystems." *Future Internet* 16, no. 3 (2024): 76.
23 Schulte, Stefan, Marten Sigwart, Philipp Frauenthaler, and Michael Borkowski. "Towards blockchain interoperability." In Claudio Di Ciccio, Renata Gabryelczyk, Luciano García-Bañuelos, Tomislav Hernaus, Rick Hull, Mojca Indihar Štemberger, Andrea Kő, Mark Staples (eds), *Business Process Management: Blockchain and Central and Eastern Europe Forum: BPM 2019 Blockchain and CEE Forum, Vienna, Austria, September 1–6, 2019, Proceedings 17*, pp. 3–10. London, New York, Berlin, Shanghai, and Tokyo: Springer International Publishing, 2019.
24 Mohanta, Bhabendu Kumar, Soumyashree S. Panda, and Debasish Jena. "An overview of smart contract and use cases in blockchain technology." In *2018 9th International Conference on Computing, Communication and Networking Technologies (ICCCNT)*, pp. 1–4. IEEE, 2018.
25 Fotiou, Nikos, and George C. Polyzos. "Smart contracts for the Internet of Things: Opportunities and challenges." In *2018 European Conference on Networks and Communications (EuCNC)*, pp. 256–260. IEEE, 2018.
26 Jamil, Faisal, Lei Hang, KyuHyung Kim, and DoHyeun Kim. "A novel medical blockchain model for drug supply chain integrity management in a smart hospital." *Electronics* 8, no. 5 (2019): 505.
27 Singh, Amritraj, Reza M. Parizi, Qi Zhang, Kim-Kwang Raymond Choo, and Ali Dehghantanha. "Blockchain smart contracts formalisation: Approaches and challenges to address vulnerabilities." *Computers & Security* 88 (2020): 101654.
28 Raj, Anu, and Shiva Prakash. "Smart contract-based secure decentralized smart healthcare system." *International Journal of Software Innovation (IJSI)* 11, no. 1 (2023): 1–20.
29 Vinayak, Muskan, Saulo dos Santos, Ruppa K. Thulasiram, Parimala Thulasiraman, and Srimantoorao S. Appadoo. "Design and implementation of financial smart contract services on blockchain." In *2019 IEEE 10th Annual Information Technology, Electronics and Mobile Communication Conference (IEMCON)*, pp. 1023–1030. IEEE, 2019.
30 Kalajdjieski, Jovan, Mayank Raikwar, Nino Arsov, Goran Velinov, and Danilo Gligoroski. "Databases fit for blockchain technology: A complete overview." *Blockchain: Research and Applications* 4, no. 1 (2023): 100116.
31 Liu, Yang, Jinlong He, Xiangyang Li, Jingwen Chen, Xinlei Liu, Song Peng, Haohao Cao, and Yaoqi Wang. "An overview of blockchain smart contract execution mechanism." *Journal of Industrial Information Integration* 14, (2024): 100674.
32 Sookhak, Mehdi, Mohammad Reza Jabbarpour, Nader Sohrabi Safa, and F. Richard Yu. "Blockchain and smart contract for access control in healthcare: A survey, issues and challenges, and open issues." *Journal of Network and Computer Applications* 178 (2021): 102950.
33 Amir Latif, Rana M., Khalid Hussain, N. Z. Jhanjhi, Anand Nayyar, and Osama Rizwan. "A remix IDE: A smart contract-based framework for the healthcare sector by using Blockchain technology." *Multimedia Tools and Applications* 81, (2020): 1–24.
34 Gupta, Meenu, Rachna Jain, Meet Kumari, and Gaurav Narula. "Securing healthcare data by using blockchain." *Applications of Blockchain in Healthcare* 83, (2021): 93–114.

35 Kumar, Adarsh, Rajalakshmi Krishnamurthi, Anand Nayyar, Kriti Sharma, Vinay Grover, and Eklas Hossain. "A novel smart healthcare design, simulation, and implementation using healthcare 4.0 processes." *IEEE Access* 8 (2020): 118433–118471.

36 Garcia, Rodrigo Dutra, Gabriel Augusto Zutião, Gowri Ramachandran, and Jo Ueyama. "Towards a decentralised e-prescription system using smart contracts." In *2021 IEEE 34th International Symposium on Computer-Based Medical Systems (CBMS)*, pp. 556–561. IEEE, 2021.

37 Faisal, Mohammad, Halima Sadia, Tasneem Ahmed, and Nashra Javed. "Blockchain technology for healthcare record management." *Pervasive Healthcare: A Compendium of Critical Factors for Success* (2022): 255–286.

38 Madine, Mohammad Moussa, Ammar Ayman Battah, Ibrar Yaqoob, Khaled Salah, Raja Jayaraman, Yousof Al-Hammadi, Sasa Pesic, and Samer Ellahham. "Blockchain for giving patients control over their medical records." *IEEE Access* 8 (2020): 193102–193115.

39 Zakzouk, Amaal, Ayman El-Sayed, and Ezz El-Din Hemdan. "A blockchain-based electronic medical records management framework in smart healthcare infrastructure." *Multimedia Tools and Applications* 82, no. 23 (2023): 35419–35437.

40 Tian, Shuo, Wenbo Yang, Jehane Michael Le Grange, Peng Wang, Wei Huang, and Zhewei Ye. "Smart healthcare: Making medical care more intelligent." *Global Health Journal* 3, no. 3 (2019): 62–65.

41 Gatteschi, Valentina, Fabrizio Lamberti, Claudio Demartini, Chiara Pranteda, and Víctor Santamaría. "Blockchain and smart contracts for insurance: Is the technology mature enough?" *Future Internet* 10, no. 2 (2018): 20.

42 Nugent, Timothy, David Upton, and Mihai Cimpoesu. "Improving data transparency in clinical trials using blockchain smart contracts." *F1000Research* 5 (2016): 1–7.

43 Petrova, Elina. "Innovation in the pharmaceutical industry: The process of drug discovery and development." In *Innovation and Marketing in the Pharmaceutical Industry: Emerging Practices, Research, and Policies*, pp. 19–81. New York: Springer New York, 2013.

44 Olatoye, Olamide. "Understanding clinicians' requirements, perception and acceptance of clinical decision support systems: User study for implementation of sepsis best practice advisory in general paediatric care." Master's thesis, University of Waterloo, 2021.

45 Chandini, A. G., and Prabhugoud I. Basarkod. "Patient-centric pre-transaction signature verification assisted smart contract based blockchain for electronic healthcare records." *Journal of Ambient Intelligence and Humanized Computing* 14, no. 4 (2023): 4221–4235.

46 Košt'ál, Kristián. "Multi-chain architecture for blockchain networks." *Information Sciences and Technologies* 12, no. 2 (2020): 8–14.

47 Tyagi, Amit Kumar, S. U. Aswathy, and Ajith Abraham. "Integrating blockchain technology and artificial intelligence: Synergies perspectives challenges and research directions." *Journal of Information Assurance and Security* 15, no. 5 (2020): 1554.

48 Krichen, Moez. "Strengthening the security of smart contracts through the power of artificial intelligence." *Computers* 12, no. 5 (2023): 107.

49 Sonko, Sedat, Kenneth Ifeanyi Ibekwe, Valentine Ikenna Ilojianya, Emmanuel Augustine Etukudoh, and Adefunke Fabuyide. "Quantum cryptography and US digital security: A comprehensive review: Investigating the potential of quantum technologies in creating unbreakable encryption and their future in national security." *Computer Science & IT Research Journal* 5, no. 2 (2024): 390–414.

5 Decentralised Identity Management in Healthcare

Akhil Sharma, Akanksha Sharma, Ashish Verma, Sunita, Neeraj Kumar Fuloria and Shaweta Sharma

Introduction

Identity and access management (IAM) covers five main areas: policy, identity management, access management, security, and monitoring. An IAM policy is needed to identify who has access to systems and data as well as appropriately define who can change functionality in information technology (IT) systems. Must include onboarding and offboarding of employees, vendors, and applications as well as what events need to be logged and monitored.

Identity Management consists of a series of processes to verify the identity of a person or device upon first contact as well as subsequent interactions. In other words, access management governs what a user is allowed to do and limits what a user can access through security controls. Logging is also necessary to capture system activity and data exchanges for an investigation into unauthorised activity, with logs monitored on a routine basis and alerts generated and investigated in the event of anomalous behaviour.[1]

Principles of Identity and Access Management in Healthcare

Figure 5.1 shows five key principles of IAM: identification, authentication, authorisation, access governance, and logging/monitoring of access and user activity.

Identification

All staff, suppliers, contractors, and subcontractors who require access to systems and data as well as the physical devices and applications used for those purposes must be identified and their true identities verified. Identification, usually done by using a unique username or IP address, is establishing the digital identity of a user, device, or system.

Authentication

Once a user or device is identified, it is necessary to authenticate to ensure that the user or device is what it claims to be. Usually, this is done through a password

DOI: 10.4324/9781003529910-5

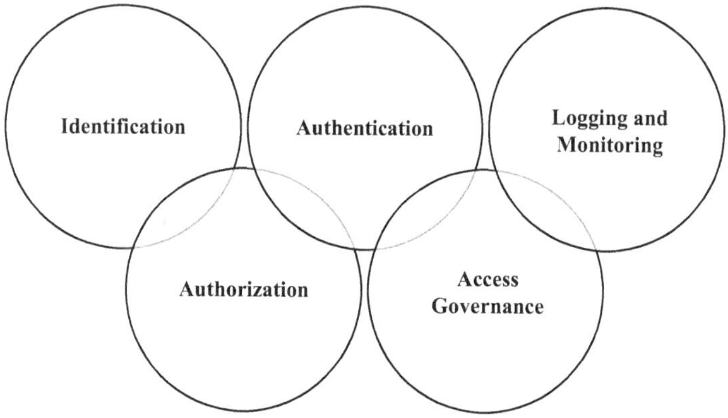

Figure 5.1 Principles of Identity and Access Management in Healthcare.

specific to the username or device. As usernames and passwords can be guessed and obtained, other forms of authentication are required.

Authorisation

After establishing user identity and performing authentication, conditional access to systems and data will be granted to the user. Authorisation should be least privileged, where every user and device must be authorised to perform specific actions, access data, or control the environment. Set the permission to the least amount of level so that user can only do their work.

Access Governance

Access governance pertains to the policies and procedures surrounding the assignment, management, and revocation of access. It ensures that the appropriate permissions have been granted to each user, device, or application via a central user repository.

Logging and Monitoring

Logs of access and system activity must be produced and analysed on a regular basis for signs of unauthorised access or abnormal behaviour that might indicate compromise or attempts at unauthorised access.[2,3]

Common Identity and Access Weaknesses in Healthcare

Cybercriminals view the healthcare industry as an easy target and commonly exploit identity and access vulnerabilities to gain a hold in healthcare networks, move laterally, steal data, and conduct highly damaging attacks that severely disrupt operations and put patient well-being at risk. Identities are difficult to manage, and access control is complex across all sectors. Still, the specific combination of factors in healthcare, such as a lack of resources, often leads to vulnerabilities that are easy to exploit. Across the healthcare sector, there are common weaknesses that malicious insiders and cyber threat actors frequently exploit, the most common of which are discussed below.[4]

Poor Identity and Access Management

At many healthcare organisations, there is little to no guarantee that a person or entity requesting access is who they say they are. With the continuous need for employees, contractors, and others to access networks, applications, and data, rapid changes in roles and responsibilities, high staff turnover, identity, and access management is a huge challenge in healthcare, and all too often, monitoring is lacking, resulting in compromises going undetected as hackers gain unauthorised access.

Access rights are more easily managed when users are clustered together in roles, so most healthcare organisations use role-based access control. This minimises the number of access policies that need to be created and maintained by acknowledging that different roles will require access to similar resources. However, this method is also highly prone to entitlement creep as users are granted access to resources they do not need with controls far less stringent than what they should be. This is particularly crucial when it comes to PHI access. Every year, there are dozens of reports about snooping in which employees gain access to patient records when they have no legitimate workplace-related reason, and investigations show that unauthorised accesses take place for months or even years.

Access rights should be monitored continuously by healthcare organisations to provide the right permissions based on roles and responsibilities; robust IAM are also essential for privileged accounts. Access controls should be based on the least privilege, and policies must be uniformly enforced throughout the organisation, with routine audits to validate the correct access levels for employees and third-party vendors. Healthcare data and systems may be compromised due to the delays in revoking access after contracts expire or employees change roles or find another job.[5]

Earlier this year, the HIMSS healthcare cybersecurity surveys found that very few healthcare organisations have even implemented IAM across the organisation, leaving wide-open doors for easy attacks to get into systems and data. The use of IAM software removes all the complexities from IAM. It enables organisations to create a secure environment simply by enabling controls for getting employees and devices seamlessly associated with IAM, making it difficult for unauthorised individuals to gain complete access to sensitive resources.[6]

Slow Migration to Zero Trust

While robust IAM are needed to limit access to systems and data, healthcare organisations should be working towards a zero-trust security framework. Traditional security is an approach that revolves around securing the perimeter, where basically anything or anyone inside the perimeter can be trusted; unfortunately, with cloud infrastructure gaining momentum, no clear perimeter exists to protect. The idea behind a zero-trust approach is that the network is already compromised. Therefore, if there is ever a security issue, an attacker should not have free access to everything within the perimeter. In a zero-trust environment, you verify and validate access to applications and data all the time before granting it. Zero trust seems to be the future of healthcare security, preventing cybercriminals from accessing health systems and data. Still, its adoption has been stagnant in the industry, with the success of the attack and any consequences felt.[7]

Poor Password Practices

Health Insurance Portability and Accountability Act (HIPAA) password requirements only require entities regulated by HIPAA to "implement procedures that allow a covered entity to verify that a person or entity seeking access to electronically protected health information is the one claimed" in addition to "procedures for monitoring log-in attempts and reporting failures," and "procedures for creating, changing, and safeguarding passwords".

Healthcare data breaches mostly happen because users do not set strong and unique passwords, reuse the same password on multiple platforms, and share their passwords. User-created passwords are frequently trivial to brute force, password reuse makes the organisation susceptible to credential stuffing attacks, and sharing a password is unconstitutional under HIPAA because user activity cannot be tracked.[8]

Employees can take the easy way out, though, by utilising shortcuts, so it is crucial to put in strong password policies. Using a password manager is one solution to the problem of developing strong passwords and employees needing to remember them. It has a built-in password generator that is secure enough to generate truly random strings of characters that are brute-force-resistant and save them in an encrypted vault.

Single sign-on (SSO) is one authentication solution that should be on the radar of businesses looking to balance workflow disruption with security and are working to eliminate some of the password-based security vulnerabilities. Instead of needing to authenticate into each system, for which the user has a different login, once authenticated, all further logins happen via security token or physical interaction. You could also use SSO solutions to gather central access logs, which can assist in unauthorised access monitoring.[9,10]

Reliance on Single-Factor Rather than Multifactor Authentication

Multi-factor authentication (MFA) is one of the most commonly recommended security improvements after a healthcare data breach. In this case, even if MFA had been used proactively to trickle alert logins, the resulting registration would have stopped the data leak. Phishing continues to account for the vast majority of healthcare data breaches, and while multifactor authentication is one of the most effective methods to protect against phishing attacks, adoption is relatively low compared to other sectors.

Multifactor authentication requires additional means of authentication other than a password to verify a user's identity. The authentication process suggests using two factors, such as something a person knows (password) and something a person possesses (physical device or token) or something unique to the user (fingerprint, face recognition, biometric data). Although any multifactor authentication is better than single-factor authentication, more phishing attacks take advantage of weak controls around multifactor authentication. The highest standard for MFA resistance against phishing is FIDO/WebAuthn authentication. Whether you choose one or the other, or a combination of both, MFA must be mandated throughout the organisation.[11,12]

Failure to Secure Third-Party Vendor Access

While hackers will attack healthcare organisations directly, it has become more common for malicious actors to target security vulnerabilities and gain access to vendor networks, using remote access tools that give unwanted entry to a healthcare organisation's network. Similar to this, supply chain attacks are introduced by wounding one vendor and letting an access point open to reach a doorway for multiple healthcare networks. Just like vendor access, employee access must be limited to the least privilege principle. Unfortunately, around half of healthcare organisations do not regularly monitor access by vendors, which is something that must be closely monitored.[13]

Insufficient Logging and Monitoring

Numerous healthcare providers find their networks invaded days, weeks, or even months after the attack has taken place; unfortunately, the intrusion is detected only when files are encrypted with ransomware. Log management and intrusion detection solutions (IDS) detect abnormal behaviour that may point towards a system breach and send alerts to notify if any suspicious activity is observed, thereby facilitating instant investigations for compromised access so as to limit the damage.[14]

Challenges in Current Healthcare Identity Systems

This is an overview of the identified challenges in health IT related to patient safety, categorised according to the stage of the health IT lifecycle in which they appear (Table 5.1).

Data Fragmentation

In the healthcare sector, patient information is frequently stored across several providers, such as hospitals, clinics, and laboratories, with minimal communication or integration among these entities. Such fragmentation makes it challenging, as

Table 5.1 Challenges in Health Information Technology (IT)-Related Patient Safety

A. Design and Development Challenges
1. Developing models, methods, and tools to enable risk assessment
2. Developing standard user interface design features and functions
3. Ensuring the safety of software in an interfaced, network-enabled clinical environment
4. Implementing a method for unambiguous patient identification[15,16]
B.Implementation and Use Challenges
5. Developing and implementing decision support that improves safety
6. Identifying practices to manage IT system safely transitions[17]
C.Monitoring, Evaluation, Optimization Challenges
7. Developing real-time methods to enable automated surveillance and monitoring of system performance and safety
8. Establishing the cultural and legal framework/safe harbour to allow the sharing of information about hazards and adverse events
9. Developing models and methods for consumers/patients to improve Health IT safety[18]

a unified system to manage the identities of patients is missing, which leads to the formation of information silos, hindering communication and collaboration across healthcare providers. This has led to a situation where clinical practitioners have not always had access to the full record of patients necessary for appropriate, timely care. Clinicians can lose access to the most important pieces of a patient's full medical history, such as prior diagnoses, treatments, allergies, and even more relevant details. The absence of medical history can put patients at high risk for medical errors, misdiagnoses, and inappropriate treatment plans, resulting in delayed interventions and adverse patient outcomes. In addition, the inconsistencies resulting from this fragmented approach not only influence the care of patients but also lead to expensive healthcare and more ineffectiveness at a health system level. Overcoming these challenges is critical in improving identity management and data integration to improve patient safety, optimise care coordination, and enable the delivery of the highest quality of care by standards that healthcare providers can achieve.[19,20]

Medical Identity Theft

Possible errors in the identification of patients during registration or while undergoing treatment represent a major challenge (misidentification risks). Such a misidentification could cause improper procedures or diagnoses to be performed and can jeopardise the safety of patients. Moreover, medical identity theft can also be done by another person using the identity of someone else to receive a healthcare service. This leads to monetary losses and creates medical hazards for both the victim and the medical service provider associated with it. Medical identity theft can have far-reaching consequences; the wrong medical records may wrongly indicate a patient's health status, leading to billing inaccuracies and creating difficulties in treatment protocols. In addition, if health care professionals administer treatment based on false information, it results in compromised health status of the patients, thus endangering the quality of care and safety of patients. To safeguard patients and healthcare organisations from these risks, enhanced identity management practices must be addressed.[21,22]

Duplicate and Inconsistent Records

A common problem in healthcare can be the failure of integration across providers, which leads to the same patient getting duplicate or inconsistent records because there are no effective mechanisms for sharing data. In the absence of a centralised system, another hospital, clinic, or lab may have different and fragmented records that do not correspond with each other, resulting in data errors. The differences may include things like different demographics, an incomplete medical history, or a lack of important health data, all of which deteriorate care. This fragmented data management causes confusion and miscommunication among healthcare providers and makes it difficult to coordinate care effectively. Furthermore, such inconsistencies lead to delays in the delivery of effective patient care as healthcare professionals may be required to authenticate information or carry out procedures repeatedly, thus ruining patient experience and attempting care outcomes. When potentially better addressed by a more integrated approach to healthcare data systems, these challenges can lead to greater fragmentation of care and increased inefficiencies in the delivery of services.[23]

Limited Patient Control

The issue with transparency in healthcare identity management is so profound that patients do not even know who is allowed to see their identity data and health records. This can create privacy concerns as well as an element of not being in control of their sensitive information. Conventional healthcare systems tend to deliver restricted access and ownership of data, lacking in enabling patients to control or transfer their identity information effectively between multiple healthcare institutions. As a result, patients experience a diminished sense of autonomy regarding their personal health information, unable to easily monitor or control how their data is being used or shared. This lack of control not only affects patients' trust in the healthcare system but also hinders their ability to engage actively in their care, underscoring the need for more transparent and patient-centric identity management solutions that facilitate better data ownership and control.[24,25]

Components of Healthcare Identity Management

Unique Patient Identifiers (UPIs)

Each patient gets a UPI that helps identify them among the entire healthcare system. Figure 5.2 is showing the components of healthcare identity management. The

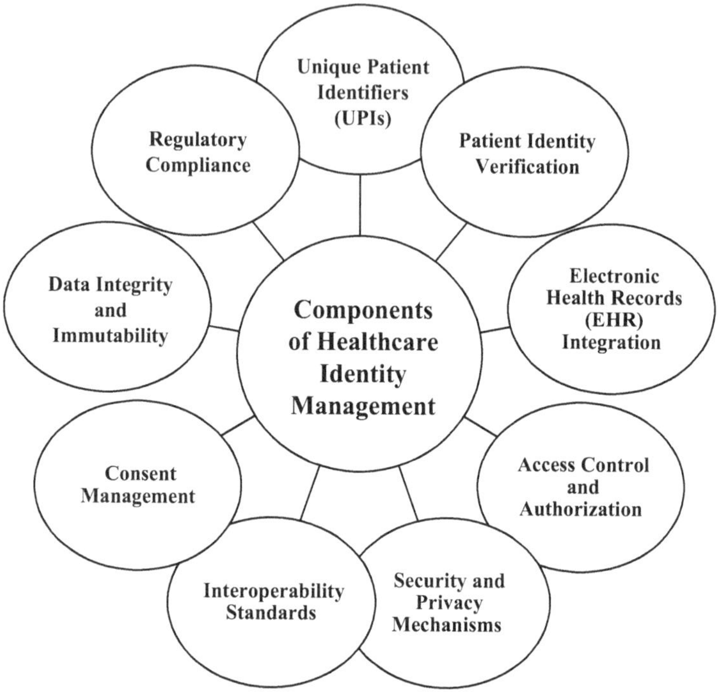

Figure 5.2 Components of Healthcare Identity Management.

main function of PID is to guarantee that every patient is identified correctly in any healthcare interaction or system to reduce errors and avoid discrepancies in patient records. UPIs can be National Health Identifiers, Social Security Numbers, or any blockchain-based Decentralised Identifiers (DIDs) that efficiently and securely manage patient identity across disparate platforms.[26]

Patient Identity Verification

Biometric Verification is an advanced method of authenticating patients that employs unique biological characteristics, such as fingerprints, iris scans, and facial recognition, to ensure accurate identification. This technology provides a potentially high level of security, as it is nearly impossible to duplicate or forge likely biometric traits, ensuring a low probability of misidentification. Document-based verification is another essential element of identity verification for patients, utilising government-issued identification documents like passports and driver's licenses (or even health care cards). These documents offer a well-established legal form of identification that can help to confirm the identity of the patient to legal identifiers. To add another layer of security, MFA is used where two or more types of identification verification are required. As an example, a healthcare provider might use both their password and biometric authentication to access systems, so even if one of those methods is compromised, the other will prevent incidental entry. Through the use of biometric verification, document-based checks, and MFA, identity management can be greatly enhanced within healthcare systems to protect patient information from manipulation, loss, or theft.[27,28]

Electronic Health Records Integration

A centralised data storage system creates a single, unified source of information where all patient identity and health data are associated with one unique identifier. Interoperability allows for the easy sharing of patient identity data from multiple providers and systems so that the information in a medical record is consistent, reliable, and made available to authorised users. To improve accuracy, records are cross-verified to avoid duplication or misidentification of patients, thus linking patient data throughout platforms.[29]

Access Control and Authorization

With role-based access, the identity data of patients is protected depending on whether a healthcare professional is either a doctor, nurse, or administrator; one can view or modify only if patients are allowed to do so. Patient-centric control gives the power of decision-making to patients by managing who can access their identity and health records through real-time consent management systems. Also, the data sharing permissions automatically actions and are governed by the same mechanism, including smart contracts that form a secure medium of access to the identity and health data of all patients.[30]

Security and Privacy Mechanisms

Encryption is one of the significant processes carried out to protect the data related to patient identity by sophisticated techniques that convert sensitive information into unreadable formats, which only authorised users will have access to decrypt. Through encryption of patient records and identity data in healthcare organisations, there can be protection against unauthorised access and breaches that ensure the privacy of patients through complying with regulatory standards. By applying blockchain technology to encrypt data, a whole new means of storing patient identity information could be implemented. Blockchain utilises a decentralised ledger whereby all information is safe, permanent, and transparent. If information about the identity of a patient is entered into the blockchain, it cannot be changed without it being evident, creating tremendous trust and integrity in data management. In addition, it helps maintain audit trails, which aid in raising accountability within healthcare identity management systems. These immutable logs track every time patient identity data was accessed or altered, yielding an unambiguous record of usage. Audit trails provide an essential level of transparency as well, and they create a tangible basis for compliance inspections and forensic investigations that an enterprise can utilise in the event of any breaches or anomalies. The combination of encryption, blockchain technology, and audit trials represents a strong foundation for secure and trustless patient identity management that addresses the privacy, security, and accountability challenges in this sector.[31]

Interoperability Standards

Fast Healthcare Interoperability Resources (FHIR) is a newer standard for exchanging healthcare information, including patient identities, across systems and platforms. FHIR describes specific resources and application programming interfaces that streamline the sharing process, expanding interoperability in such a way that healthcare providers can access and share critical patient data with greater efficiency, regardless of the technology or system in use. Besides FHIR, HL7 (or Health Level 7) still gives a full set of standards for the exchange, integration, sharing, and retrieval of information associated with patient identity data. HL7 enables interoperability among diverse healthcare ecosystems by facilitating the exchange of relevant information needed for continuous care planning and reliable patient identification. Global Health Identity Frameworks will play an important role in defining the rules for how patient identities can be locally managed and cross-border shared in a compliant manner. With growing globalisation and the desire for our patient identity information to be shared cross-border and across various healthcare systems, these frameworks are designed around standardised protocols that can be recognised across borders. Ensuring that healthcare delivers quality, patient-first care is at the heart of every healthcare organisation. Clearly, FHIR, HL7, and global health identity frameworks are all critical components on the pathway to ubiquitous interoperability and effective identity management throughout care delivery.[32,33]

Consent Management

Patient Consent Management Systems refer to tools that help patients provide (or also restrict) access to their identity and medical data in real time. This gives patients the power to manage who views their information. Granular Consent enables patients to share only precise portions of their identity data or medical records with any given entity for predictable access and utilisation. This is complemented by Blockchain-based consent registering, in which the usage or sharing of identity data can be managed with smart contracts, thus making them transparent, secure, and efficient.[34]

Data Integrity and Immutability

Data validation is one of the crucial components of ensuring that patient identity data is accurate and error-free. This means data verification at the point of entry to avoid wrong identification or treatment due to errors. Finally, it is essential to implement tamper-proof systems and technologies such as blockchain to secure patient identity data. Blockchain eliminates alteration and ensures the integrity of data, as patient identity information can only be added by entering it but not deleted without a trace. In addition, auditability through strong mechanisms enables tracking of access or modifications to identity data, enhancing transparency and security. This ability not only provides a record of changes made to data or access to sensitive information but also allows the healthcare provider systems to be more accountable and ensures that patient privacy is upheld. All of these combine to create a robust and confidence-inducing identity management model in healthcare.[35]

Regulatory Compliance

HIPAA is one of the most basic regulations that govern healthcare identity management, ensuring that it follows stringent regulations to protect patient data privacy within the U.S. HIPAA creates standards to safeguard the confidentiality of personal health information, which helps patients feel safe and confident that their medical information remains private in the healthcare system. Likewise, in Europe, the General Data Protection Regulation (GDPR) is a key concern for some healthcare organisations as its focus on data privacy includes provisions based on how to handle patient identities. Under the GDPR, organisations are required to take appropriate steps to secure personal data, which may give individuals increased control of their information. Healthcare providers need to comply with regional and global data protection laws when storing and processing personal identity data. Such laws create a foundation for responsible data practices, helping to ensure that patient data is managed safely and ethically, which helps build confidence in health systems across the globe. Altogether, these regulations emphasise the need for strong identity management practices that are built around patient privacy and the law.[36]

Blockchain in Identity Management

World Economic Forum recommended uniqueness-based digital IDs to all internet users. This digital ID would act as a digital watermark placed on every single transaction conducted by the user, using a blockchain and an all-encompassing identity validation system. Additionally, this digital ID would serve as a mechanism for verifying the user's identity. It is possible to determine the real identity of a person's sovereign state, provided that it is applied effectively and by the regulations. Step-by-step support may be offered by a crypto exchange development company during this process.[37]

The following are some examples of blockchain digital identification solutions and key benefits.

The Ease with Which Duplicate ID Evidence May Be Obtained Once the Original Is Lost

This is the simplest blockchain-based application for identity management. As mentioned, there are always people who need to find their initial identity proof paper. Patients have to go to the corresponding government branch in order to get proof of duplicate ID, but it is an extensive process. Most of the government agencies have information silos and business processes. That delays the underlying cause of the duplicate ID problem.

Homeless and those who live far away from a government service also would suffer in the disproportionate way that this system is programmed. People living in rural places might have to go to government offices many times due to the several steps needed to get duplicate ID evidence. In this case, blockchain could help because identity documents can be stored in a way that they cannot get damaged or altered. Government organisations can store ID evidence of individuals on a blockchain. There is no way to tamper with this record; it enables total safety and trustworthiness, while the security attributes of blockchain ensure its immutability. In case of loss of genuine ID proof, duplicate ID proof can be quickly issued by government officials.[38,39]

Identity of Self-Sovereignty (SSI)

The Cambridge Analytics/Facebook data scandal has revealed how technological behemoths like Facebook and Google control and manage users' digital identities and how dangerous this may be. Outdated means of digital identity management make the manual approach complex, and internet users struggle to manage their identities digitally.[40]

The concept of "Self-Sovereign Identity" (SSI) can benefit in the following ways:

- Users own and have complete control over their digital identities.
- Other parties can see this information only with the principal user's permission.
- An SSI is designed to be trustless, so relying on a third-party supplier is not necessary.
  - Hackers cannot damage SSIs since they are permanent.
  - Their portability is a significant benefit.
  - Blockchain can facilitate the development of a system through which all individuals must receive their SSIs. In practice, Hyperledger Indy is a business blockchain platform focused on digital identity use cases (under the larger Hyperledger Consortium).[41]

Identity Management in Healthcare

Identity Management in Healthcare plays a critical role in processes:

Patient Onboarding

Improving the patient identification process for not only accurate registration but also to overcome the risks of delays and errors while interacting with healthcare systems.

Telemedicine

Establishing patient and provider identities for secure genuine communication during virtual consultations helps ensure both protection of data transmission in natural healthcare workflows and builds trust between parties involved.

Medical Record Access

Allows access to electronic health records (EHRs) but prevents unauthorised personnel from accessing or altering sensitive patient information, allowing privacy and regulatory compliance.

Cross-Institution Identity Sharing

Enabling interoperability between hospitals and other providers by passing reliable patient identity data from one healthcare setting to another so that the right information accompanies the patient.[42]

Privacy and Data Security

Privacy and Data Security in healthcare identity management is crucial to protecting patient information. Figure 5.3 is representing the privacy and data security in healthcare identity management.

HIPAA and GDPR Compliance

Enable compliance with ID management systems in the regulations, which is one of the key works for patient Data integrity and data protection. Patient data privacy is fundamentally ensured through legislation like the Health Insurance Portability and Accountability Act (HIPAA) in the United States and the GDPR in Europe. HIPAA provides strict standards that govern how health information must be protected, restricting access and requiring appropriate measures to secure patient data. Similarly, GDPR offers a detailed and general structure for information assurance that accentuates the security of taking care of individual information, just as patients' rights towards their data, including access and control over them. It creates a framework that aims to make sure identity management systems comply with legal structures, but the rights of patients are also the priority. Compliance with HIPAA and GDPR helps healthcare organisations build confidence among patients, reduce data breach risks,

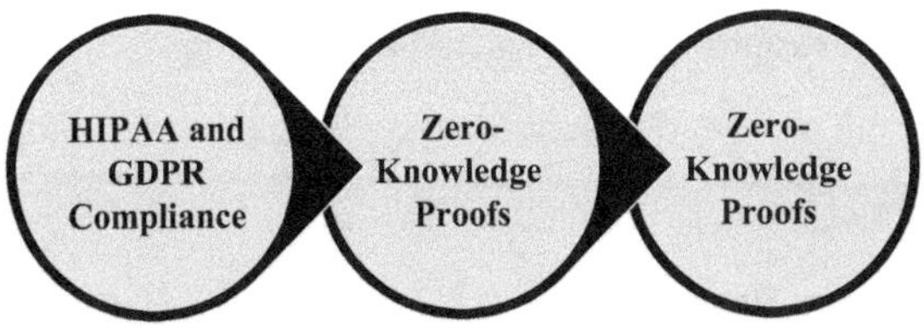

Figure 5.3 Privacy and Data Security in Healthcare Identity Management.

and encourage responsible data management. Having all that in mind, it is important to comply with these regulatory standards in order to provide a secure environment that keeps patient identities under control and, as a whole, improves quality care and privacy, which are fundamental for the efficiency of the healthcare ecosystem.[41]

Zero-Knowledge Proofs

Zero-knowledge proofs (ZKPs) is a cryptographic technique that allows for the identity verification of patients without revealing any private information. This novel method also provides increased privacy as one party may verify the identity of a patient without disclosing the underlying personal data. By using ZKPs, the healthcare provider can still be confident that the patient meets certain minimum requirements (age, valid identity, etc.) without accessing or exposing any actual details of their identity. Using this mechanism, healthcare systems can mitigate the likelihood of data breaches and unauthorised access on a much larger scale than standard processes inherently enable, as patient information is kept private under verification. With the increased demand for more decentralised and private healthcare identity management systems, this functionality will be especially critical in preserving patient trust and adherence to privacy laws. In the end, zero-knowledge proofs make for a more secure healthcare environment and allow health systems to quickly accelerate efforts to verify identities while maintaining the absolute highest patient privacy standards.[43]

Role of Encryption

Encryption is another key technology that ensures that patient identity data cannot be accessed without authorisation, whether at rest or in transit, establishing a layer of confidentiality around sensitive information. Using encryption to convert patient information into a cypher prevents unauthorised users from gaining access to or being able to read the information, keeping it safe from a breach or cyberattack. Encrypted data will stay protected even in the event of a data breach because only designated parties with the correct keys can decrypt the original information. Such security is critical in healthcare, where patient identity data are incredibly vulnerable and must remain private to comply with HIPAA, GDPR, and other regulations. In addition, encryption also provides the integrity of the rest of the healthcare information systems through a reduction in potential risks for data leaks and breaches. Through strong encryption, healthcare organisations can safeguard patient identities and trust, both of which are inherent in their commitment to patient privacy and data security.[44]

Challenges in Implementing Modern Identity Systems

Challenges in Implementing Modern Identity Systems in healthcare include several key issues:

Integration with Legacy Systems

Most systems are outdated and do not support changes that accelerate the adoption of modern identity management solutions; hence, finding seamless data exchange and interoperability with upgraded healthcare infrastructure is likely to be a very difficult journey at a huge cost.

Regulatory and Legal Concerns

Many organisations are faced with uncertainties related to privacy laws, HIPAA, GDPR, or other regional regulatory complexities, which make it difficult to adopt new systems and remain compliant. These issues can inhibit adoption and introduce legal risks for health systems.

Scalability

Handling wide amounts of identity data securely and efficiently poses a challenge. A growing number of healthcare service providers leads to the continuous growth of data on irrelevant sources. Subsequently, it makes it less easy to keep accelerating performance and security throughout many platforms.[24,45]

Future Trends in Healthcare Identity Management

The evolution of healthcare identity management is expected to revolutionise the field by integrating relevant new technologies while overcoming many existing challenges. Blockchain and AI will work together to create smart identity verification systems that improve security and verify patient identities accurately. This means that identity data will be immutable and tamper-proof owing to the decentralised aspect of blockchain, even though AI algorithms can detect anomalies and patterns, which reduces the risk of fraud or identity theft. Together, they offer a more secure, economical, and extensible identity-management solution. With the increasing globalisation of healthcare, the idea of Global Identity Management is slowly gaining emphasis. This market trend is the next stage in a future of understanding where patients can easily retrieve and control their identity data across other geographies, providing cross-border healthcare delivery unattached from the burdensome administrative and security challenges presented by existing systems. This would especially help patients who are frequently moving around or being treated in healthcare facilities abroad to make sure their identification and medical history are available no matter where the patient went. Smart Contracts for Consent Management are a novel mechanism to automate patient consent for data sharing. Powered by blockchain, these smart contracts allow patients to provide or deny access to their identity and medical data as per predefined conditions in real time. It will enable patient data to be transferred only to authorising parties under certain conditions, increasing data privacy and enforcement and regulatory compliance. When combined, these trends suggest a migration towards healthcare identity management that is safer, more patient-centric, and internationally interoperable.[46–48]

Conclusion

The secure and efficient management of identities in the future will depend on the combination of advanced technologies along with innovative frameworks that prioritise patient safety and data integrity. With the use of blockchain and Artificial Intelligence systems, the identity verification method is secured, which means there are fewer chances of fraud taking place, and security can be improved to a very large extent when it comes to patient data. Global Identity Management systems will play an important role in enabling seamless cross-border healthcare services, and patients will be able to very smoothly retain their rights over the ownership of their data sharing via smart contracts for consent management, which will help maintain privacy and regulatory compliance as well. Key to these advances is a patient-centred identity management system. This type of system focuses on the patients and their rights to information about themselves, granting them greater control over how they present their identity or medical records. It builds trust between patients and healthcare providers while also creating a more seamless healthcare system with access to accurate care information, resulting in better quality of care. Ultimately, as the healthcare landscape evolves, adopting a holistic and patient-focused identity management strategy will be essential for meeting the challenges of modern healthcare delivery while ensuring the security and confidentiality of patient information.

References

1 Anand, Darpan, and Vineeta Khemchandani. "Identity and access management systems." *Security and Privacy of Electronic Healthcare Records: Concepts, Paradigms and Solutions* 20 (2019): 61.
2 Syed, Fayazoddin Mulla, and Faiza Kousar ES. "OX compliance in healthcare: A focus on identity governance and access control." *Revista de Inteligencia Artificial en Medicina* 10, no. 1 (2019): 229–252.
3 Mohamed, Aya Khaled Youssef Sayed, Dagmar Auer, Daniel Hofer, and Josef Küng. "A systematic literature review of authorisation and access control requirements and current state of the art for different database models." *International Journal of Web Information Systems* 20, no. 1 (2024): 1–23.
4 Sookhak, Mehdi, Mohammad Reza Jabbarpour, Nader Sohrabi Safa, and F. Richard Yu. "Blockchain and smart contract for access control in healthcare: A survey, issues and challenges, and open issues." *Journal of Network and Computer Applications* 178 (2021): 102950.
5 Chen, Xu, Damon Berry, and William Grimson. "Identity management to support access control in e-health systems." In *4th European Conference of the International Federation for Medical and Biological Engineering: ECIFMBE 2008 23–27 November 2008 Antwerp, Belgium,* pp. 880–886. Springer Berlin Heidelberg, 2009.
6 Katta, Ansu. "The value of cybersecurity investment in electronic health records (EHRs)." PhD diss., Walden University, 2024.
7 Zaheer, Zirak, Hyunseok Chang, Sarit Mukherjee, and Jacobus Van der Merwe. "Entrust Network-independent zero-trust parameterisation for microservices." In *Proceedings of the 2019 ACM Symposium on SDN Research,* pp. 49–61. 2019.
8 Fedorowicz, Jane, and Amy W. Ray. "Impact of HIPAA on the integrity of healthcare information." *International Journal of Healthcare Technology and Management* 6, no. 2 (2004): 142–157.

9 Mbonihankuye, Scholas, Athanase Nkunzimana, and Ange Ndagijimana. "Healthcare data security technology: HIPAA compliance." *Wireless Communications and Mobile Computing* 2019, no. 1 (2019): 1927495.
10 Chen, Jim Q., and Allen Benusa. "HIPAA security compliance challenges: The case for small healthcare providers." *International Journal of Healthcare Management* 10, no. 2 (2017): 135–146.
11 Das, Sanchari, Bingxing Wang, Zachary Tingle, and L. Jean Camp. "Evaluating user perception of multi-factor authentication: A systematic review." *arXiv preprint arXiv: 1908.05901* (2019).
12 Gunson, Nancie, Diarmid Marshall, Hazel Morton, and Mervyn Jack. "User perceptions of security and usability of single-factor and two-factor authentication in automated telephone banking." *Computers & Security* 30, no. 4 (2011): 208–220.
13 Li, Yuchong, and Qinghui Liu. "A comprehensive review study of cyber-attacks and cyber security; Emerging trends and recent developments." *Energy Reports* 7 (2021): 8176–8186.
14 de Wasseige, Carlos, and Pierre Defourny. "Remote sensing of selective logging impact for tropical forest management." *Forest Ecology and Management* 188, no. 1–3 (2004): 161–173.
15 Hanson, Kami, and Brett E. Shelton. "Design and development of virtual reality: Analysis of challenges faced by educators." *Journal of Educational Technology & Society* 11, no. 1 (2008): 118–131.
16 Richey, Rita C., and James D. Klein. *Design and Development Research: Methods, Strategies, and Issues*. Abingdon, Oxfordshire: Routledge, 2014.
17 Ranjan, Shree, Vijay Kumar Jha, and Pralay Pal. "Literature review on ERP implementation challenges." *International Journal of Business Information Systems* 21, no. 3 (2016): 388–402.
18 Cai, Wei, Lianguo Wang, Li Li, Jun Xie, Shun Jia, Xugang Zhang, Zhigang Jiang, and Kee-hung Lai. "A review on methods of energy performance improvement towards sustainable manufacturing from perspectives of energy monitoring, evaluation, optimisation and benchmarking." *Renewable and Sustainable Energy Reviews* 159 (2022): 112227.
19 Ciriani, Valentina, Sabrina De Capitani di Vimercati, Sara Foresti, Sushil Jajodia, Stefano Paraboschi, and Pierangela Samarati. "Fragmentation and encryption to enforce privacy in data storage." In *Computer Security–ESORICS 2007: 12th European Symposium on Research In Computer Security, Dresden, Germany, September 24—26, 2007. Proceedings 12*, pp. 171–186. Springer Berlin Heidelberg, 2007.
20 Kaczmarczyk, Michal, Marcin Barczynski, Wojciech Kilian, and Cezary Dubnicki. "Reducing the impact of data fragmentation caused by in-line deduplication." In *Proceedings of the 5th Annual International Systems and Storage Conference*, pp. 1–12. 2012.
21 Judson, Timothy, Mark Haas, and Tara Lagu. "Medical identity theft: Prevention and reconciliation initiatives at Massachusetts General Hospital." *The Joint Commission Journal on Quality and Patient Safety* 40, no. 7 (2014): 291–295, AP1.
22 Ayub, Akeem Olalekan. "Factors facilitating the perpetration of Medical Identity Theft: A case of Ahmadu Bello University Teaching Hospital (ABUTH), Zaria." *Atras Journal* 5, no. 1 (2024): 84–101.
23 Terry, Nicholas P., and Leslie P. Francis. "Ensuring the privacy and confidentiality of electronic health records." *University of Illinois Law Review* (2007): 681.

24 Popescu, Catalin, Hani El-Chaarani, Zouhour El-Abiad, and Iza Gigauri. "Implementation of health information systems to improve patient identification." *International Journal of Environmental Research and Public Health* 19, no. 22 (2022): 15236.

25 Gliklich, Richard E., Nancy A. Dreyer, and Michelle B. Leavy. "Managing patient identity across data sources." In *Registries for Evaluating Patient Outcomes: A User's Guide [Internet]*. 3rd edition. Agency for Healthcare Research and Quality (US), 2014.

26 Riplinger, Lauren, Jordi Piera-Jiménez, and Julie Pursley Dooling. "Patient identification techniques–approaches, implications, and findings." *Yearbook of Medical Informatics* 29, no. 01 (2020): 081–086.

27 Jabin, Suraiya, and Farhana Javed Zareen. "Biometric signature verification." *International Journal of Biometrics* 7, no. 2 (2015): 97–118.

28 Elhoseny, Mohamed, Ahmed Elkhateb, Ahmed Sahlol, and Aboul Ella Hassanien. "Multimodal biometric personal identification and verification." *Advances in Soft Computing and Machine Learning in Image Processing* (2018): 249–276.

29 Serbanati, Luca Dan. "Health digital state and Smart EHR systems." *Informatics in Medicine Unlocked* 21 (2020): 100494.

30 Vos, Janita F. J., Albert Boonstra, Arjen Kooistra, Marc Seelen, and Marjolein Van Offenbeek. "The influence of electronic health record use on collaboration among medical specialities." *BMC Health Services Research* 20 (2020): 1–11.

31 Meingast, Marci, Tanya Roosta, and Shankar Sastry. "Security and privacy issues with health care information technology." In *2006 International Conference of the IEEE Engineering in Medicine and Biology Society,* pp. 5453–5458. IEEE, 2006.

32 Vorisek, Carina Nina, Moritz Lehne, Sophie Anne Ines Klopfenstein, Paula Josephine Mayer, Alexander Bartschke, Thomas Haese, and Sylvia Thun. "Fast healthcare interoperability resources (FHIR) for interoperability in health research: systematic review." *JMIR Medical Informatics* 10, no. 7 (2022): e35724.

33 Ayaz, Muhammad, Muhammad F. Pasha, Mohammed Y. Alzahrani, Rahmat Budiarto, and Deris Stiawan. "The Fast Health Interoperability Resources (FHIR) standard: A systematic literature review of implementations, applications, challenges and opportunities." *JMIR Medical Informatics* 9, no. 7 (2021): e21929.

34 Tith, Dara, Joong-Sun Lee, Hiroyuki Suzuki, W. M. A. B. Wijesundara, Naoko Taira, Takashi Obi, and Nagaaki Ohyama. "Patient consent management by a purpose-based consent model for electronic health record based on blockchain technology." *Healthcare Informatics Research* 26, no. 4 (2020): 265–273.

35 Ali, Aitizaz, Bander Ali Saleh Al-Rimy, Ting Tin Tin, Saad Nasser Altamimi, Sultan Noman Qasem, and Faisal Saeed. "Empowering precision medicine: Unlocking revolutionary insights through blockchain-enabled federated learning and electronic medical records." *Sensors* 23, no. 17 (2023): 7476.

36 Act, Accountability. "Health insurance portability and accountability act of 1996." *Public Law* 104 (1996): 191.

37 Liu, Yang, Debiao He, Mohammad S. Obaidat, Neeraj Kumar, Muhammad Khurram Khan, and Kim-Kwang Raymond Choo. "Blockchain-based identity management systems: A review." *Journal of Network and Computer Applications* 166 (2020): 102731.

38 Stockburger, Lukas, Georgios Kokosioulis, Alivelu Mukkamala, Raghava Rao Mukkamala, and Michel Avital. "Blockchain-enabled decentralized identity management: The case of self-sovereign identity in public transportation." *Blockchain: Research and Applications* 2, no. 2 (2021): 100014.

39 Atlam, Hany F., Ahmed Alenezi, Madini O. Alassafi, and Gary Wills. "Blockchain with internet of things: Benefits, challenges, and future directions." *International Journal of Intelligent Systems and Applications* 10, no. 6 (2018): 40–48.

40 Kuperberg, Michael. "Blockchain-based identity management: A survey from the enterprise and ecosystem perspective." *IEEE Transactions on Engineering Management* 67, no. 4 (2019): 1008–1027.

41 Lin, Jie, Wei Yu, Nan Zhang, Xinyu Yang, Hanlin Zhang, and Wei Zhao. "A survey on internet of things: Architecture, enabling technologies, security and privacy, and applications." *IEEE Internet of Things Journal* 4, no. 5 (2017): 1125–1142.

42 Morais, Eduardo, Tommy Koens, Cees Van Wijk, and Aleksei Koren. "A survey on zero knowledge range proofs and applications." *SN Applied Sciences* 1 (2019): 1–17.

43 Kyriakidou, Chalima Dimitra Nassar, Athanasia Maria Papathanasiou, and George C. Polyzos. "Decentralized identity with applications to security and privacy for the internet of things." *Computer Networks and Communications* 1 (2023): 244–271.

44 Distler, Verena, Carine Lallemand, and Vincent Koenig. "Making encryption feel secure: Investigating how descriptions of encryption impact perceived security." In *2020 IEEE European Symposium on Security and Privacy Workshops (EuroS&PW)*, pp. 220–229. IEEE, New York City, US, 2020.

45 Trinckes Jr, John J. *The definitive guide to complying with the HIPAA/HITECH privacy and security rules*. CRC Press, 2012.

46 Junaid, Sahalu Balarabe, Abdullahi Abubakar Imam, Abdullateef Oluwagbemiga Balogun, Liyanage Chandratilak De Silva, Yusuf Alhaji Surakat, Ganesh Kumar, Muhammad Abdulkarim Aliyu Nuhu Shuaibu, Aliyu Garba, Yusra Sahalu, Abdullahi Mohammed, Tanko Yahaya Mohammed, Bashir Abubakar Abdulkadir, Abdallah Alkali Abba, Nana Aliyu Iliyasu Kakumi and Saipunidzam Mahamad. "Recent advancements in emerging technologies for healthcare management systems: a survey." In *Healthcare*, vol. 10, no. 10, p. 1940. MDPI, 2022.

47 Ekramifard, Ala, Haleh Amintoosi, Amin Hosseini Seno, Ali Dehghantanha, and Reza M. Parizi. "A systematic literature review of integration of blockchain and artificial intelligence." *Blockchain Cybersecurity, Trust and Privacy* (2020): 147–160.

48 Rejeb, Abderahman, Karim Rejeb, Horst Treiblmaier, Andrea Appolloni, Salem Alghamdi, Yaser Alhasawi, and Mohammad Iranmanesh. "The Internet of Things (IoT) in healthcare: Taking stock and moving forward." *Internet of Things* 22 (2023): 100721.

6 Interoperability and Data Exchange in Blockchain Healthcare

Sunita, Shaweta Sharma, Akanksha Sharma, Ashish Verma, Shilpa Thukral and Akhil Sharma

Health Information Systems

The use of information and communication technology (ICT) in healthcare institutions has increased. Major corporations that depend on a strong IT infrastructure exhibit a similar tendency. Among the projects that affect healthcare market management and practice are web technologies, database systems, and network infrastructures.

However, there is substantial opposition to the use of electronic medical records (EMR) in e-health systems in relation to the advancement of ICT in healthcare institutions.[1] Patient Data information systems convert paper records to electronic formats in the form of files, making management easier and more efficient. But it is relevant to notice how the users seem to learn about their role in the promotion or prevention of healthcare, as well as their rights and the legal standards that have some real influence on the information systems development, which takes these issues under consideration.[2]

A health information system (HIS) is a basic line along which Health ICTs are organised; thus, it derives from the key concept of Health Information. HISs are often defined in terms of people, processes, and technology in an attempt to create a conceptual model that can support basic information processing, management, and accessibility functions that are oriented towards the improvement of healthcare services. Like other industries, the health sector has transformed itself from a stable activity to a dynamic backdrop. The evolutionary stage of HISs is its data processing tools, which are capable of serving as a processing aid towards knowledge generation and delivering information for healthcare settings. A more detailed definition might be that a HIS consists of the people, technology, processes, and assets needed to collect, process, analyse, and communicate data in order to advise planning, implementation, and evaluation of health services.[3]

HISs are primarily aimed at efficient and high-quality healthcare. These systems should further enhance their design, rationalisation, and management processes. Interoperability standards, excellent privacy and security measures, scalability, reliability, and data-wise timeliness of processing and storage periods are all necessary for HISs to achieve these objectives. They should increase the effectiveness and security of information flow and bring them closer to the health systems by

DOI: 10.4324/9781003529910-6

expediting and eliminating needless duplication of tasks (like diagnosis). These systems should also have clinical and management components, and they should be connected via connecting the various information systems that are utilised. Access to data for economic evaluation studies, case-mix consolidation, and performance monitoring will be made possible by this. Data mining will also be used to inform health planning, provider procurement, increased transparency, evidence-based policies, and better decision-making that reorganises logistical and supply chain flows.[1]

The need for point-of-care information is emerging to be thorough, homogeneous, accurate, current, and clinically relevant. Evidence comes from multiple works that demonstrate a positive impact of information systems on the quality of care, as their potential economic benefits are currently unquestionable.[4]

Health Information Systems Interoperability

Interoperability in health refers to different computer programs and HISs capacity to interact and exchange data easily, efficiently, and consistently, also the use of facts that have been shared.[1] A vital aspect of electronic health records (EHRs) is their interoperability, the extent to which communication and cooperation between diverse entities in the industry are possible, allowing for information exchange via EHRs as well as other healthcare systems. However, integrating HISs is notoriously challenging, either because there are numerous vendors offering technology and systems or because an organisation's applications must support multiple communication interfaces that need constant maintenance and modification, or because there are numerous applications that exchange administrative and clinical data. Interoperability across heterogeneous HISs is crucial since it will lower medical expenses and enhance patient care.[5]

The automated transmission of complementary diagnostic procedure findings for EMR systems is one of the levels of integration that the National Alliance for Health Information Technology (NAHIT) is considering. Other information systems ought to be able to access these findings without requiring further semantic translation or translation.[1]

Standard messages should be defined to allow interoperability between HISs. Then, the need for all manufacturers of this type of technology should be restored, which does not put the effective performance system at risk. The two most significant standards include DICOM (Digital Imaging and Communication in Medicine) and HL7 (Health Level Seven).

HL7 version 2.x, an electronic data exchange protocol based on application-to-application message interchange, is an industry standard for sending clinical and administrative data across various health applications. An object-oriented approach based on the Reference Information Model (RIM), a data model that forms the basis of the Unified Modelling Language, is used in HL7 version 3 (HL7 v3) in relation to the HL7 v2.x protocol. HL7 messages are XML documents that can be checked against the pertinent XML schemas derived from the conceptual model, making them an appropriate transport format for heterogeneous systems.[1] The HL7 Reference Information Model is a static model of the medical information domain. The rules (implementation, meaning, and drift of certain domain information models from RIM) that are used to generate XML schema definitions for a particular message type are specified while developing the standard HL7 v3. The standard HL7 RIM covers a broad variety of messaging capabilities, including envelopes that allow applications to communicate with one another.

The framework to guarantee consistency so that computer systems and their end users may comprehend the Clinical Document Architecture (CDA) is established by the Standard CDA. This standard assists the production systems industry in developing a generic model of general clinical records as part of the process of developing a universal model of centralised medical records.[1,6,7]

Electronic Health Records

EHRs are also called EMRs, so the terms EHR versus EMR are often used interchangeably by many individuals. All of the patient data that was previously entered into a paper chart is contained in an EHR. An example of a patient EHR that is owned, operated, and developed by a healthcare provider. An EHR can only be accessed and used by the medical professionals who are directly involved in the patient's care. A patient has control over and modification authority over their personal health record, or personal health record (PHR). The Health Insurance Portability and Accountability Act (HIPAA), a federal statute, provides protection for EHRs.[8,9]

This was the official definition of an EHR provided by the Health Information Management Systems Society (HIMSS) in a 2006 National Institute of Health study. EHR is a longitudinal record of patient health data generated by one or more interactions in any kind of care delivery system. Patient demographics, issues, progress notes, prescription drugs, vital signs, previous history of medical, vaccination records, and laboratory and radiological data are all included in this data. The EHR streamlines and automates the clinician's workflow. It provides a comprehensive recording of all clinical patient interactions and, either directly or indirectly through interfaces, supports other care-related activities including quality monitoring, evidence-based decision support, and outcome reporting.[8,10]

Electronic Health Records Requirement

An EHR must help a hospital or physician's office satisfy a variety of clinical and administrative requirements. Clinical decision support, quality, billing, and patient documentation will all be made possible by the EHR, which will act as the main data repository.[8]

Patient Documentation

An EHR should be capable of recording an entire face-to-face interaction between the doctor and the patient. The documentation of the process should be simple and quick because the doctor has a busy schedule and usually has a long queue of patients. Therefore, this documentation procedure must be quick and easy. Laboratory findings, radiography and X-ray reports, physician orders, pharmacy prescriptions, doctor notes, patient histories, and other medical interventions are all included in the EHR record of patients.[8,11]

Quality Assurance

Through the EHR, doctor's offices and hospitals will be able to keep track of the data they require to comply with government rules and insurance companies. Physician orders for x-rays, lab tests and other diagnostic procedures either enter a central database or are stored in the EHR, and they await follow-up. This is among many of the things that have been tracked to determine if the physician had been doing those tests associated with a condition. Providers also can submit Qualified Professional (QP) data to the federal government.[12]

Track Healthcare Expenses and Patient Utilisation

The number of tests, days of treatment, and visits in a 24-hour period, as well as almost every service offered within a hospital, are among the patient data that hospitals and other healthcare facilities spend a great deal of time tracking. The data is then used to identify trends in financial reporting, resource allocation, budgeting, and use. With an EHR, these processes may be expedited and precise, real-time data can be acquired. When combined with economic data, these utilisation statistics might be used to monitor healthcare spending and possibly increase efficiency.[8,13]

Health Record Portability

Today, 99% of health records are papers based on charts. As such, transferring a patient chart is an arduous task. When a patient transfers or observes another doctor, the chart follows them. During this significant departure, the chart is photocopied, sent to a new location, and frequently left unfinished. The hospital owns this chart and must stay with them. This issue is resolved with the aid of an EHR as the patient-related record can be delivered anywhere.[14]

Billing and Coding

In modern healthcare, correct billing and coding are of utmost importance. For example, Accurate recording of patient contacts is required by Medicare and other commercial insurance organisations. Proper medical coding accurately depicts the patient's health condition.[8] A patient's bill is driven by medical coding. This means that wrong coding translates into wrong billing. Such errors can also beset a medical provider with compliance issues with insurers and Medicare, resulting in fraud penalties. EHR technology aids in appropriate documentation and has a database of diagnoses integrated to guide billers and coders to create healthcare claims that are true reflections of clinical conditions.[15]

Patient Confidentiality

Healthcare professionals are very serious about patient confidentiality. Among these laws, the HIPAA is one of the strictest, imposing civil liability on healthcare providers that violate patient confidentiality or the security of their patient medical records, subject to difficult federal fines. EHRs should have security systems integrated to prevent unauthorised entry to a patient's health information. Bio-metrics, passwords, and network firewall security are the layers that EHRs use to keep a patient record away from unauthorised access. The question of whether paper records or EHR are safer is a highly debated topic. Most EHRs have a date and time stamp on a record, so if a personnel who is not authorised goes into the chart, an auditor can ascertain this. This method of auditing paper records is not feasible.[16,17]

Uses of Electronic Health Records

In order to assist doctors provide patients with better treatment, EHR systems have the power to transform the healthcare system from one that mostly uses paper records to one that leverages clinical and other data. Some of the application EHRs are discussed below.[18,19]

Administrative Applications

Some form of administrative application is required for each EHR. The part of the EHR that handles patient registration and other tasks is called the administrative side or application. During the registration procedure, the patient's name, sex, age, contact, and residence details are entered into the health record. Additionally, the patient's major complaint, insurance information, and employment are noted. Each healthcare provider has a distinctive patient ID number that is assigned to the patient.[20]

Computerised Physician Order Entry (CPOE)

All EHRs are required to have the CPOE application. An application called CPOE is used to place orders for radiology, laboratory, pharmacy, and other medical services. CPOE offers a number of benefits to medical providers by enabling physicians to order tests electronically, eliminating the need to order these on paper-based request forms. By informing the appropriate region that the patient must be received, it ensures that the orders are placed precisely. It also helps the healthcare professional to tell what tests need to be done. Meaningful use requirements set by the government also constitute CPOE functions.[21]

Laboratory Systems

Nowadays, lab information systems (LIS), which frequently connect with EHR, are used in most healthcare laboratories to convey test findings and patient data. Nearly all lab analysers and testing apparatus are connected to LIS. Additionally included in LISs are schedules, lab orders, test results, and other administrative duties.[8,22]

Radiology Systems

The Radiology Information System (RIS) is another departmental information system that has a connection to the EHR. RISs handle images, scheduling, patient information, and orders for each specific order that is taken, just like lab systems do. They are also associated with picture archiving communications systems. It is the management and storage system of digital radiography images. EHR apps can view and share digital radiology images.[23,24]

Clinical Documentation

Clinical documentation is an important part of the EHR as physicians, nurses, and others will capture a great deal of information about a patient. This includes all of the clinical reports, assessments, and medication administration records included in the clinical notes. Additional components of clinical documentation include discharge summaries, vital signs, transcription records, and utilisation management.[8,25]

Pharmacy Systems

The pharmacy in large hospitals is mostly automated, with robots filling prescriptions and electronically integrated med carts. Another technology with an EHR interface is these standalone pharmaceutical systems. In hospitals, persons and drugs are barcoded to guarantee that the proper patient gets the right medication at the right time. Pharmacy systems that integrate with the EHR are essential since drug allergies and interactions will be recorded in the EHR. Incorrect administration of medication is the dominant form of medical error causing harm to patients in healthcare. E-prescribing is one of the pharmacy applications that make up a significant part of an EHR. Doctors' illegible handwriting on prescriptions and other Medication orders is a single source of medication errors. This is not an issue with e-prescribing, as this sends the prescription directly and electronically to the pharmacy or retail pharmacy of the hospital. The use of EHRs is one of the tools that will contribute to reducing or even eliminating drug errors.[26,27]

Other Uses

Most EHRs have other applications filled to provide more complete and comprehensive records. One of the most prominent applications is clinical decision support. This is an instrument for nurses and physicians that helps to select the right action on a patient's status. Quality management systems are one application area covered by the meaningful use requirements. It also allows for certain tools available to healthcare providers to report patient outcomes to federal entities, as these quality management systems have been designed with such capabilities.[28]

Interoperability and Data Exchange in Healthcare

In healthcare, ICTs have progressed rapidly over the last few years, providing opportunities to manage access to patient particulars through a digitised form of health information. Applying ICTs in the health and medical field can minimise errors by physicians, improve interconnections between doctors themselves, cut down on the expense of medical care, and provide huge advances in healthcare distribution and quality. The IMIT revolution in healthcare has also added to the enormous quantity of information we currently have on patients' medical histories by diagnosing, testing, and monitoring them, treating them, managing their health, billing for their medical services, and managing their assets.[29–31]

This data is diverse, dispersed among several HISs, and kept in proprietary file formats. Healthcare practitioners need to interact with this information in a standardised manner, with full transparency and accessibility wherever and whenever required, according to the patient treatment pathway. For example, doctors will have to exchange clinical notes, observations, lab findings, diagnostic imaging reports, etc.; prescription drugs and their treatments; allergies; and letters with bills and x-rays. But this knowledge can vary in terms of vocabularies, schema, syntaxes, semantics, data types, and formats and even be constrained by the model. Such heterogeneity leads to dramatic data interoperability issues. Thus, the healthcare system is expensive, error-prone & full of knowledge mismanagement. This could lead to a high mortality rate.[30,31]

Interoperability Concept

The capacity of various software programs and ICT systems to interact and exchange data in a precise, efficient, and consistent manner as well as to use the information that has been sent is known as interoperability. Data portability is a confident interpretation of the data across the system or organisational boundaries.[31] There are generally seven distinct interoperability levels, which are discussed in Table 6.1.

In contrast, the term interoperability is not exactly defined in healthcare. However, interoperability in healthcare has been defined by NAHIT as a technology that allows various information technology systems and software applications to communicate, exchange data in an efficient, accurate, and consistent manner, and utilise information which is exchanged. Healthcare interoperability may be analysed in a variety of ways, including patient identities interoperability, coding words, clinical recommendations, healthcare business procedures, and messages (information) sent and received between healthcare apps and EHRs.

However, the syntactic and semantic interoperability layers are the two higher layers into which all of these interoperability categories may be broadly separated. Facilitating the exchange of information between two or more systems is called syntactic interoperability, also known as the messaging layer.[31,36]

Syntactic Interoperability in Healthcare

The different layers of syntactic interoperability, which plays a crucial role in blockchain healthcare, are discussed in Figure 6.1

Table 6.1 Different Levels of Interoperability

S. No.	*Levels*	*Key Functions*
1	No interoperability	No communication or transfer of data occurs between isolated systems or entities.[31]
2	Technical interoperability	Exchange of data between systems without consideration for data meaning.[32]
3	Syntactic interoperability	Exchange data following standardised formats but do not understand the meaning of the content.[33]
4	Semantic interoperability	Common understanding of data meaning to ensure correct interpretation and appropriate action on shared data.[34]
5	Process interoperability	Integration of workflows and processes between systems for seamless operations.[35]
6	Organisational interoperability	Enabling business rules, policies, and governance across organisations for data sharing.[32]
7	Strategic interoperability	Top-level collaboration, ensuring systems correlate with long-term goals and strategies.[36]

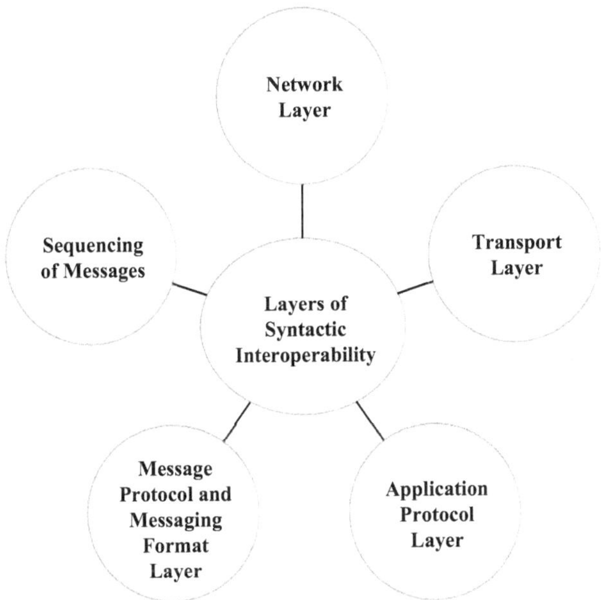

Figure 6.1 Different Layers of Syntactic Interoperability.

Network Layer

In order to move variable-length data sequences from a source host on one network to a destination host on another, the transport layer protocol asks for a specific quality of service, and the network layer provides the functional and procedural means.[37]

Transport Layer

The effective sharing of health-related data by healthcare applications is made possible via the Internet and other transport protocols. Today, the standard for communication over health messages between devices is based on the Transport Communication Protocol/Internet Protocol (Internet).[31,38]

Protocol Layer Application

End-user and application processes are supported by this layer. This layer function usually consists of identifying systems that are communicating, user authentication, and privacy. It also clarifies the limitations of data structure. It also offers application services for e-mail and file transfer. File Transfer Protocol is an example of protocols in this layer.

Messaging Format Layer and Message Protocol

Message layer is in charge of specifying the format and structure of messages sent back and forth between endpoints. The Simple Object Access Protocol is an instance of a protocol that is utilised at this layer.[31,39]

Sequencing of Messages

Healthcare sequencing of messages needs to be standardised. The expected reply message that is given in response to the message "I05 RQC Request Clinical Information"[31] is "I05 RCI (Return Clinical Information)," using Health Level 7 standards as an example.[31] There are also many kinds of messages. These messages might be a request message intended to be followed up on, an error message, or an acknowledgement message verifying that the peer has successfully exchanged a message. Nevertheless, message content must be standardised around the structure of its contents and the data items included for the receiving application to process them properly.[40]

Syntactic interoperability simply guarantees that the receiving system has received the message. On the other hand, this does not mean that the receiving system can process the information. As a result, it is determined that data and information cannot be efficiently processed or used in the absence of syntactic interoperability, which includes features like format, encoding, attributes, values, or types. Hence, in order to offer complete interoperability within the healthcare sector, it is necessary to enable semantic interoperability.[31,41]

Semantic Data Interoperability in Healthcare

The ability of information sent across systems to be comprehended at the level of clearly stated domain conceptions is known as semantic interoperability. The capacity of two or more computer systems to interact with one another in a fashion that allows the receiving system to automatically interpret the information accurately enough to produce a satisfactory result for the human users of both systems would be another way to define this. Semantic interoperability in healthcare has not yet been achieved, according to the aforementioned idea. This is solely due to the fact that, as defined, "being useful to end users"[31] refers to end users, who are able to comprehend conveyed data, even if it is erroneous, redundant, inadequately codified, or rife with ambiguity and duplications. However, computers do not have this capacity. This is because the computer does not understand the meaning of every piece of data and does not have a previous library of situations; consequently, a more clear and carefully described semantic representation is needed.[31,42]

Semantic interoperability's present issue is that information needs to be understandable to both parties on both sides of the ICT communication channel as well as to computer systems and the software that runs on them. Thus, without semantic interoperability, it is impossible to properly comprehend or negotiate the semantics of the vocabulary, metadata values, and used language.[31]

For semantic interoperability, this means needing clear interfaces that are based on published standards. There are no interfaces in systems that do not communicate. At the core are systems that use proprietary or non-standard technology; they are not based on any accepted standard yet are capable of communication. For instance, the Admission and Patient Discharge (ADT) messages or the Continuity of Care Document (CCD) standard for EHRs developed by HL7 outline certain accepted practices to establish modular design.[43]

There are distinct techniques for sharing semantic data between the data-encoding layer and the semantic meaning layer. The industry standard for encoding almost any type of data is XML. The linguistic principles that specify what each XML tag should represent or how data should be shown are absent from XML, despite the fact that it is a means of organising data. These languages, also referred to as domain-specific languages, or DSLs, specify exactly what may be expressed together with its characteristics and values. This may be accomplished by using well-known medical vocabularies such as ICD-9 and SNOMED codes, whose use is outlined in emerging standards such as HL7v3 and the CCD standard for EHRs. Apps may find it simpler to communicate data across organisational and functional boundaries if the vocabularies, web services, and transport are combined.[43–45]

Current Status of Interoperability and Data Exchange

Interoperability has several key benefits in healthcare. Firstly, systems with standard communication can help to create higher operational efficiencies, leading to less time for administrative tasks such as entering data from the faxes of patients. Interoperability may also be utilised to cut down on waste and pointless medical procedures like imaging tests and lab prescriptions. By reducing invasive procedures and radiation exposure, it can also lessen damage to patients. Finally, interoperability may facilitate better access to relevant, longitudinal clinical data at the time of care, perhaps leading to better clinical care. Although there have been mixed results from practical studies on some interoperable implementations (such state-level Health Information Exchanges, HIEs), interoperability in theory is crucial to provide complete, reasonably priced clinical care.[46]

Healthcare data interoperability itself is primarily organisational in focus with the object mappings (i.e. private clinics, hospitals, and pharmacies), and while semantic data creation tends to happen open-loop by an information system which produces siloed patient records (for instance, an EHR of hospital). Trade is easily explained via financial interest or regulatory pressure, and many initiatives have been launched to promote better liquefaction of health data. For example, due to the need for even greater investment in that field, 21CCA views the state-wide health information exchanges that HITECH pioneered as an almost inviolable principle. Because of this setup, no organisation has a comprehensive view of the health information on a specific patient, which is dispersed over several systems.

Furthermore, even if the different systems were extremely interoperable, there would still be no patient-generated lifestyle behaviour, social determinants of health, or data from personal device monitors. Since the EHR representation of a patient is often the closest thing to a complete picture that exists in one place, there has been a lot of interest in adding more data to EHRs in an attempt to get around this limitation, especially the social and behavioural determinants of health.[46]

There are also many existing interoperability challenges. Interinstitutional exchange can be difficult to operationalise and will depend on a high level of cooperation among the institutions involved. Before any exchange of data can happen, agreements of data sharing, complicated patient matching algorithms, processes, and governance rules to facilitate this need to be agreed upon between organisations. Likewise, many technical obstacles exist. For instance, entity and transaction authentication has to be strong and applied to every link between entities. It is recommended to incorporate activity and threshold monitoring in addition to anomaly detection. Finally, data sharing standards need to be set, and data exchange security is essential.[46]

However, in this context, the past few years have seen an explosion of efforts focused on making it easier for patients to obtain their health information. There is minimal disagreement on patients' health information and their ability to access it. With very few exceptions, including psychotherapy notes, HIPAA requires companies to provide individuals access to their health information when they ask for it. Even though programs like Meaningful Use (which now states that every affected person should be able to view, download, and transmit their fitness data) and 21CCA (which even mandates that APIs be required in EHR system certification) have strictly regulated access to these digital statistics, this invitation has been sent via photocopies and faxes through organisational Health Information Management offices.[46] Patients can still obtain their findings and other documents electronically through patient portals. Beyond API capabilities, VA and CMS announced other measures in October 2023 to facilitate patient access to their digital health information. Clinical data standards (such as the Fast Healthcare Interoperability Resources) and practical implementation consortiums (such as the Argonaut project) will further lower barriers to specimen exchange.[46,47]

With the emergence of broader APIs, data liquidity will matter less, and as patients gain improved access to their information electronically, they may eventually take on the role of digital stewards for their medical records. Patients will still experience much of this data generation in institutional silos. Still, now, in addition to having access to their data and the ability to share it with others, the patient will have a complete picture of their health. The transition to patient-driven interoperability will require new procedures for electronic consent, privacy settings, security requirements, and governance.[48]

Blockchain Interoperability Requirement in Healthcare

The healthcare sector is now going through a paradigm shift from conventional service delivery techniques to technology-based service delivery, as ICTs are becoming an increasingly important part of healthcare. However, with healthcare costs rising, inefficiencies persisting, and healthcare quality failures affecting patients and healthcare providers, it is critical to acknowledge the role of interoperability in data sharing and re-use among disparate healthcare applications and devices, cost reduction, and care quality improvement. The benefits of complete interoperability in blockchain healthcare are discussed below.[31,46,49]

Easy Access to Patient Records

Patients generally access care from multiple caregivers (i.e., hospitals, pharmacies, testing labs, urgent care centres, physician groups and single nurses and doctors, public health sites, and school clinics) within driving distance that are near them with good attitudes and give them the highest quality of care. This has caused patients' information to be divided between proprietary heterogeneous systems among healthcare organisations. This makes it hard to get important information in these systems and prevents them from providing a full and accurate picture of the patient. In an outpatient clinic, a similar study found that 81% of cases had missing patient information, with an average of four items per case. The entire medical record was unavailable 5% of the time.[31]

Moreover, patients' data is often available in non-standard, unstructured, and uncoded formats, which becomes a hurdle in information exchange. This fragmentation leads to inefficient shared resources, unnecessary suffering, and lost lives for both patients and the system. Furthermore, inadequate communication among healthcare professionals results in preventable fatalities and injuries every year. Also, communication breakdowns between healthcare providers lead to thousands of preventable deaths and injuries each year. However, healthcare professionals need more thorough and accurate patient data from several systems to guarantee the safe and efficient delivery of healthcare services.[32]

However, with health information exchange and interoperability, physicians may easily access patient longitudinal records that are kept in private heterogeneous systems. Healthcare procedures will be accelerated by giving care providers the relevant patient data they require in order to provide useful advice on a case. The second advantage of full healthcare interoperability is that people will be able to control their health by accessing the various medical records kept by their healthcare providers. An ongoing healthcare chain is provided by interoperability.

Regardless of the geographic location of patients and healthcare providers, the main benefit of interoperability in healthcare is that it facilitates easy access to health information held in diverse systems.[31,48–50]

Easy Comprehension of Medical Terms

In the healthcare industry, interoperability is used to help caregivers understand terminology and concepts when data is transferred from one system to another while maintaining both content and meaning. Through the provision of precise definitions of medical words to systems that interact with one another, interoperability will improve therapy. For the purpose of diagnosis and decision-making, it, therefore, enables doctors to quickly examine the information from all joining systems.[31,44]

Decrease in Medical Errors

Healthcare delivery frequently mobilises the locus of care across varied providers and sites. This results in patient records being spread across multiple doctors' offices, laboratories, and hospitals. As a consequence of non-interoperable healthcare systems, this process is often error-ridden. For instance, according to an inpatient research, a lack of patient information was responsible for 18% of medical mistakes that resulted in an adverse medication event. Therefore, medical errors are a huge problem for healthcare organisations, so they have become the sixth leading cause of death from hospital-based studies. Furthermore, at least 44,000 and maybe as many as 98,000 Americans lose their lives to medical errors every year, making them a leading cause of mortality in hospitals. Additionally, every year, over a million patients are harmed due to faulty healthcare processes and system breakdowns. All of these improve patient safety by avoiding medical errors. The format of health-related data such that various computer systems can understand the structure and content of the shared information is known as interoperability in healthcare, according to the International Organization for Standardization (ISO).[31,51]

Decreased Cost of Healthcare

The main issue that healthcare is struggling with is rising expenses. In the United States of America, healthcare costs as a share of GDP were estimated to be 14.9%, or $1.6 trillion, in 2002 and $1.9 trillion in 2005. They are also expected to grow from $3.0 trillion to $3.6 trillion by 2014 in the United States. Nationally, interoperability among healthcare ICT systems would save 77.8 billion dollars annually. Therefore, one of the factors that will contribute to reducing the cost of healthcare is the efficient exchange of data, information, and expertise across health network stakeholders.[51]

Health-Related Records Integration

The healthcare system is an information-intensive operation that generates enormous volumes of data from its several subsystems, such as operating rooms, wards, labs, wearable and wireless technologies, and primary care groups. On the other hand, combining knowledge from independently developed applications is challenging because these applications are typically not designed for cooperation and often rely on different conceptualisations. However, interoperability across health systems and organisations requires the ability to share, aggregate, and integrate information. One of the most significant benefits of interoperability is that it allows different applications that fall in diverse healthcare facilities to understand each other. When healthcare companies integrate data from many applications, including surgical software suites, registration, lab, and core measure tracking, they tremendously benefit from this interoperability. Furthermore, a healthcare system may work with other national organisations, healthcare providers, vendors, and organisations thanks to interoperability.[52]

Improved Support in Chronic Conditions Management

Many doctors and other healthcare professionals are involved in the majority of chronic illnesses. Currently, half of US citizens are afflicted with a chronic ailment. An integrated healthcare system will assist people in learning the knowledge they need to prevent chronic illnesses, though, because many of them are preventable. To enhance their way of life and guard against chronic sickness.[31,45]

Application of Interoperability and Data Exchanges

A blockchain can be viewed as a new digital marketplace where the market itself is already operational without a typical intermediary. Numerous systems may include health data, and data exchange requires numerous points of interoperability between institutions. The evolution of interoperability from being primarily provider-focused to more patient-centric means we can leverage the use of blockchain to support this exchange, as well as provide patients with additional consumer control over their data. Figure 6.2 represents the different applications of interoperability.

Digital Access Rules

An important use case for blockchain is the management of digital access rules, which might promote patient-driven interoperability. The challenging process of securing appropriation permits for the distribution of healthcare data is overseen by the silo's owner. A single distributed repository for managing permission and authentication rules pertaining to data is offered by blockchains. For example, a blockchain controls the ownership of Intelligence Properties, which allows for clean ownership of digital property. Because the blockchain explicitly represents the data custodian, like the patient, who can then set permissions and access limitations for their data, sharing is made simple.[46]

Data Aggregation

One way that cryptocurrencies and blockchain technology may support patient-led interoperability is through data availability. Setting up an API link to each system that has information that patients wish to access will be one of the first things

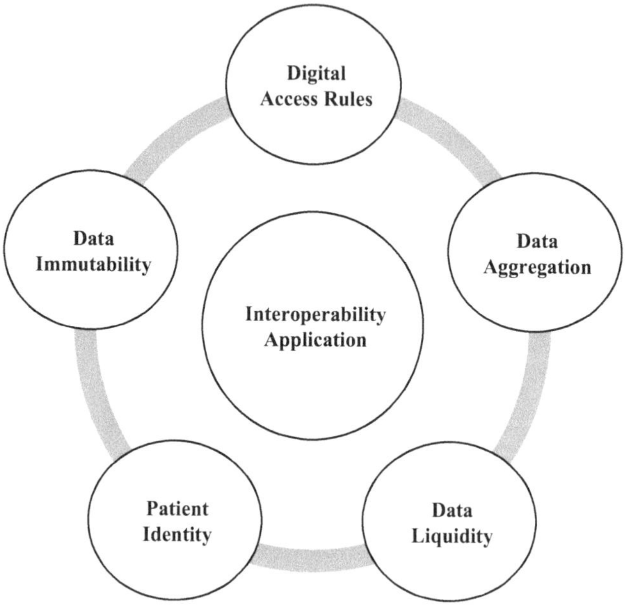

Figure 6.2 Application of Interoperability.

they must do when they begin to take greater control of their health information.[46] Patients can then gather and compile their health data as needed after they have made these connections. If this were left up to the patient, it would be a cumbersome task. However, a blockchain platform might enable this, especially if paired with rules for digital access enforced by blockchain. For example, Clinical encounters could annotate what is happening securely and be published to the network and associated with a patient breaking digital anonymity. Then, suppose this was the paradigm for all clinical encounters at all institutions. In that case, the patient only needs to interface with one platform because all health data will also be wrapped using a common protocol and standard. Furthermore, patients could be able to upload their own PGHD (Patient-Generated Health data) to a blockchain network. A PGHD may provide activity monitoring or other private health information gathered outside of formal medical settings with consent from the patient.[38,46]

Data Liquidity

The speed at which healthcare data may be retrieved is another significant way that blockchain technology may enhance interoperability in a patient environment. Since the immutable ledger makes it obvious who has permission for what data and, once established, permits parties to move and trade the data, this is immediately evident for data stored in permission blockchains. If the primary data had meta-data, such as time or location, but was not stored on the blockchain, it would be easy to obtain. Inquiring about a patient's prior imaging study completion at a hospital is helpful since it enables us to verify that resource even in the event that the imaging study is unavailable. In this sense, blockchain improves data availability and liquidity while also making it simpler for patients to exchange their data with other parties.[46,49]

Identity of Patient

The patient as an entity for driving interoperability around their identity appears like an assisted transition. There is no one national patient identity in the United States, and clinical information systems may contain many records for the same person. These records undergo entity resolution, a very active area of research and practice that can become complex when carried out on a wide scale. For example, while transferring clinical data, each clinical system has to associate the patient with an internal identifier. Public-key infrastructure (PKI) and blockchain technology have been used to provide a central means of identification, or a single public key from the individual, which may provide ways to link the patient's data across institutions. In the event that each institution knew a patient's public key and that key was linked to their internal identifier (for example, the patient linked their public key to their patient-portal account when they registered), subsequent clinical events broadcast to the blockchain network could use that public key as a patient reference, simplifying patient matching.[46,52]

Data Immutability

The benefit of traditional, institution-driven interoperability is that the entity that generates the data bears the responsibility for data security and storage, so patients don't have to worry about that. Even if they are accepting a release on behalf of the organisations, putting patients at the centre of interoperability may replace real data control from the institutions. This is especially important when dealing with interfaced data that is not primarily produced by the entities. Due to the immutability of blockchains, data added to them will stay there. It provides an audit trail (for example, to guard against dishonest actors), reduces the danger of loss, and guarantees that all participants have access to the whole digital history (if the appropriate access constraints are in place).[4,53]

Conclusion

The integration of blockchain technology into healthcare has the property to revolutionise HISs by addressing existing challenges related to interoperability and data exchange. HER sin HISs are necessary tools that help to document patients, provide quality assurance, track costs, and ensure healthcare portability effectively. Seamless and secure EHR systems are vital throughout EHR functions, from patient confidentiality to billing and more in coding reserved works and administrative CPOE type tasks, as well as clinical documentation. Healthcare interoperability is a seamless exchange, perception, and use of data across many systems and devices. This includes syntactic and semantic levels of interoperability. Syntactic interoperability ensures the technical structure of data exchange across various network layers, such as transport, messaging protocols, and many other layers. Semantic interoperability provides a deeper layer to standardisation, which is that the healthcare provider or system accepting exchanged information not only understands what the data means but can use patient data accurately and efficiently. Data silos, inter-system incompatibility, and inefficiencies in data sharing plague healthcare systems today. Blockchain, with its decentralised and secure nature, offers a solution to these issues by providing a framework for transparent, immutable, and readily accessible health data. Blockchain also allows for digital access rules, data aggregate, patient ID management, and liquidity with immutability and security at all steps of application in eHealth interoperability. Healthcare interoperability must adopt blockchain at this scale to reduce access to patient records, allow a simple understanding of medical terms, and reduce the rate of medical errors while lowering healthcare costs and managing chronic diseases. Moreover, via blockchain technology, an exceptional degree of security is granted, which protects the confidentiality of patients yet enables the amalgamation of diverse health data. Advanced interoperability and data exchange solutions will be needed in healthcare, and blockchain may play an intriguing role. It has the potential to change how HISs work together and can enable more efficient use of care delivery resources by allowing better access to real-time data. Blockchain-led transformation can deliver significant improvements necessary for patient record management, cost control, and quality assurance in the healthcare domain without compromising patient safety and confidentiality.

References

1 Buntin, M. B., Burke, M. F., Hoaglin, M. C., & Blumenthal, D. The benefits of health information technology: A review of the recent literature shows predominantly positive results. Health Affairs, 30, no. 3 (2011): 464–471. https://doi.org/10.1377/hlthaff.2011.0178.1220.

2 Braa, Jørn, Esselina Macome, João Carlos Mavimbe, José Leopoldo Nhampossa, João Leopoldo da Costa, Bonifacio José, Aurélia Manave, and António Sitói. "A study of the actual and potential usage of information and communication technology at district and provincial levels in Mozambique with a focus on the health sector." The Electronic Journal of Information Systems in Developing Countries 5, no. 1 (2001): 1–29.

3 Mamlin, Burke W., and William M. Tierney. "The promise of information and communication technology in healthcare: Extracting value from the chaos." The American Journal of the Medical Sciences 351, no. 1 (2016): 59–68.

4 Gubala, Vladimir, Leanne F. Harris, Antonio J. Ricco, Ming X. Tan, and David E. Williams. "Point of care diagnostics: Status and future." Analytical Chemistry 84, no. 2 (2012): 487–515.

5 Cresswell, Kathrin, and Aziz Sheikh. "Organizational issues in the implementation and adoption of health information technology innovations: An interpretative review." International Journal of Medical Informatics 82, no. 5 (2013): e73–e86.

6 Barbarito, Fulvio, Francesco Pinciroli, John Mason, Sara Marceglia, Luca Mazzola, and Stefano Bonacina. "Implementing standards for the interoperability among healthcare providers in the public regionalised Healthcare Information System of the Lombardy Region." Journal of Biomedical Informatics 45, no. 4 (2012): 736–745.
7 Dolin, Robert H., Liora Alschuler, Calvin Beebe, Paul V. Biron, Sandra Lee Boyer, Daniel Essin, Elliot Kimber, Tom Lincoln, and John E. Mattison. "The HL7 clinical document architecture." Journal of the American Medical Informatics Association 8, no. 6 (2001): 552–569.
8 Seymour, Tom, Dean Frantsvog, and Tod Graeber. "Electronic health records (EHR)." American Journal of Health Sciences 3, no. 3 (2012): 201.
9 Anshari, Muhammad. "Redefining electronic health records (EHR) and electronic medical records (EMR) to promote patient empowerment." IJID (International Journal on Informatics for Development) 8, no. 1 (2019): 35–39.
10 Bradley, Betsy W. "The impact of the electronic medical record on health information management staff in two southeastern states." (2014). Memphis, TN: University of Tennessee Health Science Center UTHSC Digital Commons.
11 Baxter, Sally L., Helena E. Gali, Michael F. Chiang, Michelle R. Hribar, Lucila Ohno-Machado, Robert El-Kareh, Abigail E. Huang, Heather E. Chen, Andrew S. Camp, Don O. Kikkawa, Bobby S. Korn, Jeffrey E. Lee, Christopher A. Longhurst, Marlene Millen. "Promoting quality face-to-face communication during ophthalmology encounters in the electronic health record era." Applied Clinical Informatics 11, no. 01 (2020): 130–141.
12 Burton, Lynda C., Gerard F. Anderson, and Irvin W. Kues. "Using electronic health records to help coordinate care." The Milbank Quarterly 82, no. 3 (2004): 457–481.
13 Silow-Carroll, Sharon, Jennifer N. Edwards, and Diana Rodin. "Using electronic health records to improve quality and efficiency: The experiences of leading hospitals." Issue Brief (Commonw Fund) 17, no. 1 (2012): 40.
14 Detmer, Don E., Elaine B. Steen, and Richard S. Dick, eds. "The computer-based patient record: An essential technology for health care." (1997). Washington, DC: National Academies Press.
15 Rudrapatna, Vivek A., Benjamin S. Glicksberg, Patrick Avila, Emily Harding-Theobald, Connie Wang, and Atul J. Butte. "Accuracy of medical billing data against the electronic health record in the measurement of colorectal cancer screening rates." BMJ Open Quality 9, no. 1 (2020): e000856.
16 Benaloh, Josh, Melissa Chase, Eric Horvitz, and Kristin Lauter. "Patient controlled encryption: Ensuring the privacy of electronic medical records." In Proceedings of the 2009 ACM Workshop on Cloud Computing Security, pp. 103–114. 2009.
17 Smith, E., and Jan HP Eloff. "Security in health-care information systems—Current trends." International Journal of Medical Informatics 54, no. 1 (1999): 39–54.
18 Birkhead, Guthrie S., Michael Klompas, and Nirav R. Shah. "Uses of electronic health records for public health surveillance to advance public health." Annual Review of Public Health 36, no. 1 (2015): 345–359.
19 https://www.coursehero.com/file/31556555/Discussion-3docx/
20 Ehrenstein, Vera, Hadi Kharrazi, Harold Lehmann, and Casey Overby Taylor. "Obtaining data from electronic health records." In Gliklich, R. E., and Leavy, M. B. (eds), Tools and Technologies for Registry Interoperability, Registries for Evaluating Patient Outcomes: A User's Guide, 3rd edition, Addendum 2 [Internet]. Agency for Healthcare Research and Quality (US), Dreyer, NA, 2019.

21 Kuperman, Gilad J., and Richard F. Gibson. "Computer physician order entry: Benefits, costs, and issues." Annals of Internal Medicine 139, no. 1 (2003): 31–39.
22 Wilkerson, Myra L., Walter H. Henricks, William J. Castellani, Mark S. Whitsitt, and John H. Sinard. "Management of laboratory data and information exchange in the electronic health record." Archives of Pathology and Laboratory Medicine 139, no. 3 (2015): 319–327.
23 Rebelo, Luís, Filipe Fidalgo, and Ângela Oliveira. "Radiology Information System (RIS)." In 2022 17th Iberian Conference on Information Systems and Technologies (CISTI), pp. 1–6. IEEE, 2022.
24 Sanderson, Amy L., and Jeffrey P. Burns. "Clinical documentation for intensivists: The impact of diagnosis documentation." Critical Care Medicine 48, no. 4 (2020): 579–587.
25 Boogie, Daniel T., Jennifer J. Howard, and Armen I. Simonian. "Pharmacy information systems." In Philip O. Anderson Susan M. McGuinness Philip E. Bourne (eds), Pharmacy Informatics, pp. 111–124. Boca Raton, FL: Taylor & Francis Group, 2009.
26 Collen, Morris F., and Stuart J. Nelson. "Pharmacy Information (PHARM) Systems." The History of Medical Informatics in the United States 2(2015): 611–657.
27 Ayaz, Shamim, Athar Naqvi, and Geof Branch. "The role of E-prescribing in health care." In 2015 Internet Technologies and Applications (ITA), pp. 315–319. IEEE, 2015.
28 Romano, Max J., and Randall S. Stafford. "Electronic health records and clinical decision support systems: Impact on national ambulatory care quality." Archives of Internal Medicine 171, no. 10 (2011): 897–903.
29 Aceto, Giuseppe, Valerio Persico, and Antonio Pescapé. "The role of Information and Communication Technologies in healthcare: Taxonomies, perspectives, and challenges." Journal of Network and Computer Applications 107 (2018): 125–154.
30 Torab-Miandoab, Amir, Taha Samad-Soltani, Ahmadreza Jodati, and Peyman Rezaei-Hachesu. "Interoperability of heterogeneous health information systems: A systematic literature review." BMC Medical Informatics and Decision Making 23, no. 1, (2023): 1–13.
31 Iroju, Olaronke, Abimbola Soriyan, Ishaya Gambo, and Janet Olaleke. "Interoperability in healthcare: Benefits, challenges and resolutions." International Journal of Innovation and Applied Studies 3, no. 1 (2013): 262–270.
32 Robkin, Michael, Sandy Weininger, Benjamin Preciado, and Julian Goldman. "Levels of conceptual interoperability model for healthcare framework for safe medical device interoperability." In 2015 IEEE Symposium on Product Compliance Engineering (ISPCE), pp. 1–8. IEEE, 2015.
33 Tolk, Andreas. "Conceptual alignment for simulation interoperability: Lessons learned from 30 years of interoperability research." Simulation 100, no. 7 (2024): 709–726.
34 Arvanitis, Theodoros N. "Semantic interoperability in healthcare." In Integrating Information Technology and Management for Quality of Care, pp. 5–8. Amsterdam, The Netherlands: IOS Press, 2014.
35 Perugu, Bharath, Varun Wadhwa, Jin Kim, Jenny Cai, Auey Shin, and Amar Gupta. "Pragmatic approaches to interoperability–surmounting barriers to healthcare data and information across organisations and political boundaries." Telehealth and Medicine Today 8, no. 4 (2023): 1–22.
36 Dixon, Brian E., Saurabh Rahurkar, and Nate C. Apathy. "Interoperability and health information exchange for public health." Public Health Informatics and Information Systems no. 3 (2020): 307–324.
37 Umberfield, Elizabeth E., Catherine J. Staes, Teryn P. Morgan, Randall W. Grout, Burke W. Mamlin, and Brian E. Dixon. "Syntactic interoperability and the role of syntactic

standards in health information exchange." In Brian E. Dixon (ed), Health Information Exchange, pp. 217–236. Florida: Academic Press, 2023.

38 Dogac, Asuman, Tuncay Namli, Alper Okcan, Gokce Laleci, Yildiray Kabak, and Marco Eichelberg. "Key issues of technical interoperability solutions in health and the ride project." Software R&D Center, Dept. of Computer Eng., Middle East Technical University, Ankara 6531 (2007): 1–11.

39 Miranda, Filipe Manuel Mota, and Cecilia Coimbra. "Message system to healthcare interoperability." In José Machado (ed), Big Data Analytics and Artificial Intelligence in the Healthcare Industry, pp. 289–309. Hershey, Pennsylvania, New York, NY, Beijing, China: IGI Global, 2022.

40 Adams, John, Jamie Bartram, and Yves Chartier, eds. Essential Environmental Health Standards for Health Care. World Health Organization, 2008.

41 Seo, Kyung-Min, Kwang-Phil Park, and Bum-Jik Lee. "Achieving data interoperability of communication interfaces for combat system engineering." IEEE Access 5 (2017): 17938–17951.

42 Cardoso, Jorge. "The syntactic and the semantic web." In J. Cardoso (ed), Semantic Web Services: Theory, Tools and Applications, pp. 1–23. Hershey, Pennsylvania, New York, NY, Beijing, China: IGI Global, 2007.

43 Gaynor, Mark, Feliciano Yu, Charles H. Andrus, Scott Bradner, and James Rawn. "A general framework for interoperability with applications to healthcare." Health Policy and Technology 3, no. 1 (2014): 3–12.

44 Rabadi, Yousef E., and Joan Lu. "Building a secured XML real-time interactive data exchange architecture." In Research Anthology on Architectures, Frameworks, and Integration Strategies for Distributed and Cloud Computing, pp. 270–357. Hershey, Pennsylvania, New York, NY, Beijing, China: IGI Global, 2021.

45 Spooner, S. Andrew, and Judith W. Dexheimer. "Standards for interoperability." Pediatric Biomedical Informatics: Computer Applications in Pediatric Research, no. 2, (2016): 37–55.

46 Gordon, William J., and Christian Catalini. "Blockchain technology for healthcare: Facilitating the transition to patient-driven interoperability." Computational and Structural Biotechnology Journal 16 (2018): 224–230.

47 Sieck, Cynthia J., Jennifer L. Hefner, and Ann Scheck McAlearney. "Improving the patient experience through patient portals: Insights from experienced portal users." Patient Experience Journal 5, no. 3 (2018): 47–54.

48 Gunawardana, Suranga Ruwan Sampath. "Balancing interoperability and data sensitivity: A design science approach to building a zero-knowledge API for healthcare data." Uppsala University (2023): pp. 1–91.

49 Hussain, Sharif, Hameedur Rahman, Ghaida Muttasher Abdulsaheb, Haneen Al-Khawaja, and Osamah Ibrahim Khalaf. "A blockchain-based approach for healthcare data interoperability." International Journal of Advances in Soft Computing & Its Applications 15, no. 2 (2023): 87–98.

50 Holmgren, A. Jay, Moritz Esdar, Jens Hüsers, and João Coutinho-Almeida. "Health information exchange: Understanding the policy landscape and future of data interoperability." Yearbook of Medical Informatics 32, no. 01 (2023): 184–194.

51 Bauer, Ursula E., Peter A. Briss, Richard A. Goodman, and Barbara A. Bowman. "Prevention of chronic disease in the 21st century: Elimination of the leading preventable causes of premature death and disability in the USA." The Lancet 384, no. 9937 (2014): 45–52.

52 Faisal, Mohammad, Halima Sadia, Tasneem Ahmed, and Nashra Javed. "Blockchain technology for healthcare record management." Pervasive Healthcare: A Compendium of Critical Factors for Success (2022): 255–286.

53 Yaqoob, Ibrar, Khaled Salah, Raja Jayaraman, and Yousof Al-Hammadi. "Blockchain for healthcare data management: Opportunities, challenges, and future recommendations." Neural Computing and Applications, no. 3 (2022): 1–16.

7 Tokenomics

Incentivising Data Sharing and Security

Ashish Verma, Akhil Sharma, Shaweta Sharma, Akanksha Sharma, Sunita and Shivkanya Fuloria

Introduction to Tokenomics in Healthcare

Tokenomics, a combination of the words token and economics, is the study of the economic systems and incentive schemes that tokens create. Blockchain in the Healthcare tokenomics model builds trust and creates a sharing data system and patient empowerment and efficiency of healthcare. The key features of the blockchain (immutability, cryptographic security, and decentralisation) make it a good fit for the healthcare industry, which requires privacy and accountability in database management. Tokenomics is fast shaping up to be a game-changing school of thought in the blockchain healthcare space, addressing decades-old issues such as data interoperability and privacy and incentivising all participants in the healthcare ecosystem.

One major drawback of traditional healthcare systems is that the data usually resides in silos within an institution and does not interconnect across providers. This area fragmentation hinders efficient and complete patient care. Healthcare Data Management on the Blockchain: Tokenised Incentives Tokenomics creates a structure where the shared data is secure, and even patients, healthcare providers, researchers, and insurers are able to use this organised platform for seamless decision-making and better outcomes. Here, the key innovation comprises cryptographic tokens ranging from patient health records (PHRs) to rewards for sharing information or participating in clinical trials.[1]

Role of Tokens in Blockchain Ecosystems

Tokens serve as a foundational element in blockchain ecosystems, facilitating various economic activities and interactions among participants. Table 7.1 describes the role of tokens in blockchain ecosystems, focusing on their various types and functions in healthcare:

Utility Tokens

Utility tokens often power the healthcare blockchain ecosystem. They are designed to give access to the services and interact between parties for transactions. For

DOI: 10.4324/9781003529910-7

Table 7.1 Describes the Role of Tokens in Blockchain Ecosystems, Focusing on Their Various Types and Functions in Healthcare

Types of Tokens	*Description*	*Function*
Utility tokens	Any kind of token that gives users access to a service or product within the ecosystem of a blockchain.	Unlock healthcare services (telemedicine or electronic health records, etc.), Enable transactions for services in healthcare platforms, and provide an incentive to patients to engage with the purpose of sharing data.[2]
Security tokens	Ownership-backed tokens, also called position tokens, operate under regulation.	Enable fractional ownership into a healthcare venture or technology that offers to fund strategic breakthroughs.[3]
Governance tokens	Tokens that allow holders to vote on decisions within a blockchain network.	Empower stakeholders to engage in decision-making for platform governance and policies.[4]

example, in healthcare, utility tokens could be used to buy access to PHRs or pay for telemedicine services; they might even be used to purchase personalised treatment recommendations. In some use cases, patients might receive utility tokens by joining the research process and voluntarily providing their health data. Researchers can then utilise these tokens to unlock anonymised datasets that provide value for, for example, medical studies, drug development, or predictive analytics.

Utility tokens make patient data management easier and more centred around patients. Patients have control over the circulation of their personal health and medical data, as opposed to intermediated or highly centralised institutions. With utility tokens, you can use smart contracts to automate data transfer so that users only have access when some predetermined conditions (i.e., patient consent) are satisfied. This decentralisation helps secure patient data and ensures that individuals can decide who can see their sensitive medical records.[5]

Security Tokens

Security Tokens are a traditional financial asset backed by regulatory bodies. For example, in healthcare, security tokens can be used to represent fractional ownership of healthcare infrastructure/technologies/platforms. This creates pathways for capital raise opportunities, especially for startups and health tech innovations. A case in point is considering a decentralised healthcare network issuing security tokens to investors as equity. These tokens provide liquidity for previously illiquid assets, with the added benefit of enabling investors to exchange their stakes on secondary markets without violating legal and regulatory frameworks, e.g., the Health Insurance Portability and Accountability Act (HIPAA).

Health Centres will be able to align incentives across all stakeholders (healthcare centres, hospitals, and investors) while retaining the transparency of ownership and governance by using security tokens. Such a tokenised model of ownership stimulates innovation and infrastructure, leading to better care delivery.[6]

Governance Tokens

Tokens that allow holders to cast votes within decentralised networks and governance tokens offer stakeholders the ability to influence how and in which direction healthcare blockchain ecosystems evolve. As an example, a healthcare blockchain platform could issue governance tokens to its users, allowing them to participate in decision-making processes concerning data ownership policies, resource distribution, or new features. Such a democratised style of governance can be seen as the complete opposite of common healthcare models, where decision-making is closed and top-down. Governance tokens in blockchain ecosystems make sure that all stakeholders have a say regarding how the platform evolves, promoting trust and collaboration between participants.

Governance tokens can help to safeguard the ethical management of data in healthcare. As data is extremely sensitive, especially in healthcare, governance tokens enable communities to set and enforce policies around how the data can be shared while being aligned with patient rights, data sovereignty, and compliance. Here, token holders would be given the ability to propose, discuss and vote on software upgrades or governance structure changes within the platform, transforming it into an ever-evolving organisation that could withstand the rising tides of changing regulatory environments and ethical expectations.[7]

Importance of Data in Healthcare

Data has been viewed as a key asset in the health sector, serving as the backbone of informed decisions, research, and personalised patient care. With the shift in healthcare strategies towards value-based care and precision medicine, high-quality, reliable data is growing in importance. Improving clinical outcomes is but one function it serves; however, it also drives innovation in treatment modalities, operational efficiencies, and patient engagement strategies. Nevertheless, this opens up a whole host of new challenges around privacy, security, and access to healthcare data.[8]

Data as a Critical Asset

In modern healthcare, data ranges from myriad sources such as electronic health records (EHRs), patient-reported outcomes, and genomic information to real-time monitoring of biological markers via wearable devices. While this large amount of data, commonly known as big data, has the potential to advance clinical decision-making and enhance healthcare outcomes for patients, for example, predictive analytics that leverages historical patient data can assist clinicians in anticipating disease progression and delivering more relevant interventions accordingly. In addition, insights based on data are critical for public health initiatives in which healthcare organisations need to recognise trends and direct resources while taking proactive steps against emerging health threats.

Aggregating data across different sources offers a comprehensive view of health and moves care from reactive to proactive. However, for data to be used effectively, it has to be of good quality: accurate, complete, and up-to-date. As a result, healthcare organisations recognise the importance of data governance frameworks and analytics capabilities in deriving value from these invisible assets in order to help deliver better care and improve patient satisfaction.[9]

Current Challenges in Healthcare Data Management

Healthcare data is one of the most critical resources that a healthcare organisation has; yet managing it effectively comes with challenges that can hinder successful utilisation. A key challenge is the ubiquity of fragmented data isolated in different systems and platforms. Numerous healthcare organisations rely on heterogeneous EHR systems, laboratory information systems, and administrative databases that have low interoperability. This fragmentation makes it difficult for providers to share information easily, leading to incomplete patient records and a disjointed experience of care. Inability to Access Complete Patient Data Clinicians are assisted in clinical care by tools such as computer-generated decision support paragraphs, which can risk their safety and quality of care if faced with a complete, accurate picture.[10]

The increase in the amount and type of data sources, such as the ones from telehealth, remote monitoring, and genomics, adds to this complexity. As the amount and type of data produced grow exponentially, health organisations experience challenges not only in storage or retrieval but also in how to combine heterogeneous types of data. The complication comes when we need to be over into one data architecture because it may be in different formats and standards. Still, it should also have a meaningful analysis of the data.[9,10]

Privacy, Security, and Accessibility Issues

There are privacy and data security issues surrounding the management of healthcare data. Patient data contains protected health information, so it is inherently sensitive; it may be required to comply with regulations such as HIPAA. Healthcare organisations must ensure adherence to these regulations to retain the patient trust and avoid legal consequences. Yet, data breaches have never stopped being a unique point in the digital world when cybercriminals run after medical institutions. Such breaches can lead to more than just financial losses; in fact, they may put patients at risk and tarnish the reputation of an organisation.

The availability of healthcare data is a double-edged sword. Data sharing between healthcare providers can support more efficient coordination of care and thus may lead to better health outcomes for patients. Still, it also presents new opportunities for unauthorised access to or misuse of data. This raises the challenge among healthcare organisations to facilitate data sharing purposes and ensure security, too. Moreover, lack of access to health care data among certain populations can increase inequities in the way care is delivered and retained. These initiatives to enhance the accessibility of data need to be done responsibly, ensuring that vulnerable populations are not further marginalised in terms of digital health.[11]

Blockchain and Tokenisation in Healthcare Data Security

The last few years have seen the proliferation of digital health technologies that have never been experienced in the healthcare sector before. This has necessitated data management frameworks that prioritise security and patient privacy. The decentralised and immutable nature of blockchain technology provides powerful benefits to meet these pressing needs. Blockchain can redefine the security of huge healthcare databases through data integrity, secure access, and patient empowerment. Together with tokenisation, in which sensitive data is replaced by a non-sensitive equivalent called a token, these technologies provide a solution punch for improving both privacy and access management in healthcare.[12]

Role of Blockchain in Healthcare Data Security

Blockchain is a kind of distributed ledger technology (DLT) that allows transactions to be recorded in a safe, transparent, and immutable way. Blocks of data, where each block represents a transaction, are connected to the previous one using cryptographic hashes in such a way that they cannot be altered without also modifying all subsequent blocks, therefore making it virtually impossible to manipulate this data. This architecture greatly reduces the risk of security breaches, data leaking, and single failure points that centralised data repositories are prone to. The nature of these risks has significant implications given the amount of sensitive patient data involved in the healthcare context, making it a compelling consideration for the implementation of blockchain.

Blockchain has the potential to strengthen data integrity in healthcare. The nature of data, once recorded, cannot be changed without the agreement of the parties in the network, which prevents malicious tampering or manipulation. This unchangeable nature of blockchain assures that patient records are true and reliable, thus establishing trust between the healthcare providers, patients, and regulators. In addition to that, blockchain is transparent and enables compliance with authorised stakeholders to access audit transaction data and confirm transactions without knowing patient identity.

Blockchain allows for the automation of patient identity verification and access control. Conventional approaches mostly depend on the use of older, bulky systems for identifying patients, which could result in mistakes and ineffectiveness. Identity solutions based on blockchain utilise cryptographic methods to offer digital identities that are more secure and easily verifiable. Patients are able to control their own identities. In fact, they can permit specific healthcare providers to access their health records while keeping the rest of their data private. This not only enhances security but also gives the patient more power to manage his health data as per his privacy standards.[13]

Tokenisation as a Solution for Data Access and Privacy

Tokenisation is an additional tool that helps to solve some of the data access and privacy issues through the capabilities of blockchain. Tokenisation involves replacing sensitive data with unique, non-sensitive equivalents (tokens) that still maintain the essential information about the original data without compromising its security, enabling healthcare organisations to reduce their exposure to potential breaches while allowing access to patient information in a controlled manner. In the event that access to those tokens is granted outside of proper channels, tokenisation protects the underlying sensitive data because the tokens have no personally identifiable information present.

Utility tokens have more than one use in a tokenised healthcare ecosystem. For example, some may be used as currency to pay for health records, to take part in clinical trials, or even to provide medical data for researchers/employers. Through this model, patients are incentivised to provide their health data for research purposes, which creates a culture of data shared by stakeholders. This token can be given to patients in exchange for their consent, allowing them access to some of their data, which, in turn, they can later redeem against healthcare services, helping it tie value around the sharing of data.

Tokenisation improves data privacy not only by reducing the amount of sensitive data in use but also by inherently allowing for additional access controls. This is where smart contracts come in and automate the entire process of validating tokens and managing access permission. A smart contract might, for example, specify that a certain healthcare provider may access patient data only for certain treatment purposes and only during a specific time window. Embedding the rules in tokenisation ensures that therapeutic data complies with ethical manners and regulatory bodies while keeping patient identity safe within a hospital.

By using tokens, data can be interoperable across disparate healthcare systems. Standardised tokens representing health data can help achieve interoperability among different EHR systems.[14] This interoperability not only facilitates greater data sharing but also enables complete and longitudinal PHRs, leading to enhanced clinical decision-making and better patient outcomes.[15]

Tokenomics Framework for Data Sharing in Healthcare

With the rapid pace of data generation in healthcare, including various forms– digital health technologies, EHRs, wearable devices, and patient-generated health data, the term "data as a commodity" is making rounds. Due to this paradigm shift, a strong mechanism is in place to enable the secure and effective data exchange between all stakeholders within the healthcare ecosystem. Tokenomics has conceived a reasonable solution to these aspects, with its focus on some core concepts: while data are considered a commodity, sharing of patient data and smart contracts for the execution of transactions involving data, which are also illustrated in Figure 7.1.

Data as Commodity

With the growth of the digital age, data has shifted from being simply a by-product of operations to an important asset tackled under the banner of "data as a commodity."[16] Patient data is valuable for healthcare providers, researchers, pharmaceutical

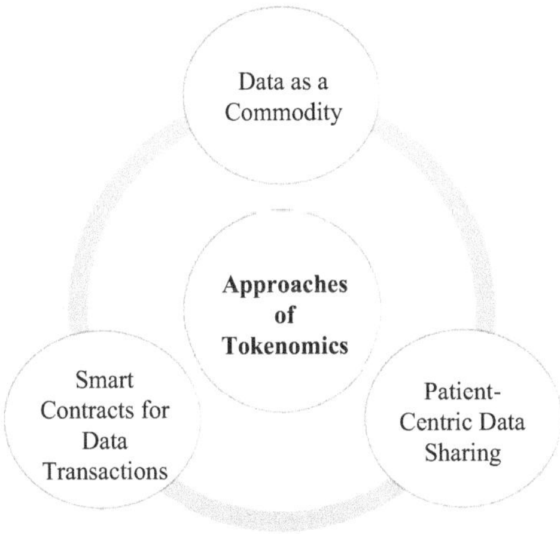

Figure 7.1 Approaches of Tokenomics in Healthcare.

companies, and insurance companies. With the novel approach of this transformation also comes the need to rethink how data is viewed and controlled: data has become a vital resource that not only serves as an asset for patients' betterment but also a lucrative asset for generating revenue.

Commoditisation of health care data means treating health care data as a trading commodity. It allows data to be sold and or purchased in a manner using tokenomics, which makes exchanging smooth through an exchange. Healthcare data can be transformed into tokenised assets (digital tokens on a blockchain) that allow accurate and verifiable tracking of their ownership rights, usage rights, transaction history, etc. This enables a marketplace for health data with patients, providers, and researchers interacting in an open landscape.

When data is referred to as a commodity, it relates to creating value propositions for sharing the data. Patients can be rewarded for sharing their data as a result of receiving compensation or by providing the patients with tokens. It's a win-win as not only does this encourage patients to contribute, but it also enables researchers with access to the vital datasets required to develop solutions that will drive medical science and public health forward. Yet such commodification raises ethical issues concerning privacy, consent and data ownership that need to be considered in order to protect the responsible and equitable use of health data.[17]

Patient-Centric Data Sharing

The tokenomics framework for data sharing is grounded in the concept of patient-centricity. In the past, patients have been passive receivers of healthcare services, having little or no control over their health data. Blockchain technology and tokenomics, on the other hand, have empowered patients to play a proactive role in maintaining their health information. Not only does this enable patients, but it also builds a trusting relationship between patient and provider.

Data sharing in the patient-centric approach focuses on informed consent, ownership of data, and privacy. Within a tokenomics framework, patients are part of the ecosystem, not just subjects. Users may opt-in to share their data and allow access for particular groups, but they would also have the right to withdraw it at any time. Such control over personal health data increases patient trust and incentivises people to take part in initiatives that require them to share their data.[18]

Smart Contracts for Data Transactions

Smart contracts are self-executing contracts with the agreement terms written directly in code. They are fundamental to blockchain technology and act as intermediaries that enable secure data transactions within the tokenomics model for health data exchange. Smart contracts automate everything about a data access request: they allow anyone to submit requests, notify the owner of a dataset, and automatically execute upon agreement by both parties.

In healthcare, for example, smart contracts could be used to program the terms of data access and usage. For example, a smart contract can specify that a researcher may only access the health data of a patient under certain conditions, such as gaining direct consent from the patient. This automated enforcement of consent guarantees ethical and law-compliant data sharing while decreasing the risk of unauthorised access and misuse of sensitive health information.

With the help of Smart contracts, real-time data transaction tracking becomes possible. This means that every interaction with health data can then be recorded on the blockchain, where an unchangeable audit trail adds a layer of accountability and transparency. As a result, stakeholders would be able to authenticate data ownership, track its use, and check if regulatory compliance requirements were followed, thus minimising risks of data breaches or fraud. In short, the tokenomics of tokens and smart contracts form a solid and secure environment for healthcare data sharing. Patients, providers, and researchers can confidently exchange data among all parties involved in the transactions, relatively assured that their rights are preserved with clearly delineated terms prescribed interactively binding to the wheelhouse of each of the participants involved. Such data sharing works to further the trustfulness of participants past this, resulting in improved patient outcomes and healthcare innovations.[19,20]

Enhancing Data Security with Tokenomics

Blockchain ecosystems, blended with the concept of tokenomics, have transformative capabilities regarding data safety in healthcare settings. With the healthcare sector struggling against constant threats of data breaches, patient privacy, and data integrity concerns, tokenomics provides a decentralised approach to alleviating these factors. With the incentive to provide high-quality data, the element of a distributed continual storage mechanism, and a privacy guarantee for users' data, tokenomics is able to protect any sensitive health information.

Incentivising Data Integrity and Security

In the healthcare industry, any inaccuracies can lead to adverse effects at both the patient safety level and clinical outcomes, making it essential to maintain data integrity. Tokenomics adds a framework where all different stakeholders can be incentivised to keep up with high standards of data quality and security through mechanisms that reward or punish truthful and false reporting, respectively. Forty-three participants inside a blockchain ecosystem get rewarded with tokens for validating and verifying the health data. In such a decentralised network, healthcare providers can be rewarded with utility tokens for every validated health record and outcome data they submit. This model creates a good correlation between the financial interest of the data provider and its quality, making the overall data stored in the blockchain more trustworthy. On top of that, tokens can be used to establish a reputation system whereby stakeholder contributions of higher quality are rewarded and given access privileges over more resources or data.

Through the introduction of penalties for non-compliance or data manipulation, tokenomics creates a mechanism of accountability. As a concrete example, if a healthcare provider is determined to have submitted fictitious data, they will face token forfeiture, creating an economic disincentive for harmful actions. Rewards and penalties will ensure ethical use of data while fostering a sense of accountability among the participants, which in turn guarantees the integrity of health information.[21,22]

Distributed Data Storage and Security

Tokenomics has also become a decisive factor for improved data security through distributed data storage. Traditional healthcare systems are built to use centralised databases, which exposes them to central points of failure as well as cyberattacks. Conversely, blockchain technology distributes data across a network of nodes, so there is less vulnerability with centralised data repositories. Every single data point gets encrypted and published in a distributed way, which increases its resistance to access breaches.

In this distributed architecture, tokenomics rewards stakeholders for providing storage back to the network by making it a requirement for stakeholders with tokens to host a node that has at least partial copies of the health data, which will help to increase redundancy/security and accessibility. This incentivisation enhances the overall robustness of the network. Also, it democratises data storage by enabling smaller healthcare providers or even solo practitioners with minimal infrastructure to help secure the ecosystem as a whole.

The use of decentralised storage mechanisms such as InterPlanetary File System (IPFS) in conjunction with tokenomics further increases security. Tokens can enforce access control and permissions, while IPFS stores and fetches data in a decentralised way. Smart contracts can help narrow access to sensitive health data so that only specified parties can read or make changes to it. This reinforces the security of data while also enabling patients to determine who gets access to their health records, promoting privacy and individual independence.[23]

Data Privacy

Data privacy is traditionally an important issue in the healthcare market, where patient information is considered to be more sensitive and comes with greater regulation. Tokenomics lays out the groundwork for solving privacy issues through privacy-preserving technologies like ZKPs (zero-knowledge proofs) and other cryptographic tricks. They enable users to verify transactions or data without revealing the details behind them, thus maintaining privacy while still demonstrating data validity.

By using ZKPs, a healthcare provider would be able to check if the patient is eligible for treatment without having access to or revealing the whole medical history of the patient. Tokens can enable these interactions by incentivising data holders to leverage ZKPs to use patient information while still being confidential for legitimate purposes. Such a novel approach not only maintains privacy but also builds trust among the patients to share their data for research and development. Decentralised identity management systems that leverage tokenomics will also be helpful in improving the privacy of our data. The underlying token acts as an access key, giving patients the power to control their digital identities and determine which health information to share with whom. This infinite control reduces the chance of information leaks and allows patients to enter into data-sharing agreements solely with entities they want.[24]

Token Models for Healthcare Systems

Since the introduction of blockchain technology in the health sector, different token models have revolutionised it. These models allow stakeholders access to diverse interactions, protect data, and make healthcare services more efficient. This discussion differentiates various types of token models applicable to healthcare systems, as illustrated in Figure 7.2.

Token-Based Access to Health Records, Treatments and Telemedicine

Tokenised access to health records utilises the distributed nature of blockchain to give patients ownership of their health data in the form of encrypted tokens. They act as gateways to access EHR, ensuring that sensitive medical data is only retrieved by trusted parties. The introduction of the utility token will provide healthcare providers with a safe way to share health records between unconnected systems. This creates a patient-centric ecosystem where patients can earn tokens for granting access to their data for clinical research or personalised treatment solutions.

The use of tokens in combination with telemedicine platforms can help improve the patient-provider experience. Patients could use tokens to pay for virtual consultations, easing transactions but maintaining anonymity. These tokens work thanks to smart contracts where appointments can be made, payments processed, and records maintained by both parties observing the established agreements. It reduces the cost of rendering telemedicine services while ensuring patients are informed and consenting, thus maintaining ethicality in healthcare provision.[25]

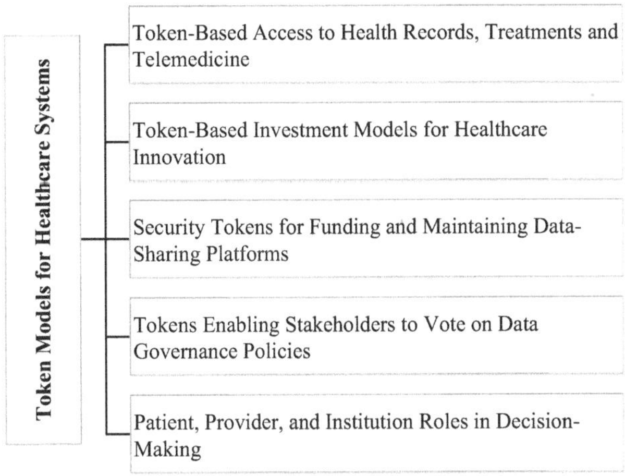

Figure 7.2 Token Models for Healthcare Systems.

Token-Based Investment Models for Healthcare Innovation

Tokenised investment setups offer a new manner in which stakeholders can share resources to invest in healthcare innovation, considerably lowering traditional barriers to entry. Diverse investors can finance health tech innovations through initial coin offerings (ICOs) or token sales. To democratise healthcare investment, investors buy tokens which entitle them to a stake in the company or a share of its future revenue.

Such tokens can be monetised for their appreciation in value tied to the performance of the underlying technology or service, thereby giving investors a motive to back up innovative projects. These investment models, in turn, also help ensure that the interests of different stakeholders are aligned, whether it is a patient who will need innovative therapy or technology or a healthcare provider wishing to improve their service offering. The inherent transparency of the blockchain ensures that all records are immutable, which creates trust and accountability in the whole investment process.[26]

Security Tokens for Funding and Maintaining Data-Sharing Platforms

The context of the healthcare ecosystem offers strong grounds for utilising or funding and sustaining their data-sharing platforms through security tokens. So, in the case of these security tokens, they adhere to regulatory standards and give holders a share of an asset or profit. Healthcare companies can issue security tokens to protect themselves from the risk of not following legal frameworks such as Securities and Exchange Commission rules in America while obtaining investment capital.

Security tokens are not only an incentive in the funding stage but will continue to generate profits via profit-sharing. As an example, a healthcare data exchange platform may distribute some of the revenues earned through using the platform to token holders, providing strong incentives for long-term investment and participation in the network. Additionally, security tokens could improve the governance model around healthcare platforms with holder voting rights on important decisions (e.g., operational changes and data-sharing policies) in exchange for stakeholder engagement and accountability.[27]

Tokens Enabling Stakeholders to Vote on Data Governance Policies

Governance tokens help ensure that everyone involved in the health ecosystem has a vote for data governance. Participants can use these tokens for decentralised decision-making activities. Through the distribution of governance tokens proportioned by user activity or contribution, healthcare organisations can create a more equitable governance system.

Governance tokens enable stakeholders to propose, discuss, and vote on several aspects of data management, including access protocols, data-sharing policies, and ethical considerations. This participatory perspective contributes to greater transparency while allowing the individual to take ownership of their health data and related rights. As a result, governance tokens can propagate community-first standards in line with the behaviour of all participants whose interests are represented, helping to build a culture of trust and collaboration for data-sharing.[28]

Patient, Provider, and Institution Roles in Decision-Making

Token models in healthcare reform the decision-making process that patients, providers, and institutions do together. Decision-making has long been a top-down approach, with providers and health systems controlling patients, who often must rely on those same institutions to get care or obtain their data. Tokenomics, on the other hand, encourages the collective ability of patients to have agency in deciding over their own health information and treatment paths.

When patients are incentivised through tokens, this beneficially influences patient involvement with health data and management, rendering a new block of clinical research outcomes from patient-centric initiatives. Patients can opt-in with informed consent to use their data in tokenised ecosystems, receive compensation for their contributions, and help dictate which research is prioritised based on their needs/preferences. Token models can earn a lot in the healthcare space as well because patient data used to optimise care delivery and improve operational efficiency is priceless. The tokenised setup provides practitioners with access to real-time health data and insights generated from the patient population at scale for making clinical decisions. In addition, token-based payment systems simplify billing and reduce administrative overhead, enabling providers to devote more time to patient care.

Focusing on the hospitals and health systems, proper governance of tokenised ecosystems is a key role of institutions. They have to implement and manage token-based solutions, ensure compliance with regulatory standards, and maintain patient data security. Governance tokens can empower institutions to engage with their stakeholders and make sure that the decision-making process is harmonious between respecting patient autonomy and achieving organisational objectives.[29]

Future Directions and Innovations in Tokenomics in Healthcare

The intersection between blockchain technology, tokenomics and artificial intelligence (AI), machine learning (ML), and personalised medicine signals a new paradigm for healthcare. Access to these innovations allows the healthcare sector to move towards improving interoperability between data, support cross-border health assistance networks, and encourage personalised medicine by allowing for proper decentralised incentivised data sharing. This section explores the future directions and innovations in tokenomics in healthcare, highlighting the integration of AI and ML, the establishment of interoperable systems, and the potential for personalised medicine.[30]

AI and ML Integration

Bringing AI and ML into the analysis of tokenised healthcare data will create never-before-seen opportunities to improve the quality of care, impact patient outcomes, and drive operational efficiencies. With this, AI algorithms can analyse massive datasets created from multiple focus points, such as healthcare providers, patients, and wearable devices, enabling them to discover patterns and insights that are mostly impossible for human analysts to detect. These solutions can enable predictive analytics powered by advanced statistical models and neural networks, helping to determine which populations are at greater risk of impairment, the best treatment protocols per patient type, and care plans per need.

Tokenised healthcare data can be an abundant resource for training AI models that create algorithms based on longitudinal datasets while using cryptographic techniques to protect patient identities. For example, federated learning enables AI models to train on decentralised data without the need to transfer that sensitive data away from where it originated, making it easier to comply with relevant data protection laws. Such an approach not only protects patient confidentiality but also helps the AI models gain additional generalisability by acquiring diverse data reflecting different demographics and clinical contexts.

When tokenisation technology is coupled with AI in healthcare settings, operational efficiency can also become better immediately. ML algorithms for predictive analytics can provide automated decision support systems that benefit healthcare providers by making more data-driven decisions, optimising resource allocation, and reducing costs caused by unnecessary interventions. By utilising AI-powered predictive analytics, you can manage the flow of patients and forecast the need for healthcare services so that providers can just-in-time capacity management optimise operations and improve service delivery.

Natural language processing (NLP) deployment in the tokenised ecosystem can help turn these unstructured data sources into actionable insights, such as clinical notes and research articles. The power of NLP techniques allows health organisations to analyse clinical narratives and research studies systematically, improving clinical decision-making while gaining deeper insights into patient engagement.[31,32]

Interoperability and Global Healthcare Networks

The future of healthcare depends on interoperable systems that facilitate the exchange of data across various platforms and stakeholders. By manufacturing commonplace tokens that may be recognised through multiple healthcare ecosystems, tokenomics is central to creating interoperability. The idea of trust networks relies on unique non-fungible tokens that serve as secure, standardised protocols for the transfer of value and information between providers, payers, and patients, improving interoperability within health by creating a third-party analytic mechanism.

Interoperable systems can eliminate silos in healthcare and allow for data to be pulled from across multiple sources and analysed. For example, a blockchain HIE (health information exchange) enables different health institutions to share patient records securely, furnishing everyone concerned with holistic and latest health data. Smart contracts increase interoperability as self-executing agreements that automate data-sharing protocols in compliance with regulations; this means faster and more secure access to patient data.

One way that tokenomics can enhance the networks spanning national borders found in global healthcare is by encouraging the establishment of partnerships. The tokenisation of data can help promote international research collaborations and the ability for organisations to access a wider variety of datasets, which is particularly useful for clinical trials and epidemiological studies. In this way, one can create a token economy that incentivises data sharing and stakeholder participation in global health initiatives, contributing to collective knowledge while promoting global health equity.

Creating interconnected systems also requires action on data standards and compliance with rules. Through tokenomics, this can make a set of industry standards for data formats, privacy protocols, and security measures that all players follow while maintaining trust with patients. The evolution of regulatory frameworks will also be imperative, as how tokenomics integrates with interoperable systems will determine how we navigate this complex landscape together and provide the basis for a culture of collaboration among stakeholders.

Tokenomics in Personalised Medicine

Personalised medicine is a new paradigm for the delivery of health care that aims to personalise treatment strategies based on individual patient characteristics, including genetic, environmental, and lifestyle factors. Tokenomics can then improve personalised medicine by incentivising patients, healthcare practitioners, and researchers to move their data between them. Such token-based ecosystems can incentivise stakeholders to share their data for research purposes into targeted therapies and precision medicine.

By rewarding patients to take part in clinical trials or sharing their health data, tokenised incentives could also help build the sense of a collaborative culture necessary for us to move towards personalised treatment. More specifically, patients might earn tokens in return for contributing genomic data, wearable health metrics, or answers to health-related questionnaires. These tokens could be exchanged for healthcare services, educational materials, or access to specialised treatment, benefitting patients and providers alike.

Tokenomics can promote the unification of different data types – EHRs, genomic databases, patient-reported outcomes, etc. When these data types are tokenised, analyses that span broader dimensions of health can be performed and ultimately culminate in patient-specific biomarker signatures and treatment pathways. By addressing both biological and psychosocial factors, this broad-spectrum method can substantively augment treatment regimen effectiveness, subsequently increasing the quality of life for affected individuals.

Throwing some Tokenomics behind creating dynamic treatment plans that evolve with real-world data. Patients transmit their health data, and healthcare providers tailor treatment protocols according to the latest information about the patient. This flexibility in treatment options can ultimately result in chronic disease management, minimise hospital visits, and increase patient satisfaction.[33]

Conclusion

Tokenomics is a unique way to encourage data sharing and security in the health sector. With tokenomics, an entire ecosystem can be built upon blockchain technology where healthcare stakeholders can facilitate the complexities of data management by leveraging different types of tokens (utility, security, and governance) for their respective privileges. Tokens are essential to enable access to health services; they also empower patients and provide them with control over their data, as well as promote the collaboration between providers, researchers, and patients.

The importance of data in healthcare is undeniable, as it has never been more significant in the COVID era. It is an invaluable resource responsible for creating better patient outcomes and improving research efficacy and healthcare processes when properly managed. However, a new breed of privacy, safety, and accessibility challenges must be addressed to create effective solutions. Blockchain technology solves these challenges by offering a secure and decentralised infrastructure for managing healthcare data. This framework is further strengthened by tokenisation, which facilitates patient-centric data exchange and allows the design of automated smart contracts that automate transactions while adhering to regulations governing privacy.

With the limitless possibility of commoditised health data with a patient-centric strategy, stakeholders build an ecosystem in which patients are encouraged to record their health data so that it can then contribute to the creation of a databank benefiting all stakeholders equally. In addition, incentivising integrity, promoting distributed storage, and ensuring privacy tokenomics will play an important part in creating a secure environment for healthcare data management.

Looking ahead, In the future, opportunities for tokenomics in healthcare will be endless as AI and ML develop further, interoperable global healthcare networks emerge, and personalised medicine becomes a focus. With the evolving scenery, the thoughtful use of tokenomics should help eliminate obstacles to data exchange and increase overall system efficiency, ultimately leading to a more just and effective healthcare sector.

Consent for Publication

All authors are given their consent for publication. The authors authorised Mr. Ashish Verma for all correspondence.

Conflict of Interest

The authors have no conflict of interest.

Acknowledgement

Authors are highly thankful to their Universities/Colleges for providing library facilities for the literature survey.

References

1 Bourque, Pierre. "Tokenomics-economics of blockchain-based systems: Analyzing token economics models and incentives mechanisms in blockchain-based systems to ensure network participation and sustainability." *Journal of Artificial Intelligence Research and Applications* 3, no. 2 (2023): 1–10.

2 Adhami, Saman, and Giancarlo Giudici. "Initial coin offerings: Tokens as innovative financial assets." *Blockchain Economics and Financial Market Innovation: Financial Innovations in the Digital Age* (2019): 61–81.

3 Cunningham, James, Nigel Davies, Sarah Devaney, Søren Holm, Mike Harding, Victoria Neumann, and John Ainsworth. "The application of distributed autonomous organisation governance mechanisms to civic medical data management." *IET Blockchain* 4 (2024): 483–724.

4 Lee, Chi Kin. "Blockchain application with health token in medical & health industrials." In *2nd International Conference on Social Science, Public Health and Education (SSPHE 2018)*, pp. 233–236. Atlantis Press, 2019.

5 Urkude, Shubhangi V., Himanshu Sharma, Seethamsetty Uday Kumar, and Vijaykumar R. Urkude. "Anatomy of blockchain implementation in healthcare." In *Blockchain Technology: Applications and Challenges*, pp. 51–76. Cham: Springer International Publishing, 2021.

6 Moro Visconti, Roberto, and Donato Morea. "Healthcare digitalisation and pay-for-performance incentives in smart hospital project financing." *International Journal of Environmental Research and Public Health* 17, no. 7 (2020): 2318.

7 Yaqoob, Ibrar, Khaled Salah, Raja Jayaraman, and Yousof Al-Hammadi. "Blockchain for healthcare data management: Opportunities, challenges, and future recommendations." *Neural Computing and Applications* 34 (2022): 11475–11490.

8 Subbiah, Vivek. "The next generation of evidence-based medicine." *Nature Medicine* 29, no. 1 (2023): 49–58.
9 Molli, Vijaya Lakshmi Pavani. "Blockchain technology for secure and transparent health data management: Opportunities and challenges." *Journal of Healthcare AI and ML* 10, no. 10 (2023): 1–15.
10 Udegbe, Francisca Chibugo, Ogochukwu Roseline Ebulue, Charles Chukwudalu Ebulue, and Chukwunonso Sylvester Ekesiobi. "Precision medicine and genomics: A comprehensive review of IT-enabled approaches." *International Medical Science Research Journal* 4, no. 4 (2024): 509–520.
11 Liu, Paul Tak Shing. "Medical record system using blockchain, big data and tokenisation." In *Information and Communications Security: 18th International Conference, ICICS 2016, Singapore, Singapore, November 29–December 2, 2016, Proceedings 18*, pp. 254–261. Springer International Publishing, 2016.
12 Zubaydi, Haider Dhia, Yung-Wey Chong, Kwangman Ko, Sabri M. Hanshi, and Shankar Karuppayah. "A review on the role of blockchain technology in the healthcare domain." *Electronics* 8, no. 6 (2019): 679.
13 Bernabe, Jorge Bernal, Jose Luis Canovas, Jose L. Hernandez-Ramos, Rafael Torres Moreno, and Antonio Skarmeta. "Privacy-preserving solutions for blockchain: Review and challenges." *IEEE Access* 7 (2019): 164908–164940.
14 Schwiderowski, Jan, Asger Balle Pedersen, and Roman Beck. "Crypto tokens and token systems." *Information Systems Frontiers* 26, no. 1 (2024): 319–332.
15 Pithadia, Hirsh, Enzo Fenoglio, Bogdan Batrinca, Philip Treleaven, Radu Echim, Andrei Bubutanu, and Charles Kerrigan. "Data assets: Tokenization and valuation." Available at SSRN 4419590 (2023).
16 Liao, Wen-Ling, and Fuu-Jen Tsai. "Personalized medicine: A paradigm shift in healthcare." *BioMedicine* 3, no. 2 (2013): 66–72.
17 Shukla, Rashmi G., Anuja Agarwal, and Vidhu Shekhar. "Leveraging blockchain technology for Indian healthcare system: An assessment using value-focused thinking approach." *The Journal of High Technology Management Research* 32, no. 2 (2021): 100415.
18 Madir, Jelena. "Smart contracts-self-executing contracts of the future?" *International In-house Counsel Journal* 13 (2020): 1.
19 Freni, Pierluigi, Enrico Ferro, and Roberto Moncada. "Tokenomics and blockchain tokens: A design-oriented morphological framework." *Blockchain: Research and Applications* 3, no. 1 (2022): 100069.
20 Khatoon, Asma. "A blockchain-based smart contract system for healthcare management." *Electronics* 9, no. 1 (2020): 94.
21 Kyriakakis, Anthony. "The missing victims of health care fraud." *Utah Law Review* 3 (2015): 605.
22 Toufaily, Elissar. "An integrative model of trust toward crypto-tokens applications: A customer perspective approach." *Digital Business* 2, no. 2 (2022): 100041.
23 Gasimova, Nurana. "Developing tokenomics framework: Conceptual framework for self-sustaining tokenomics." *Digital Vetenskapliga Arkivet*, (2023): 1–60.
24 George, Liz, and Jubilant J. Kizhakkethottam. "Unleashing the future of healthcare in the metaverse: The pivotal role of blockchain in data privacy." In Pradeep Nijalingappa, T. Gururaj, S. B. Goyal, Vinod Shukla and Alessandro Bruno (eds), *Examining the Metaverse in Healthcare: Opportunities, Challenges, and Future Directions*, pp. 77–102. Hershey, PA: IGI Global, 2024.

25 Trypidakis, Georgios. "Evolution of public token sales: The next generation of ICOs." Master's thesis, European University of Cyprus (Cyprus), 2021.
26 Zhang, Aiqing, and Xiaodong Lin. "Towards secure and privacy-preserving data sharing in e-health systems via consortium blockchain." *Journal of Medical Systems* 42, no. 8 (2018): 140.
27 Jaiman, Vikas, and Visara Urovi. "A consent model for blockchain-based health data sharing platforms." *IEEE Access* 8 (2020): 143734–143745.
28 Cornwall, Andrea, Henry Lucas, and Kath Pasteur. "Accountability through participation: Developing workable partnership models in the health sector." *IDS Bulletin* 31, no. 1 (2000): 1–13.
29 Samir Damani, Vishal Verma, Raleigh Harbour, Jeremy Gross, Tanuj Nigam, Umesh Lalwani, and Eric Daniels. "Aligning Stakeholders in a New Healthcare Ecosystem." MintHealth, Inc. (2018): 1–45.
30 Selvaraj, Sivachandran. "Empowering patients with AI-driven personalized care: The transformative power of generative AI and healthcare data integration."
31 Raja, Kalpana, and Siddhartha Jonnalagadda. "Natural language processing and data mining for clinical text." *Healthcare Data Analytics* 36 (2015): 219.
32 Salunkhe, Vishwasrao. "Transforming healthcare research with interoperability: The role of FHIR and SMART on FHIR." In Vijit Chaturvedi, Prashant Singh, Anandhi Ramachandran and Divya Aggarwal (eds), *Healthcare Administration and Managerial Training in the 21st Century*, pp. 211–248. Hershey, PA: IGI Global, 2024.
33 Lavallee, Danielle C., Kate E. Chenok, Rebecca M. Love, Carolyn Petersen, Erin Holve, Courtney D. Segal, and Patricia D. Franklin. "Incorporating patient-reported outcomes into health care to engage patients and enhance care." *Health Affairs* 35, no. 4 (2016): 575–582.

8 Blockchain and AI Integration in Patient Care

Akanksha Sharma, Sunita, Akhil Sharma, Ashish Verma, Shaweta Sharma and Neeraj Kumar Fuloria

Introduction

Blockchain technology has probably become common and recognised all over the world for about ten years. After the technology was signed into use, the researcher pivoted to examining its key insights. This is the digital currency or cryptocurrency concept that Nakamoto talked about. These digital currencies rely on decentralised systems, and the underlying technology of these currencies is called blockchain. Blockchain is a disruptive and revolutionary technology with many promising applications, working as a distributed ledger. Even in the beginning of all communities around here, it was believed that bitcoin was blockchain and myths about what technology is and how that will impact business applications. Subsequently, developers, industry experts, and academics in several fields (Banking, Healthcare, and Government) came to realise that there is a core technology/solution much deeper than Bitcoin driving this revolution.[1,2]

The basic definition of Blockchain is several blocks containing transactions followed one after the other. However, Blockchain is decentralised and distributed in nature based on a Peer-to-Peer (P2P) network. Every participant in it can control the network. A blockchain network includes many connected computers, and the part of the block cannot be changed without assembly over the entire framework. The block is just a wrapper for the data. In the blockchain network, computers are referred to as nodes, and each node has a copy of this digital ledger.[3]

Patient care systems have also started to use blockchain technology to secure electronic health records (EHR) while providing improved data security, privacy, and interoperability. A prominent example is the ACTION-EHR system developed in recent years, where a permissioned blockchain framework facilitates patient-centred sharing of core components of EHR data across multiple healthcare institutions. It allows patients to manage their health records. Also, it keeps HIPAA compliant with its elements by storing data that is sensitive off-chain and only keeping metadata on the blockchain utilising encryption.[4]

In healthcare, the new idea of the decentralised nature of blockchain is very beneficial as it facilitates access to data and that too without central intermediaries by enhancing patient confidentiality with reduced chances of data breaches. Blockchain can enable secure communication among various entities in the healthcare

DOI: 10.4324/9781003529910-8

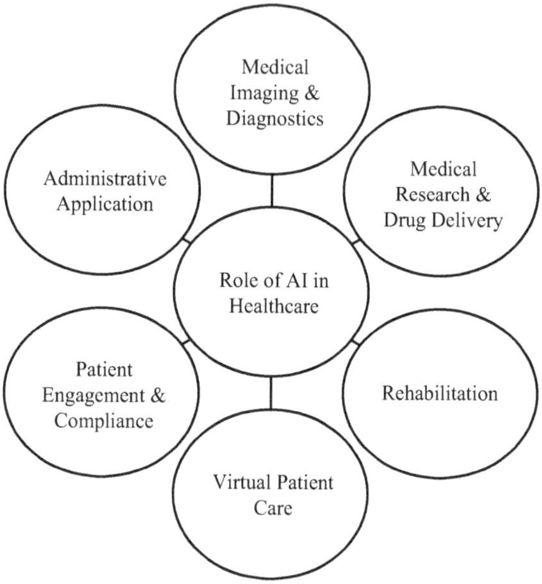

Figure 8.1 Role of AI in Healthcare.

sector through smart contracts and crypto techniques, where only authenticated personnel can access sensitive medical data. In addition, the transparency and immutability of blockchain may also help in building trust between patients and providers by creating a trustworthy audit trail for all transactions involving health data.[5]

Besides enhancing EHR management, blockchain can facilitate applications in remote patient monitoring as well as supply chain management with pharmaceuticals and health insurance claims processing. Efforts focused not just on increasing operational efficiencies but also on placing patients in more control of their health information. The integration of blockchain technology is about to take centre stage in the ever-changing landscape of healthcare, playing a key role in long-standing issues relating to data security and patient privacy.[6]

Role of AI in Healthcare

Figure 8.1 is depicted the role of artificial intelligence in healthcare system for managing various tasks.

Medical Imaging and Diagnostic Services

Radio-diagnosis is one of the key applications for AI-based early disease diagnosis and minimising diagnostic errors. Used in ECG and echocardiography chart analysis to assist with decision-making. Using body imaging modalities, AI has demonstrated promising early results for various diseases, including breast and skin cancer, eye disease, and pneumonia. Its analysis can also use speech patterns to predict psychotic events and identify characteristic features of neurological disease. The various AI techniques that have proven to be a great help in the fight against COVID-19 are in their early diagnosis. This describes medical image analysis using a transformer as a deep learning model, which is applied to various modalities, such as registration, detection/classification, image-to-image translation/completion, segmentation, and video-based. We then propose a hybrid chest CT-built method via wavelet Renyi entropy and a three-segment biogeography-grounded optimisation algorithm for automatic COVID-19 detection.[7]

Virtual Patient Care

Recent advancements in wearable technology and the implementation of machine learning (ML) and artificial intelligence (AI) techniques in the healthcare industry have resulted in virtual patient monitoring and management. Wearable sensors are also where AI has its hands full in controlling chronic disease. A smart sensor system that integrates a combined sensor network to monitor the physiological variables will supply data for elderly care. The use of wearable digital devices may also facilitate accurate diagnosis, as demonstrated in a case report where atrial fibrillation was identified as a potential explanation for stroke in the patient. More innovative models need to be developed through future research.[8]

Medical Research and Drug Discovery

Medical research and drug development entail analysing enormous, complicated datasets – along with the right type of AI, it can facilitate drug innovation and drug development. It can apply predictive analytics to risk-assess, prospectively identify viable candidates for clinical trials, and create precision models of biological systems. Improving participant management with natural language processing in clinical trials is well established, but demonstrated improvements to trial quality and experience are unknown. Generative AI can be used to create synthetic data that helps enhance the datasets and diversity, while metaverse applications help make it easier to collaborate for research virtually.[9]

Patient Engagement and Compliance

Patient engagement and compliance are 'the last mile' challenges in healthcare and the final barrier to better vs poorer health outcomes. Non-compliance refers to a patient not following a treatment regimen or taking prescribed medicines. If patients have good health outcomes (>healthcare utilisation, cost, and patient experience), then they are engaged in healthcare. In a survey of healthcare leaders and executives, they indicated that in fewer than half the cases, their patients were deeply involved in shared decision-making with them on treatment options. If there is an acute or chronic health issue to address, healthcare providers rely on their clinical experts to devise treatment plans designed to restore health. But, for the most part, it is irrelevant when the patient blows off the necessary behavioural modifications like losing weight, scheduling a follow-up appointment, and adhering to a treatment regimen. These conditions led to the successful implementation of AI with real-time interventions for improved patient engagement. Over time, ML and workflow engines are increasingly being leveraged to support driving composite interventions across the care spectrum. Research is getting the auspicious pitch through messaging alarms and appropriately tailored content that triggers adoption at the right times.[10,11]

Rehabilitation

AI and robotics are revolutionising rehabilitation by changing methods, attitudes, and skills. AI includes both physical and virtual aspects, while ML, a subset of AI, is applied to perioperative medicine, brain-computer interface technology, myoelectric control, and neuroprosthetics. ML methods are similarly used in the musculoskeletal system for the assessment of patient data, supportive clinical decision-making, and diagnostic imaging. Applications like smart homes, wearable devices in rehabilitation to monitor adherence during exercise, and inertial sensors are some examples of how such approaches can combine health assessment and reported improvement with smart actuation, showing the promise that lies within the use of both wearables devices, ML-driven analysis of behaviour change.[12]

Administrative Applications

AI can automate the extraction and processing of data from clinical notes, patient records, and other unstructured sources reducing unnecessary administrative burdens in healthcare. For instance, the W. Lee Hedges School of Nursing has found that U.S. nurses dedicate almost a quarter of their time to regulatory and administrative activities, which AI-based voice-to-text transcription could streamline. Rule-based systems exist in most EHR but are less accurate than ML-based methods. To address this issue, solutions like Amazon's ML tools have been developed to derive meaningful information from unstructured parts of EHR. BEHRT, is a deep neural model for better modelling future clinical events based on the long-term history of patients. The flexibility of BEHRT also made it possible to incorporate other heterogeneous data, such as assessments, diagnoses, and medications, which increased the accuracy of the predictions. Moreover, hierarchical BEHRT (Hi-BEHRT) achieves enhanced performance over all-task BEHRT on risk prediction of chronic diseases like diabetes, heart failure, and stroke in patients with lengthy medical histories. These models have been shown to perform better than traditional deep-learning systems for several healthcare tasks.[13,14]

Combined Benefits of Blockchain and AI In Healthcare

The combined benefits of blockchain and AI in healthcare create a powerful synergy that enhances patient care, data security, and operational efficiency.

Enhanced Data Security and Integrity

The immutable and decentralised characteristic of blockchain protects patient data from being changed or hidden due to its secure record-keeping, therefore lowering the chance of data breaches. AI algorithms then generate analyses that can lead to diagnosis and treatment planning within this secure framework that relies on trusted datasets. These technologies in place enable sensitive health information to be protected but still accessible to those with the appropriate authorisation.[15]

Improved Interoperability

Healthcare systems have struggled for decades with interoperability, but the intersection of blockchain and AI promises a solution. Blockchain allows the secure sharing of health records between providers. AI could even analyse this data to find patterns in medical history and predict potential medical conditions allowing for more personalised treatment plans. Such smooth data switching also helps collaborate with other health providers, which results in better outcomes for patients.[16]

Streamlined Clinical Trials and Drug Development

Blockchain could increase transparency and trust in clinical trial data by providing a secure decentralised ledger for participant consent and tracking of trial progress. This use of AI could process such large amounts of data from these trials to narrow down the best drug candidates more quickly. This synergy not only expedites drug development processes but also enhances confidence in research outcomes owing to improved data integrity.[17]

Optimised Supply Chain Management

Supply chain management is important to make sure that medications and medical supplies are available in time, especially for healthcare. Blockchain comes with a transparent record of the supply chain, while AI will help in ideal inventory management and anticipate market demand in a timely manner. Their combined function minimises the possibility of fake medicines and enables the prompt distribution of required medical commodities.[18]

Enhanced Telemedicine Capabilities

It also promotes the integration of blockchain and AI, which positively impacts telemedicine by allowing medical data to be securely transferred from patient to provider and vice versa. AI-based remote monitoring systems can detect any anomalies in patient data in real time and notify healthcare professionals when required. The decentralisation of blockchain places the control in the hands of patients when it comes to their medical data, enhancing consent management.[19]

Secure Patient Data Management

A robust framework for safeguarding patient data implementing Secure patient data management that involves blockchain and AI. One of the most crucial roles blockchain provides in security is unalterable records or data, which cannot be changed as they are stored and written across an immutable ledger, therefore ensuring the integrity of the data. With this, the data is divided across many nodes in a decentralised storage architecture, further improving security by lessening the risks of single-point failure. This is exactly where AI comes in handy, as it can facilitate data processing methods like anonymisation, which removes personally identifiable information to ensure patient privacy. Moreover, the blockchain enables data to be stored in an encrypted format that AI algorithms are still capable of analysing (e.g., through predictive modelling and optimisations for treatments) without violating digital security.[20,21]

Smart contracts automate patient consent management, enabling patients to grant access and revoke it securely. Every consent action is transparent and recorded by the blockchain, ensuring that the data can only be accessed by authorised third parties. With the integration of AI, blockchain can also act as an end-to-end data encryption solution, ensuring top-notch security that secures your data. At the same time, it is being stored, transmitted, and processed. The combination of these technologies offers an unbreakable solution, keeping patient data private and giving patients back control of their health records.[22] Secure patient data management, including its benefits and challenges, is shown in Table 8.1.

Personalised Patient Care and AI-Driven Insights

Predictive Analytics

Using AI and Blockchain tech, it checks patient records for better disease prediction. The use of blockchain enables the secure and immutable storage of patient data, resulting in a reliable source of data for AI models. By analysing the historical health records of patients along with real-time information on various patterns, AI is able to read not-so-visible signals and predict the start of a disease. For example, longitudinal data to monitor changes in a patient's vital signs could predict health risks over time. Similarly, tracking genetic markers can also help in predicting health risks. Such early identification allows for prompt medical treatment, thus decreasing the risk of complications and enhancing patient prognosis.[32]

Tailored Treatments

A vital aspect of having patient data utilised to create increasingly AI-powered care plans is the ability to store this information securely, which tends through blockchain. Patients can use blockchain to keep their medical records and preserve the integrity of data for AI-supported precision medicine. It is capable of processing genetic, lifestyle, and environmental factors and forming highly customised

Table 8.1 Representation of Secure Patient Data Management

Aspect	*Description*	*Benefits*	*Challenges*
Data encryption	Uses cryptographic techniques to protect patient data.	Ensures confidentiality and integrity of sensitive information.	Complexity in encryption management and key distribution.[23]
Access control	Defines who can access patient data through permissions.	Enhances security by restricting access to authorised personnel.	Balancing user access with necessary data availability.[24]
Blockchain technology	Employs a decentralised ledger for storing health records.	Provides transparency and tamper-proof data management.	Integration with existing healthcare systems can be complex.[25]
Patient data ownership	Allows patients to control their medical records.	Empowers patients and increases trust in data sharing.	Requires patient education and awareness.[26]
Real-time monitoring	Continuously tracks patient health metrics through IoT devices.	Enables timely interventions and personalised care.	Managing vast amounts of data securely in real-time.[27]
Data interoperability	Ensures seamless data exchange between different systems.	Facilitates coordinated care and comprehensive patient profiles.	Achieving compatibility across diverse healthcare technologies.[28]
Audit trails	Keeps records of data access and modifications.	Enhances accountability and helps in compliance audits.	Managing and analysing large audit logs can be resource-intensive.[29]
Compliance with regulations	Adheres to laws like HIPAA to protect patient data.	Ensures legal protection and promotes best practices.	Staying updated with evolving regulations and standards.[30]
Data backup and recovery	Implements strategies for data preservation and recovery.	Protects against data loss and ensures continuity of care.	Developing robust backup systems can be costly and complex.[31]

treatment plans. For instance, AI-integrated solutions can utilise genomic data to treat targeted therapies with a known high level of improved efficacy over standard therapeutic options for a specific subtype or phenotype of cancer and an associated reduction in exposure to unnecessary side effects, thereby improving the quality of treatment.[33]

Real-Time Monitoring

Internet of Things (IoT) data secured by blockchain and AI models provide predictive insights into real-time patient monitoring. Blockchain will ensure the health metrics gathered by IoT devices, including heart rate, glucose data, physical activity records, etc., are protected from manipulation. Then, the AI algorithms can analyse this data and predict a potential health incident (like cardiac arrest or diabetic emergency) before it occurs. LifeTracker™ – Tracking the patient's health status continuously through wearable devices. This tremendous progress in technology enables providers to react proactively by changing treatment and preventing acute conditions, as well as providing better management of chronic diseases.[34]

Automation and Operational Efficiency

Smart Contracts for Healthcare Automation

Smart contracts are another huge step forward in automating healthcare processes, especially with insurance claims and routing patients to specialists. These are self-executing contracts based on Blockchain technology, which allow a claim to be executed automatically by processing defined conditions, thus eliminating delays and errors associated with manual handling. Smart contracts improve operational efficiencies by eliminating mid-level human interventions in administrative roles which reduces errors and accelerates payment to service providers. Such automation not only enhances operational efficiency but also enables healthcare professionals to spend more time on quality patient care rather than wrangling administrative paperwork. Figure 8.2 is representing a healthcare model assisted by blockchain technology.[35]

AI-Powered Decision-Making

Real-time blockchain data analysis models are AI-powered, which further improves clinical decision-making support. These AI systems can provide real-time insights and allow healthcare providers to make more informed decisions at the point of patient interaction. In addition, AI algorithms compare our medical history with huge databases of cases to create automated prescriptions and treatment recommendations. With this ability, patients can be treated with novel treatment plans

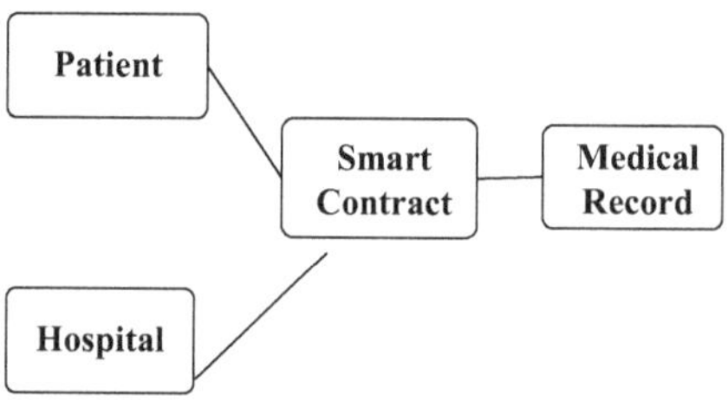

Figure 8.2 Blockchain Healthcare Model.

suited to their individual needs, ensuring improved outcomes and eliminating the possibility of adverse reactions or ineffective therapy.[36]

Streamlined Supply Chain

This is a method of ensuring that the goods are delivered transparently and traceably. Using the immutable ledger of blockchain, all stakeholders can monitor tracking for every stage in the entire lifecycle of pharmaceuticals from production to delivery. Combined with AI predicting demand for the same, it makes adjusting inventory much easier and reduces shortages or overstock. These technologies, together with the supply chain solutions they provide, contribute to increasing operational efficiency through optimal resource allocation along with on-time availability of required medications against minimum stock-out scenarios.[37]

Blockchain Transforms Patient Data Management

Blockchain technology can redesign traditional paradigms, irrespective of the sector, through industrial and scales of companies. It makes health data unchangeable to the patient, and collaboration is done more transparently. Top ways for blockchain to transform the process of managing patient data.

High Interoperability

Blockchain maintains the complete confidentiality of the data to be shared. It ensures the sharing of seamless and secure data, maintaining interoperability in the process. It enables healthcare solution providers to communicate and collaborate more effectively. It also holds the patient's privacy and consent.[38]

Streamlined Trials

An automated method of storing data for trials in a blockchain-based system will be able to ensure safety in the process so that it becomes seamless. It supports audibility, thereby strengthening the idea of transparency while being sensitive about the confidentiality of data with the patient. Better streamlined clinical trials also better safeguard the privacy of the patient.

Enhanced Medical Supplies

Blockchain solution developers support pharmaceutical and healthcare industries in their supply chain management. The system gives end-to-end tracing of drugs and surgical material, thus reducing drug counterfeits.

Secure Records

When it comes to creating secure and tamper-proof patient records, it is the most suitable and powerful option available with this technology. Such secure patient records can ensure data integrity by preventing unauthorised access or unwanted manipulation.[39]

Fraud Detection

This revolutionary technology can provide users with a transparent and immutable audit trail of online transactions, which helps organisations prevent healthcare fraud like insurance fraud and identity fraud, saving them many bucks.

Data Monetisation

Research initiatives and blockchain-based data marketplaces can be good options for monetising health data. Patients can participate in such possibilities. Thanks to blockchain, they can get incentives for data sharing without compromising their privacy.

Regulatory Compliance

Two large data protection regulations are HIPAA in the United States and the General Data Protection Regulation in the EU. Legal issues, such as regulatory compliance (e.g., 45 CFR parts 160 and 164) surrounding Protected Health Information privacy policies, are also addressed within blockchain-based health applications.

In fact, reputed mobile app development companies can help you integrate blockchain-based features into your dedicated healthcare application. These functionalities can help you to manage patient data.[40]

Patient-Centric Healthcare

Patient-centric healthcare refers to an approach in which the needs, preferences, and values of patients are also prioritised along with medical services. It focuses on the partnership of patients and their healthcare professionals, with an emphasis that patients play a role in deciding their own care. This design aims to improve the experience of patients by offering tailored care management, open channels of communication, and streamlined access to medical records. It encompasses respect for patient autonomy, the application of technology (e.g., digital health applications and data analytics), and a holistic conception of wellness. Patient-centred healthcare is intended to provide each patient with optimal surroundings thus improving health outcomes and levels of satisfaction among the patients.[41]

Patient Data Ownership

Blockchain technology allows patients to have access and control of their own medical records, supporting a decentralised and secure way of storing this data. Usually, most healthcare systems are organised with a centralised approach whereby healthcare providers have the power to access patient data. In blockchain systems, patients can choose who is allowed to see their health information. Patients can provide or revoke access to relevant data for a limited time when it matters most, which greatly improves privacy and builds trust. The almost complete ownership of their records can empower patients to have more control over decisions regarding their healthcare and increase patient-centeredness.

Personalised Health Alerts

AI models continuously monitor the patient data received to identify critical changes in health status that require early intervention. In conjunction with patient health records, AI can send customised alerts to patients and their physicians about possible issues such as elevated blood pressure levels or preferential heart rhythmic patterns. Along with these notifications can also be AI-based suggestions for lifestyle or treatment modifications, such as changing medication dosages, diet, or increasing physical activity. This proactive strategy assists in stopping things from turning into worse situations, making sure that responses are timely and enabling better long-term results with health issues.

Empowering Patients

Patient-centric healthcare and empowering individuals with a transparent, real-time view of health records will help people feel like they are in control of their own healthcare process. Using blockchain, health information is updated over time so that patients watch lab results or write down the latest medication history or clinical notes. Through this transparency, patients are made aware of their treatment plans and encouraged to take part in their healthcare management. Access to health records in real-time makes communication with healthcare providers much easier and allows for better decision-making and personalised treatments.[42]

Challenges and Considerations

Scalability

Scalability is a major issue for plug-and-play blockchain and AI technologies, especially with healthcare producing large amounts of data in the process every day. Blockchain systems should be able to deal with big data without lagging speed and even performance. Likewise, a vast computational infrastructure is needed to digest this data properly for AI models. One must tackle the performance bottlenecks in this case, using a distributed computing framework or optimising algorithms for both blockchain and AI systems to keep growing inevitably.

Both blockchain and AI technologies have scaling challenges. As more transactions take place, the blockchain networks can get congested, which slows down transaction processing time. Likewise, data usage can also demand more complex computational challenges that AI models may be forced to handle in order to cope with the vast scales of information. Scalable solutions that can handle the increasing volume of patient data, and facilitate real-time processing, are important for successful implementation.

Integration with Legacy Systems

The other big challenge is the integration of blockchain and AI systems with existing healthcare infrastructure. Healthcare organisations tend to hold onto legacy systems that may not work with newer technologies. It requires meticulous planning and execution; you need to make sure that data can flow between old systems and new without any leakage of information or functionality. Meanwhile, resistance to change can sometimes become an impediment to smooth operation, so staff training also needs to be considered when implementing these new technologies.[43]

Cost and Resource Considerations

Blockchain and AI systems have pretty high initial setup costs, which usually drive organisations away from leveraging them. Building Infrastructure, Developing Software, and Training Staff – these investments can be costly for healthcare providers to budget for the implementation of data and analytics partnerships as smaller providers may have limited budgets. The initial costs may be steep, but the savings brought on by more efficient processes and automation will pound down these higher upfront investments over time. Orgs need to balance these costs with any expected gains to weigh the decision of whether or not they should embrace both game-changing technologies.

Data Privacy and Security

Decentralisation and cryptography provide a high level of security for data centres, but there are still questions about the protection of patient privacy when using blockchain. When embedding AI systems that investigate large datasets, it is imperative to protect sensitive health information from being disclosed and kept safe. The United States has a regulation called HIPAA (Health Insurance Portability and Accountability Act) that ensures that health data is being handled automatically under very strict guidelines. Thus, organisations must carefully decide whether to share data for AI insights or preserve privacy in order to achieve those insights.[44]

Interoperability

Blockchain and AI systems must be able to fully integrate with current healthcare technologies such as EHRs and other data repositories. Interoperability across varied systems and standards can be challenging and expensive. The presence of multiple integration technologies creates silos, as without standard protocols and frameworks, the same cannot be integrated easily, which makes it difficult to access and analyse data.

Data Quality and Bias

AI relies heavily on high-quality data to generate accurate insights. If the data stored on the blockchain is incomplete, inaccurate, or biased, it can lead to erroneous predictions and recommendations. Additionally, biases in AI algorithms if trained on non-representative datasets can perpetuate health disparities among different populations. Ensuring the quality and representativeness of data is essential to mitigate these risks.[45]

Regulatory and Compliance Issues

The regulatory environments for blockchain and AI in the healthcare industry are still evolving. Compliance requirements are often complex to address, and different rules and regulations apply to diverse regions and jurisdictions. Ensuring that blockchain implementations comply with regulatory standards while using AI in clinical decision-making adds more layers of complexity to implementation efforts.

Stakeholder Buy-In and Education

The adoption of blockchain and AI in patient care requires buy-in from providers, payers, patients, and regulators. Some people may resist the adoption of these new technologies due to a lack of understanding or from simply fearing change. The adoption of these innovations in healthcare settings will require trust-building and educational initiatives between different stakeholders.[46]

Ethical Considerations

Several ethical considerations arise in the healthcare landscape regarding data ownership, consent, and accountability entailed by the integration of AI alongside Blockchain technologies. Patients should know how their data is used and have control over their PHI. Additionally, both ethical guidelines and practical protocols must be created to facilitate sound usage of AI in clinical decision-making so that technology empowers rather than hinders the practice of medicine.[47]

Future Prospects and Innovations

AI and Blockchain for Predictive Healthcare

AI and blockchain tech integration will revolutionise predictive healthcare using AI rather than centralised networks. Leveraging blockchain ensures the data leveraged for predicting healthcare trends is more reliable and safe to use. It offers a secure environment for data that makes it tamper-proof, transparent, and secure. AI can detect trends and predict occurrences like disease outbreaks, patient admissions, and treatment results using more open health data across the blockchain in anonymised forms. Such an ability to anticipate helps in better allocation of healthcare resources, taking preventative measures, and proactively implementing interventions to improve patient care.[48]

AI-Blockchain Integration with IoT

AI, blockchain, and the IoT are promised to provide safe and secure patient monitoring in a real-time manner via integrated medical devices. With the decentralisation and secure structure of blockchain, it is possible to store data collected from wearables and smart medical devices without any effect on human privacy. AI algorithms can process this information in real time, identifying important changes in health and delivering relevant insights to patients and healthcare professionals. Additionally, the rise of decentralised AI system – those that function without a central authority – has enabled P2P cooperation through healthcare networks. This encourages creative thinking and the sharing of ideas, thereby improving the generation of AI solutions to meet a variety of patient demands more efficiently.[49,50]

Conclusion

The adoption of blockchain technology and AI in patient care represents a significant move forward to an advanced, secure, efficient, and patient-centric health system. The integration of blockchain's decentralised, tamper-proof data management with AI's advanced analytics would provide new possibilities in predictive healthcare, personalised treatments, and real-time monitoring. These combined methods ensure data is secure and help provide patient-level engagement through ownership of their data, while also ensuring interoperable healthcare networks. Yet, to unlock all the potentials of blockchain and AI integration, we must overcome a few significant challenges, such as data privacy issues, interoperability challenges, scalability issues, and ethical considerations. While the potential of AI-powered decision-making in healthcare is great, we need to create regulatory mechanisms, educate stakeholders, and train algorithms on diverse and high-quality datasets to minimise bias as the healthcare landscape changes. Decentralised AI, integration of AI with Blockchain employing IoT, and P2P collaboration are other future innovations that will help to build smarter, stronger, and more resilient health systems. However, properly integrating these technologies will be crucial to propel precision medicine and patient empowerment.

References

1 Komalavalli, C., Deepika Saxena, and Chetna Laroiya. Editors: Saravanan Krishnan, Valentina E. Balas, E. Golden Julie, Y. Harold Robinson, S. Balaji, Raghvendra Kumar. "Overview of blockchain technology concepts." In *Handbook of Research on Blockchain Technology*, pp. 349–371. Cambridge, MA: Apple Academic Press, 2020.

2 Monteiro, Ana Carolina Borges, Reinaldo Padilha França, Yuzo Iano, and Rangel Arthur. "An overview of blockchain technology concepts from a modern perspective." *Blockchain for Healthcare Systems*, 1st Edition, (2021): 27–41.

3 Gamage, H. T. M., H. D. Weerasinghe, and N. G. J. Dias. "A survey on blockchain technology concepts, applications, and issues." *SN Computer Science* 1 (2020): 1–15.

4 Krishnan, Saravanan, Valentina Emilia Balas, E. Golden Julie, Harold Robinson Yesudhas, S. Balaji, and Raghvendra Kumar, eds. *Handbook of Research on Blockchain Technology*. Cambridge, MA: Academic Press, 2020.

5 Pilkington, Marc. "Blockchain technology: Principles and applications." In F. Xavier Olleros, Majlinda Zhegu (Eds), *Research Handbook on Digital Transformations*, pp. 225–253. Cheltenham: Edward Elgar Publishing, 2016.

6 Kitching, John, and Robert Blackburn. "Intellectual property management in the small and medium enterprise (SME)." *Journal of Small Business and Enterprise Development* 5, no. 4 (1998): 327–335.

7 Secinaro, Silvana, Davide Calandra, Aurelio Secinaro, Vivek Muthurangu, and Paolo Biancone. "The role of artificial intelligence in healthcare: A structured literature review." *BMC Medical Informatics and Decision Making* 21 (2021): 1–23.

8 Chase, J. Geoffrey, Jean-Charles Preiser, Jennifer L. Dickson, Antoine Pironet, Yeong Shiong Chiew, Christopher G. Pretty, Geoffrey M. Shaw, Balazs Benyo, Knut Moeller, Soroush Safaei, Meeryn Tawhai, Peter Hunter, Thomas Desaive. "Next-generation, personalised, model-based critical care medicine: A state-of-the-art review of in silico virtual patient models, methods, and cohorts, and how to validation them." *Biomedical Engineering Online* 17 (2018): 1–29.

9 Sinha, Sandeep, and Divya Vohora. "Drug discovery and development: An overview." *Pharmaceutical Medicine and Translational Clinical Research* (2018): 19–32.

10 Wilkerson, R. Gentry, Youssef Annous, Eli Farhy, Jonathan Hurst, and Angela D. Smedley. "Home pulse oximetry monitoring during the COVID-19 pandemic: An assessment of patient engagement and compliance." *Health Policy and Technology* 12, no. 3 (2023): 100776.

11 Tewari, Shuchita Pant, Richa Misra, Kritika Nagdev, and Himani Sharma. "Role of online health communities in patient compliance: A social support perspective." *Journal of Systems and Information Technology* 26 (2024): 562–585.

12 Cullen, Francis T. "Rehabilitation: Beyond nothing works." *Crime and Justice* 42, no. 1 (2013): 299–376.

13 Feldman, Robin C., Ehrik Aldana, and Kara Stein. "Artificial intelligence in the health care space: How we can trust what we cannot know." *Stanford Law & Policy Review* 30 (2019): 399.

14 Bohr, Adam, and Kaveh Memarzadeh. "The rise of artificial intelligence in healthcare applications." In *Artificial Intelligence in Healthcare*, pp. 25–60. Cambridge, MA: Academic Press, 2020.

15 Alzoubi, Mahd M. "Investigating the synergy of Blockchain and AI: Enhancing security, efficiency, and transparency." *Journal of Cyber Security Technology* (2024): 1–29.

16 Haddad, Alaa, Mohamed Hadi Habaebi, Md Rafiqul Islam, Nurul Fadzlin Hasbullah, and Suriza Ahmad Zabidi. "Systematic review on AI-blockchain based e-healthcare records management systems." *IEEE Access* 10 (2022): 94583–94615.

17 Tagde, Priti, Sandeep Tagde, Tanima Bhattacharya, Pooja Tagde, Hitesh Chopra, Rokeya Akter, Deepak Kaushik, and Md Habibur Rahman. "Blockchain and artificial intelligence technology in e-Health." *Environmental Science and Pollution Research* 28 (2021): 52810–52831.

18 Nanda, Saroj Kumar, Sandeep Kumar Panda, and Madhabananda Dash. "Medical supply chain integrated with blockchain and IoT to track the logistics of medical products." *Multimedia Tools and Applications* 82, no. 21 (2023): 32917–32939.

19 Nwankwo, Ejike Innocent, Ebube Victor Emeihe, Mojeed Dayo Ajegbile, Janet Aderonke Olaboye, and Chukwudi Cosmos Maha. “Integrating telemedicine and AI to improve healthcare access in rural settings.” *International Journal of Life Science Research Archive* 7, no. 1 (2024): 059–077.
20 Ghadi, Yazeed Yasin, Tehseen Mazhar, Tariq Shahzad, Muhammad Amir khan, Alaa Abd-Alrazaq, Arfan Ahmed, and Habib Hamam. “The role of blockchain to secure internet of medical things.” *Scientific Reports* 14, no. 1 (2024): 18422.
21 Saleh, Ahmed M. Shamsan. “Blockchain for secure and decentralized artificial intelligence in cybersecurity: A comprehensive review.” *Blockchain: Research and Applications* 5 (2024): 100193.
22 Molli, Vijaya Lakshmi Pavani. “Blockchain technology for secure and transparent health data management: Opportunities and challenges.” *Journal of Healthcare AI and ML* 10, no. 10 (2023): 1–15.
23 Raparthi, Mohan, Swaroop Reddy Gayam, Bhavani Prasad Kasaraneni, Krishna Kanth Kondapaka, Sandeep Pushyamitra Pattyam, Venkata Siva Prakash Nimmagadda, Mohit Kumar Sahu, Siva Sarana Kuna, Sudharshan Putha, and Praveen Thuniki. “Quantum cryptography and secure health data transmission: Emphasizing quantum cryptography’s role in ensuring privacy and confidentiality in healthcare systems.” *Blockchain Technology and Distributed Systems* 2, no. 2 (2022): 1–10.
24 Samarati, Pierangela, and Sabrina Capitani De Vimercati. “Access control: Policies, models, and mechanisms.” In *International School on Foundations of Security Analysis and Design*, pp. 137–196. Berlin, Heidelberg: Springer, 2000.
25 Yaqoob, Ibrar, Khaled Salah, Raja Jayaraman, and Yousof Al-Hammadi. “Blockchain for healthcare data management: opportunities, challenges, and future recommendations.” *Neural Computing and Applications* 34 (2022): 11475–11490.
26 Dubovitskaya, Alevtina, Furqan Baig, Zhigang Xu, Rohit Shukla, Pratik Sushil Zambani, Arun Swaminathan, Md Majid Jahangir, Khadija Chowdhry, Rahul Lachhani, Nitesh Idnani, Michael Schumacher, Karl Aberer, Scott D Stoller, Samuel Ryu, Fusheng Wang. “ACTION-EHR: Patient-centric blockchain-based electronic health record data management for cancer care.” *Journal of Medical Internet Research* 22, no. 8 (2020): e13598.
27 Pramanik, Pijush Kanti Dutta, Bijoy Kumar Upadhyaya, Saurabh Pal, and Tanmoy Pal. “Internet of things, smart sensors, and pervasive systems: Enabling connected and pervasive healthcare.” In Nilanjan Dey, Amira S. Ashour, Chintan Bhatt, Simon James Fong (Eds), *Healthcare Data Analytics and Management*, pp. 1–58. Cambridge, MA: Academic Press, 2019.
28 Popescu, Andrei. “Interoperability in medical device software: Standards, challenges, and opportunities for seamless integration.” *Advances in Computer Sciences* 5, no. 1 (2022): 1–7.
29 Rübsamen, Thomas. “Evidence-based accountability audits for cloud computing.” University of Plymouth, United Kingdom (2016): 1–423.
30 Tripathi, Pranav Mani. “Impact of AI on regulatory compliance in information security.” *International Journal of Computer Engineering and Technology (IJCET)* 16, no. 1 (2025): 108–124.
31 Abualkishik, Abedallah Zaid, Ali A. Alwan, and Yonis Gulzar. “Disaster recovery in cloud computing systems: An overview.” *International Journal of Advanced Computer Science and Applications* 11, no. 9 (2020): 702–710.

32 Johnson, Kevin B., Wei-Qi Wei, Dilhan Weeraratne, Mark E. Frisse, Karl Misulis, Kyu Rhee, Juan Zhao, and Jane L. Snowdon. "Precision medicine, AI, and the future of personalized health care." *Clinical and Translational Science* 14, no. 1 (2021): 86–93.
33 Shiwlani, Ashish, Murad Khan, Abdul Mannan Khan Sherani, Muhammad Umer Qayyum, and Hafiz Khawar Hussain. "Revolutionizing healthcare: The impact of artificial intelligence on patient care, Diagnosis, and treatment." *Jurihum: Jurnal Inovasi dan Humaniora* 1, no. 5 (2024): 779–790.
34 Jeddi, Zineb, and Adam Bohr. "Remote patient monitoring using artificial intelligence." In Adam Bohr, Kaveh Memarzadeh (Eds), *Artificial Intelligence in Healthcare*, pp. 203–234. Cambridge, MA: Academic Press, 2020.
35 Chang, Shuchih Ernest, YiChian Chen, MingFang Lu, and Hueimin Louis Luo. "Development and evaluation of a smart contract–Enabled blockchain system for home care service innovation: Mixed methods study." *JMIR Medical Informatics* 8, no. 7 (2020): e15472.
36 Stecyk, Adam, and Ireneusz Miciuła. "Harnessing the power of artificial intelligence for collaborative energy optimization platforms." *Energies* 16, no. 13 (2023): 5210.
37 Haq, Ijazul, and Olivier Muselemu Esuka. "Blockchain technology in pharmaceutical industry to prevent counterfeit drugs." *International Journal of Computer Applications* 180, no. 25 (2018): 8–12.
38 Belchior, Rafael, André Vasconcelos, Sérgio Guerreiro, and Miguel Correia. "A survey on blockchain interoperability: Past, present, and future trends." *ACM Computing Surveys (CSUR)* 54, no. 8 (2021): 1–41.
39 Shojaei, Parisasadat, Elena Vlahu-Gjorgievska, and Yang-Wai Chow. "Security and privacy of technologies in health information systems: A systematic literature review." *Computers* 13, no. 2 (2024): 41.
40 Bayle, Aurelie, Mirko Koscina, David Manset, and Octavio Perez-Kempner. "When blockchain meets the right to be forgotten: Technology versus law in the healthcare industry." In *2018 IEEE/WIC/ACM International Conference on Web Intelligence (WI)*, pp. 788–792. IEEE, 2018.
41 Oyeniyi, Johnson. "The role of AI and mobile apps in patient-centric healthcare delivery." *World Journal of Advanced Research and Reviews* 22, no. 1 (2024): 1897–1907.
42 Hägglund, Maria, Brian McMillan, Robyn Whittaker, and Charlotte Blease. "Patient empowerment through online access to health records." *BMJ* 378 (2022): 1–5.
43 Singh, Navdeep, and Daisy Adhikari. "Challenges and solutions in integrating AI with legacy inventory systems." *International Journal for Research in Applied Science and Engineering Technology* 11, no. 12 (2023): 609–613.
44 Zhang, Rui, Rui Xue, and Ling Liu. "Security and privacy for healthcare blockchains." *IEEE Transactions on Services Computing* 15, no. 6 (2021): 3668–3686.
45 Steimers, André, and Moritz Schneider. "Sources of risk of AI systems." *International Journal of Environmental Research and Public Health* 19, no. 6 (2022): 3641.
46 Khezr, Seyednima, Md Moniruzzaman, Abdulsalam Yassine, and Rachid Benlamri. "Blockchain technology in healthcare: A comprehensive review and directions for future research." *Applied Sciences* 9, no. 9 (2019): 1736.
47 Rubeis, Giovanni. "Ethical implications of blockchain technology in biomedical research." *Ethik in der Medizin* 36 (2024): 1–14.
48 Alabdulatif, Abdulatif, Ibrahim Khalil, and Mohammad Saidur Rahman. "Security of blockchain and AI-empowered smart healthcare: Application-based analysis." *Applied Sciences* 12, no. 21 (2022): 11039.

49 Jadhav, Jayendra S., and Jyoti Deshmukh. "A review study of the blockchain-based healthcare supply chain." *Social Sciences & Humanities Open* 6, no. 1 (2022): 100328.

50 Gad, Ahmed G., Diana T. Mosa, Laith Abualigah, and Amr A. Abohany. "Emerging trends in blockchain technology and applications: A review and outlook." *Journal of King Saud University-Computer and Information Sciences* 34, no. 9 (2022): 6719–6742.

9 Cybersecurity Threats and Mitigation Strategies in Blockchain Healthcare

Akanksha Sharma, Ashish Verma, Sunita, Akhil Sharma, Shilpa Thukral and Shaweta Sharma

Blockchain Innovation in Healthcare

Blockchain is a peer-to-peer (P2P) distributed ledger system that is decentralised by nature and allows one to store data in time-stamped blocks without the need for intermediaries. It is similarly important because data can be viewed simultaneously by participants without waiting for an individual to receive and relay. Since this changes the documents in real-time, hence the procedure is one-of-a-kind and clear; blockchain innovation consists of three significant parts: blocks, nodes as well and miners. A block contains data, hash, and nonce. Including a timestamp and transaction data to link to its preceding block, a block makes use of an algorithm point – also known as a cryptographic linking point. This algorithm pointer, or hash point, of the previous block links to the blocks that come after, therefore rendering the blockchain unchangeable and forbade modification between those blocks.[1–3]

Now, we know that every transaction in the blockchain can only be connected after its verification through a consensus mechanism on whether data in my transaction is valid or not. Two basic forms of blockchain technology are permissionless blockchains (like Ethereum and Bitcoin) and permission blockchains (like Ripple, Eris, and Hyperledger). Blockchain is one developing technology that might affect online shopping. Apart from privacy, security, e-government, and finance, blockchain innovation can find use in many other domains.[3]

Blockchain is the new disruptive technology that could transform traditional identity management employed in the majority of healthcare applications. Its ability to secure medical data is the leading reason why tech companies have begun investing in it. Blockchain technology is changing legacy systems, therefore improving efficiency and lowering costs and expenses in the healthcare industry. Health apps, blockchain technologies, raw data sources, and health stakeholders are the four conceptual tiers of blockchain-based healthcare solutions.[3,4]

Labs and medical equipment are among the several sources of raw data that progressively turn into big data. Blockchain-based healthcare depends critically on this vast volume of data, which forms the first tier of the stack. Built upon raw data, blockchain technology is the pillar for building a four-layered, safe healthcare system. Every blockchain platform offers unique consensus mechanisms and protocols. Blockchain stages are useful for creating and managing user transactions.

DOI: 10.4324/9781003529910-9

Table 9.1 Blockchain Innovation in Healthcare

S. No.	*Blockchain Innovation in Healthcare*	*Importance*
1	Data management	Electronic health records, Data management, Data storage, and worldwide scientific data exchange for the advancement of knowledge.[8]
2	Internet of medical things	Pharmaceuticals, Clinical trials.
3	Smart contract medical app	Medical devices, Healthcare IoT infrastructure and data security.[9]

Many blockchain based-platforms, including Ethereum and Hyperledger, have emerged over the last few years.[3,5]

Some of the key elements of blockchain systems include signatures, smart contracts, wallets, digital assets, and more. Several protocols can be used to connect between various blockchain networks or initiatives, such as decentralised, P2P, and distributed. Depending on the size of the requirements, stakeholders may adopt public, private, or consortium blockchain. Making sure that all of this incorporates the applications into the whole system comes next once blockchain technology has established the platform. Three domains under which blockchain applications in the healthcare space fall include data management, smart contract medical apps, and Internet of Medical Things (IoMT) apps. Globally scientific data interchange is used in electronic medical records, bulb management, preservation, and research and development. Smart contracts-based medical applications for pharmaceuticals and clinical trials IoMT, or IoT for medical devices and healthcare, IoT infrastructure for healthcare, and data security.[3,6,7]

Blockchain innovation in healthcare are shown in Table 9.1. A stakeholder layer at the top might include anyone using crypto-based healthcare apps including researchers, doctors, patients, and so on. Users of this layer are mainly concerned with sharing and managing data while maintaining its safety and privacy.

Overview of Cybersecurity in Blockchain Healthcare

In the healthcare context, technology may extend, maintain, and enhance life. These technologies comprise storage of electronic health records (EHRs); devices monitoring health and delivering medicines (including general purpose devices, wearables, and technology incorporated into the human body); and telemedicine technology offering care remotely even across countries. Patients also use their mobile apps more and more; if combined with telemedicine or telehealth, they might be included in the medical Internet of Things, therefore enabling group illness management and care coordination.[10,11]

With the increasing evolution of the interconnectivity of healthcare devices, they have traditionally been independent, but many are now in the hospital network. In the hospital, many connected devices/beds are available. There are many benefits of interconnection including, but not limited to, efficiency, reduced errors, automation, and remote monitoring. These benefits are altering the treatment for both acute and chronic long-term conditions. Extended technology allows medical personnel to monitor implanted devices and change them without resorting to invasive surgeries or hospital visits. EHRs increase the availability of health information, which can lead to better patient care. Interconnection, however, poses unique cybersecurity threats. The cybersecurity field deals with protecting networks and information associated with computers from being penetrated or infected systematically or maliciously. Already, medical information confidentiality and integrity resilience have failed among growing concerns that healthcare cyber security is far from sufficient.[11,12]

Cyber-attacks refer to those attacks targeting online users who lack security awareness either with the help of a computer network or are used as instruments for criminal acts (cyberstalking or insider attack, etc.). This digital era has made cybersecurity a hell of a task as the cyber-attacks are increasing day by day. Healthcare Cyberattacks A lot of cyber-attack challenges have come across healthcare as one of the larger industries. EHRs hold sensitive patient data like names, prescription histories, test results, payment information, contact details, and home addresses and must be shared among healthcare providers needing a strong barrier against breaches. Although the healthcare industry currently has a consistent cybersecurity architecture to guard data, there are various weaknesses in it that make EHRs open to hackers. It is not only necessary to replace the conventional cybersecurity platform of the healthcare sector with blockchain-based security, which is surely one of the best defences against cyberattacks.[3,13,14]

Internet technologies have long existed. However, there have always been some particular aspects of healthcare assessment services that involve the analysis of medical records. Using Internet technology for its advantages, like quickly fetching healthcare services, leads to high dependence on IT technologies and renders greater risk to the secrecy and protection of documents in medical information systems. EHR means electronic health records or electronic medical records, which are high-privacy medical data, and they are clinical data used by healthcare workers to heal patients with diseases and illnesses. Still, sometimes, they have trouble facing a lot of messing with cyber-attacks. Usually presenting themselves as DDoS (Distributed Denial-of-Service), vulnerabilities on IoMT, insiders, etc., these cyberattacks or threats show up. Thus, blockchain technology projects that provide a cybersecurity boost effort must be transformed to counter these cyber threats in the healthcare industry. Blockchain Technology is the winning solution that different sectors in various domains are excited about. With its capability of solving both practical problems and making people's digital transformation more efficient, blockchain technology has been implemented. At the same time, the operation needs high security and privacy because, overall, the density platform has a distraction weakness in centralised data storage that hot or cold weapons can use.[15,16]

Security is a major issue in the healthcare vertical, primarily due to the emergence and sophistication of cyberattacks via the internet. Unauthorised access and assault that infects with and executes malware attacks are among healthcare security's most frequent threats. Denial of Service (DoS) attacks have a single source that bombards the target system with requests instead of using multiple hosts to target a victim, as in DDoS assaults. That makes it less straightforward to identify where the attack came from. These attacks can harm patients and cause reputational damage to healthcare organisations.

One additional main hazard to the healthcare industry is malware, with virtually new strains coming onto the landscape all the time. One type of malware that is raising the alarm for healthcare organisations is ransomware. Ranked second among CISO issues, 17% of respondents to a Healthcare Information and Management Systems Society poll on cybersecurity threats to healthcare companies claimed they have been the victim of ransomware.

In recent years, cybercriminals have hit healthcare businesses with some very high-profile attacks. One example is the 2021 ransomware attack on the Irish Health Service Executive that brought healthcare services to a halt. As in, the WannaCry ransomware outbreak caused the National Health Service (NHS) in the UK to postpone operations and reschedule appointments in over 150 nations in 2017. This means healthcare institutions must implement strong cybersecurity measures to prevent them and protect sensitive patient data. However, a lot of healthcare institutions still do not have good security measures to guard against such intrusions. A Ponemon Institute study found only 44% of healthcare businesses implement a well-thought-out security policy. [17,18]

Significance of Health Information and Possible Damage from Vulnerabilities

The golden data of the healthcare sector makes it a prime goal for cybercrime. This data can range from health information & payroll data to personally identifiable information that is exploited for profit or evil intent. Data breaches in healthcare can lead to other major disasters for patients and healthcare institutions.[19]

Firstly, identity theft and fraud will arise from compromised personal health information. Cybercrime can use this data to create false identities and illegally get prescription medications or medical treatment. It endangers patients and exposes healthcare organisations to legal and financial consequences.[19,20]

Second, medical facilities come across financial details as well. From theft or system and infrastructure damage, breaches could cause financial loss. Not to mention, the standing of medical establishments can suffer much. Patients will lose faith in the institution to maintain their data safe, therefore lowering patient satisfaction and generating a loss of business. Also, breaches in data can affect a lot of factors that involve patient care and safety. For example, a hacker could obtain access to some online medical records and then alter or destroy important clinical details for patients, which could result in wrong diagnoses or treatments and thereby endanger patient safety. The harms mentioned above also make a case for why healthcare organisations should take cybersecurity seriously. In conclusion, the health sector remains one of the most targeted areas for cyberattacks due to its data value.[19,20]

Abuse of personal health information, financial records, pictures, and any other type of data can be done for either profit or evil intent. Finally, the growing digitalisation of healthcare systems and the interlinkage of different parties in healthcare expose these systems to new risks. While technologies in the health field are holding promise for a new precision of healthcare, we still need to build better cybersecurity measures. One of the top three businesses targeted by hackers worldwide, data breaches in the healthcare sector have grown since 2010, according to IBM and the Ponemon Institute.

The high value of its data (which includes personal health records and financial records), alongside the increasing degree of digitisation and interconnectedness in healthcare systems, makes this sector a prominent target for cyberattacks. Of course, this is why efforts to improve cybersecurity in the healthcare industry cannot wait as they strive to safeguard patient data and financial records while also ensuring the safety of one's care.[19,21]

Understanding Cyberattacks

Cyberattacks are described as intentional exploitation in the form of unauthorised access and data loss or theft that could cause disruptions of computer systems, technology-dependent businesses, and networks. Cyber-attacks use malicious code to modify computer code, logic, or data that disrupt access to or the use of your data and have the potential for exposing it; this can become cybercrimes in information thefts and identity thefts as well. These days, cybercriminals have employed various advanced methods to ensure they remain undetected as they silently infiltrate corporate networks to execute their evil deeds like stealing sensitive data. They encode their attacks using complex algorithms to bypass detection and intrusion prevention systems. The attackers will next attempt to download and install malware into the hacked system following their penetration and exploitation of a target (Table 9.2).[22]

Categories of Cyberattack in the Healthcare Industry

A flow diagram (Figure 9.1) presenting the different categories of cyberattack in healthcare industry

Table 9.2 Steps Involved in Cyberattacks

Step I	Reconnaissance: Hacker research information about their target organisation and scan for loopholes.[23]
Step II	Attack: Attackers access the organisation's network by gaining elevated access.
Step III	Expansion: Hackers attempt to attack every system on the network by engaging in malicious code.[24]
Step IV	Obfuscation: Attacker hides their tracks to mask the origins of the attack and confuse the forensic expert.[25]

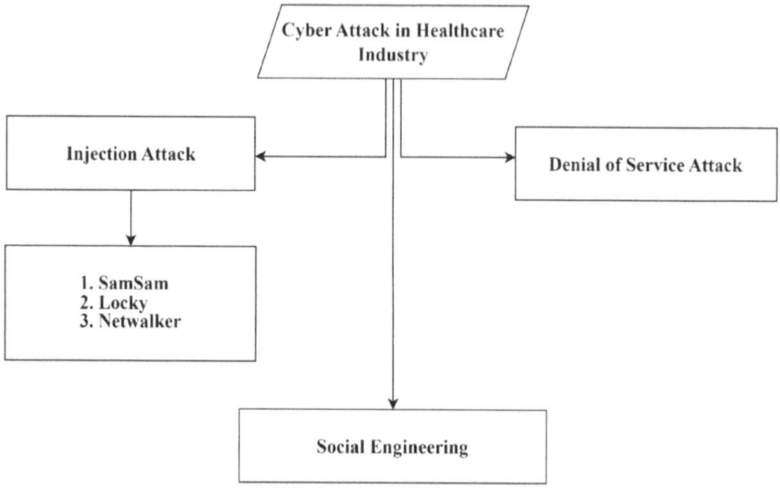

Figure 9.1 Categories of Cyberattack in Healthcare Industry.

Injection Attack

An attacker might incorporate malicious data into a web application, causing it to work differently (by sending it commands that change its workflow). Injection constitutes one of the most ancient forms of web-based attacks. An injection attack is all about malware. Malware refers to any computer code that is written for illicit access to digital devices and IT infrastructures. This is accomplished by circumventing the security mechanisms that safeguard them and exploiting vulnerabilities in security. Three categories of malware are discussed further below.[25,26]

SamSam

It is a ransomware malware that chiefly strikes the healthcare industry. For initial access to victims' machines, SamSam exploits vulnerabilities in Remote Desktop Protocol (RDP), File Transfer Protocol (FTP), and Java-based web servers.

Locky

Initially launched in 2016, it is a ransomware variant that employs a hybrid cryptosystem. The way it works is by looking for certain types of files on a victim's drives like network drives and encrypting them with Rivest–Shamir–Adleman (RSA) and Advanced Encryption Standard (AES).

Netwalker

This is referred to as the mailto attack, wherein the perpetrator exploits the victim's network to encrypt and compromise all Windows devices. The assailant can launch an attack utilising phishing emails and executable programs that propagate over the networks.[25,27]

Social Engineering

This strategy involves an attacker exploiting human interactions to manipulate the victim's psychological vulnerabilities, persuading them to disclose sensitive information. Phishing is a type of social engineering employed by hackers to entice individuals into divulging personal information, including usernames, passwords, and bank account details.[25]

Denial of Service Attack

This is a resource-draining cyberattack type that primarily targets memory, computing power, etc. This attack can be done through a wireless network or a cable. An instance of a DoS assault aimed at websites is the DDoS attack. In a DDoS assault, an assailant compromises numerous computers, each equipped with a malicious script, to target a single victim.[28]

The first and foremost threat to blockchain healthcare is the DoS. Currently, the healthcare infrastructure can be put out of service for hours and even days due to the non-availability of these services because connected objects have already grown tremendously and are implemented everywhere. According to Arbor Networks, with a capacity of traffic-generating devices ordered up to 400 GB/s, the entire hospital infrastructure will come out. The DoS is the extension of common DDoS. Attackers use DDoS using a botnet, consisting typically of infected clients' computers and IoT devices, such as medical equipment and appliances, to turn off the services. Therefore, it is not only possible that DoS occurs at hospitals; however, networked medical devices can be turned into targets and used as botnets, so DoS is said to have been distributed if the attack source >1. One of the critical services is that classroom health data will be unavailable, with at least one target health centre critical server if remote access to remote health records is used. Subsequently, there will be an extended and simple propagation of the infecting agent through the flooding traffic, finalising with devastating effects (particularly in chronic disease patients or those programmed for surgery intervention or surgical procedures). One common example of this type of cyber-attack is Memcached.[29]

Effects of Cyberattacks on Healthcare Providers, Patients and the Economy

The consequences of cybersecurity threats to healthcare organisations include more than financial repercussions and operational disruptions. Cyberattacks on healthcare organisations impact patients directly. That means their personal health information may be stolen, and this can lead to identity theft and financial fraud through sensitive healthcare data. Cyberattacks can disrupt clinical care, jeopardising patient safety and compromising the quality of healthcare services provided.

Furthermore, cyber-attacks on the healthcare industry adversely affect the economy. Financial damage is in the billions when hackers target hospitals for ransomware attacks. The harmful effects of cyber threats on the healthcare sector highlight that there is a pressing demand for improved cybersecurity measures.[19,30]

Hospitals and healthcare systems are a category of critical infrastructure essential to the economy. When cyberattacks disrupt them, the result is often economic harm in remediation costs, reputational damage, and a less secure healthcare environment. Example: Perhaps when a healthcare organisation experiences a cyberattack, it may lose critical patient data and be faced with costly litigation or reputational damages to the organisation. The interconnection and complexity of healthcare systems render them an attractive target for cybercriminals.

As healthcare organisations have access to large amounts of sensitive and valuable patient data (personal information, as well as medical records), they are attractive targets for cyber criminals looking to profit from the sale of this information. Cyber threat is any action that targets a system reinforced by information technology, which affects the functionality of networks. The repercussions of cyber threats experienced in the healthcare sector are complex and involve patients, healthcare providers, and the economy. In light of these impacts, this calls for health sector stakeholders to embrace relevant cybersecurity practices through appropriate leadership styles that ensure in public health organisations.[19,31]

The Function of the Health Insurance Portability and Accountability Act in Cybersecurity

The HIPAA is one of the most important components of US legislation. It ensures the confidentiality, integrity, and security of patient health information. HIPAA has delineated the measures required to preserve electronic Protected Health Information (ePHI) and specified the appropriate administrative, physical, and technical safeguards that healthcare organisations must adopt to maintain the confidentiality, integrity, and availability of ePHI.

The HIPAA lays the groundwork for regulatory compliance in healthcare, especially regarding cyber security. It lays down the national baseline of privacy security for medical data and helps healthcare processes prevent access to or breach of patient information. To address cybersecurity threats, healthcare insurance and the Portability & Accountability Act emphasise risk assessments, protective measures, staff training, and contingency planning. The American Recovery and Reinvestment Act of 2009 also tackled privacy and security concerns alongside the Health Information Technology for Economic and Clinical Health Act.[19,32,33]

Key Elements of Management of Cybersecurity in Blockchain Healthcare

Organisations should take several steps once they start to plan how to manage cybersecurity risks. There are a few key steps i.e. identify the relevant stakeholders at a facility and delineate cybersecurity roles and responsibilities within your staff.

The biomedical engineering department largely handles device-specific issues, as individual hospitals have their IT department for the hospital network infrastructure. The integration of much more functionality and IT capabilities into medical devices means that these two departments need to work together on protecting their devices against cyber threats. For instance, you might run into trouble when you need to install an operating system upgrade. Implementing an upgrade may result in a slight disruption to the operation of certain medical equipment. Consequently, a protocol must be instituted to guarantee that the rationale and execution are communicated clearly before its commencement. Attention must be directed towards the labelling of a medical device and the potential impact of specific software updates or patches on the device's regulatory status or intended applications. Moreover, addressing cybersecurity vulnerabilities in medical devices necessitates the involvement of additional departments, including risk management, safety committees, and hospital board members. Cybersecurity issues also impact others, so increasing the number of people who are educated on this topic within the company can improve cooperation and assist in identifying resources to utilise to remediate current threats.[34,35]

There are a few common methods that can be employed to protect the network of the facility from being exposed and potentially harmed through cybersecurity attacks. As an illustration, access to the equipment could be limited by a virtual local area network (VLAN). VLAN is an access control list that permits communication between certain ports and some systems but not with the main network. A robust, updated antimalware can identify and put any threat to the network under quarantine. Merely safeguarding the network from external users is insufficient. The process commences with a stringent and effective authentication system, after which users will obtain little access to perform their tasks. It may be prudent to instruct all device users on fundamental security standards, encompassing the use of personal mobile devices and USB flash drives.[35]

Organisations should familiarise themselves with ANSI/AAMI/IEC 80001-1, a significant standard covering hospital network security. This standard was established in 2010, and it addresses how to manage the safeguarding of a hospital information technology network. In particular, It encompasses directives on change management, risk assessment, and the allocation of duties. Even by using the risk management methodologies presented in ANSI/AAMI/IEC 80001-1, healthcare organisations can only help themselves.

An effective device management strategy commences at the procurement stage. It is essential to ensure that the equipment possesses robust safety features and that the manufacturer offers continuous support prior to purchase. An instance would involve an organisation soliciting the maker Disclosure Statement for Medical Device Security form from the device maker. This article will address compatibility with pertinent third-party software and the costs associated with the installation of security patches and software updates. This confirms that the manufacturer endorses software operating on the device and has maintained validation of updates pertinent to the respective operating system and antimalware system.[35,36]

It is also important to have a reporting mechanism for cyber security incidents. Under the HITECH Act, if loss of protected health information occurs or is reasonably believed to occur, then notification to the Office for Civil Rights is enforced. Incidents about a device should be communicated to the device manufacturers and relevant reporting agencies (FDA, Industrial Control Systems Cyber Emergency Response Team, or ECRI Institute) as ongoing information exchange and education within the healthcare sector is one of the most effective strategies for mitigating cybersecurity risks.[35,37]

Mitigations Strategies in Blockchain Healthcare

To reduce the chances of exposing private data or spoofing devices, healthcare organisations need to operate under a zero-trust model that challenges every system and process based on the belief that their IT infrastructure could be kludged at any level. Zero-trust says no device or network traffic should be thought about by default as trusted; therefore, all the transport needs to be encrypted, and it needs to be continuously monitored, which will guarantee the protection of data. The zero-trust implementation extends into its contribution to overarching cyber hygiene practices and security control equipment that protects digital assets. Recommended cyber hygiene best practices from the industry include but are not limited to secured communications, data protection, access control, authentication best practices, timely patching, security training, and controls backed up.[38]

Communication system security should be considered both externally and internally. Firewalls are very important from an external threat perspective, and depending on the topology and use case, proper network architecture allowing to segment devices behind DMZs is a key element of a customer setup as it helps minimise lateral movement of an attacker in instances of a worst case where there is a breach. In addition, the Intrusion Detection Systems (IDS) and Intrusion Prevention Systems (IPS) are fundamental for detecting incidents that are trying to occur against the system. The healthcare environment has the most stringent need for data protection, such as encryption when in use, at rest, and in transit unless actively being processed. Encryption and access protection are necessary for secure storage systems, but more so when the systems are based on the cloud. There needs to be judicial access controls both in terms of physical and data access, with strict authentication and authorisation processes being followed. It is important for IT managers to maintain patch levels on all physical devices and software and to stay abreast of emerging zero-day vulnerabilities that can be issues for an organisation. Training for the staff and mock drills decrease the chances of internal security threats by educating them about phishing and malware.[39]

There are several aspects to administrative security controls, including minimising privilege, where people only get access to things they need and nothing more; segregation of duties so that no single person has total control over a system; role-based and rules-based access, which helps in categorising and granting privileges according to the requirements of their access. MFA helps minimise the chances of stolen credentials being used for system access, so it should always be implemented if possible. In addition, whatever access or service account is used needs to be controlled intensely.

The other main component of data breach/cyber-attack management, outside of access control, is the establishment of incident response plans, including disaster recovery steps as needed. Backups should also be monitored and routinely tested to ensure recovery at defined recovery objectives. Log collection and analysis through SIEM systems are key components of detective security controls to help identify access attempts or potential breaches. Repeatedly should monitor servers, firewalls, gateways, and logs of the other communications in addition to the IDS and IPS devices. Email scanning and data loss prevention technology should be used to help prevent scam emails from reaching the victim in the first place, while data loss prevention software must stop the transmission of exploitable sensitive data. Appropriate physical security control needs to be implemented so that data centres and access to paper records are protected and only permitted for authorised personnel. There should be a wireless access policy as part of technical controls that states any non-public access points are secured with WAP3 on the off chance that existing equipment supports it. There should also be a requirement that all end-user workstations and servers have antivirus malware protection software installed.[40,41]

Therefore, blockchain could go a long way in reducing the cybersecurity threat risks to healthcare. Implementing blockchain technology security, as well as fostering a cybersecurity culture, are critical to protection against target data and reducing an organisation's risk of exposure from a cyber-attack. A further approach to addressing cybersecurity concerns is to keep interdisciplinary protection due to aggressive strategies in the area, such as hearth gemstones from enemies, gap policies, and a rack of human detector systems. Figure 9.2 Mitigation Strategies for Cyber Threats in Healthcare illustrates a range of technical, administrative, and physical safeguards designed to protect sensitive health data from unauthorized access, breaches, and other cyber threats.

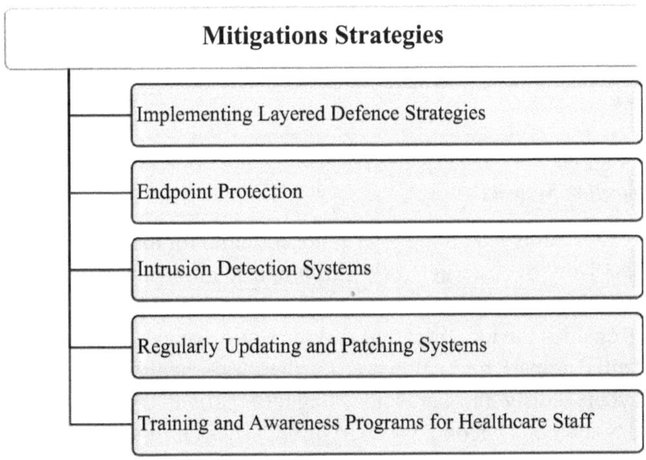

Figure 9.2 Mitigations Strategies in Blockchain Healthcare.

Implementing Layered Defence Strategies

The deployment of layered defence is essential for reducing the cybersecurity risk in healthcare. In layered defence strategies, an organisation implements numerous security protocols across different tiers of its technological infrastructure, such as a firewall, anti-virus and anti-malware software at minimum, intrusion detection systems, and employee training about not clicking on phishing emails between other methods. In addition, periodic security audits and vulnerability assessments should be undertaken to ensure any weaknesses in the system are quickly identified and resolved. By taking a layered defence approach, healthcare can create multiple walls that hackers have to breach, making it much harder to break into the system.[19,42]

Endpoint Protection

Endpoint protection serves as the foundation of a layered defense strategy. Endpoints laptops, desktop PCs, mobile devices, and the like are among the most common entry points for cyber-attacks. This means that endpoint protection needs to be strong in healthcare. The implementation of firewalls, antivirus programs, and stringent access controls may be essential to prevent unauthorised access to confidential information. Additionally, healthcare professionals must routinely inspect for malware and other malicious software, as well as update endpoint devices with the latest security patches. Proactive endpoint protection can assist healthcare organisations in reducing their systems' susceptibility to assaults.[19]

Blockchain healthcare is partitioning its networks into smaller, isolated pieces. Network segmentation can be achieved by categorising depending on the organisation's departments or functions, including administrative, clinical, and research divisions. Network segmentation enables healthcare organisations to limit the impact of a cyber-attack. For example, a hacker can only access one segmented network part; thus, that hacker will just be confined there and cannot spread out between other networks. This can reduce exposure from a breach and curtail malicious actors from moving laterally and accessing sensitive data throughout the enterprise.[19,43]

Intrusion Detection Systems

In healthcare, intrusion detection systems are essential for identifying and thwarting cyber-attacks. They oversee network traffic and identify any anomalous or detrimental activity that may indicate an ongoing cyber-attack. Utilising intrusion detection systems enables the identification and mitigation of cybersecurity threats prior to their potential impact on healthcare. Furthermore, healthcare must go towards enhanced cybersecurity measures to safeguard patient data and ensure safety. These security methods encompass encryption, access limits, and routine upgrades to mitigate vulnerabilities. Furthermore, the healthcare sector should prioritise the establishment of personnel training programs focused on cybersecurity.[19]

This will foster a culture of security awareness and diminish the probability of human error, if healthcare provides training for employees on common cyber risks and data protection best practices. The healthcare industry wants to recognise that great cybersecurity is not simply the best. Then again, it has to be no longer solely for information safety but for multidisciplinary operations of healthcare. As cyber-attacks become more frequent and severe in the healthcare sector, healthcare needs to refocus on cybersecurity. Implementing these procedures is crucial to safeguarding patient information's privacy and security while maintaining the trust and credibility of healthcare.[19,44]

Regularly Updating and Patching Systems

The second major component of cybersecurity in healthcare is keeping systems up to date with patches. Consistently updating software and systems with the most recent security patches helps mitigate vulnerabilities and safeguard healthcare startups from cyber-attacks. Healthcare organisations must have a clearly defined patch process to protect against cyber-attacks. To do this, they require a VLAN, authentication and de-authentication methods, a data breach response strategy, cloud-based computing for enhanced accessibility and security, and staff trained to recognise cybersecurity hazards. Organisations can also utilise AI technologies like machine learning and deep learning to strengthen their cyber security. They can provide a real-time response and are much quicker and more accurate than human beings in spotting dangers.[19]

Training and Awareness Programs for Healthcare Staff

Cybersecurity in healthcare is significantly dependent on employee training and awareness programs. In cybersecurity, however, employees are known to be the weakest link more often. They can become easy targets for phishing attacks or can easily leak sensitive information out of negligence. Healthcare offers comprehensive training programs that educate personnel on prevalent cybersecurity dangers and strategies for safeguarding sensitive data. Additionally, healthcare needs to up-tick this training regularly as threats change and evolve. In addition, healthcare should implement systematic internal audits and freezes to uncover possible weaknesses in its cybersecurity architecture. Ideally, these steps should form part of a wider cyber risk management approach that incorporates ongoing monitoring, incident response, and ongoing improvement.[45]

Mobilisation and Coordination for Cybersecurity in Healthcare

Similar to combating a lethal virus, addressing a cyber-attack necessitates the coordination and mobilisation of technologies among numerous public and private entities, including hospitals, IT vendors, medical device manufacturers, and various levels of government – state, local, tribal, territorial, and federal – to effectively mitigate and minimise the repercussions of a malicious assault on healthcare.[46]

Thus, cybersecurity is an organisational concern that affects the mission, operations, and programs of the entity, extending beyond information technology. In the healthcare sector, the paramount concern is patient safety and the continuity of care. Cybersecurity transcends mere technological and tactical challenges; it necessitates enhancing awareness across all facets of healthcare organisations, including nurses, administrators, health practitioners, front-line staff, cybersecurity professionals, and both IT and non-IT specialists, thereby engaging them in a mission that extends beyond technology alone.[46]

Combating this threat entails a whole-of-government and private-sector approach involving multiple organisations. The U.S. Department of Health and Human Services (HHS) is extremely committed to achieving these goals. It collaborates with various stakeholders to enhance cybersecurity inside the department and beyond the healthcare and public health sectors.[46,47]

Furthermore, HHS adopts a comprehensive 360-degree approach to guarantee the effective deployment of its cybersecurity resources under the "One Team, One Fight" ethos, while also fostering collaborations with partners from academia, medical research, and technology to enhance coordination. This extensive coalition strategy was initiated as part of the CSA in 2015. The CSA 405(d) Task Group was established under Section 405(d), Aligning Health Care Industry Security Approaches: A Status Update to the HHS Cybersecurity Program, to formulate a consensus-driven and frequently voluntary framework of guidelines, practices, methodologies, procedures, and processes aimed at enhancing cybersecurity measures within healthcare organisations.[46,48]

To facilitate the effective implementation and collaboration of the public-private development process, HHS, in conjunction with national officials, convened diverse healthcare and cybersecurity experts from both sectors to generate ideas. Participation was evident and voluntary. This collaboration developed Health Industry Cybersecurity Practices (HICP): Managing Threats and Protecting Patients a publication that provides vetted cybersecurity practices that raise awareness of specific threats and help organisations move towards greater consistency in mitigating the most relevant cyber danger to patient safety.[46,49]

Future of Blockchain Healthcare Cybersecurity

The future of cybersecurity in the realm of healthcare is expected to fall along the lines of exploration technology, modified facets of standards and regulations, and initiatives from government facilities and private corporations. The expansion of internet-enabled medical devices and the heightened utilisation of cloud computing, as well as a rise in cost-effective technology-enabled patient care solutions, also pose both opportunities and challenges for healthcare cybersecurity. While these advancements provide new opportunities for improving healthcare delivery and patient outcomes, they also introduce new risks and a new set of attack vectors. With the continued shift towards technology in healthcare and digital innovations being a prerequisite for ongoing success, the demand for security demands extraordinary coverage.[19]

This indicates the necessity to establish new industry standards and laws for healthcare cybersecurity. These would be patient-centric standards designed to protect the most vulnerable areas of everchanging healthcare systems and devices. Moreover, these standards should stress the need to include cybersecurity in the design and integration of new healthcare technologies from the start.[19,50]

Augmenting Dependence on Telehealth

Patients can now obtain medical consultations and treatment remotely due to the increasing prevalence of telehealth services. While telehealth enhances accessibility and convenience in healthcare, it simultaneously introduces novel cybersecurity challenges. These risks encompass unauthorised access to confidential patient information, breaches of telehealth platforms, and the interception or alteration of virtual consultations.[19] Higher risk of telehealth fraud and breach of patient data. In summary, growing dependence on Telehealth calls for a renewed emphasis on information security composure to safeguard person-identified features and trustful confidence in the block of emulation. That said, healthcare cybersecurity is likely to evolve in response to new technology, regulatory pressures, and the need for continued telehealth access.

Predictions About Future Threats and Vulnerabilities

The rapid advance of technology and digitalisation of the care process will undoubtedly lead to new cybersecurity threats or vulnerabilities. Such threats include advanced malware and ransomware attacks, hacking of medical devices, data breaches and social engineering techniques used by health professionals and patients. Healthcare organisations should take active steps to ensure their cybersecurity strategy adapts and responds to these emerging threats of the future.

One forecast involves cybercriminals focusing more on medical devices, especially implantable devices, and internet-connected wearable health technology. It is problematic because if these devices are compromised, the effects on patient safety and well-being can be tragic. Thus, the exclusivity of cybersecurity must be present in the design and development of new healthcare technologies by healthcare organisations. Furthermore, the sudden increase in remote work from IoT devices during COVID-19 is another cybersecurity threat. Potential dangers may encompass illegal access to sensitive patient data, heightened vulnerabilities in network infrastructure, and cyberattacks aimed at distant employees. Also, with the rising penetration of new technologies and platforms into the healthcare industry, including but not limited to artificial intelligence and machine learning, a strong emphasis is required on cybersecurity measures to help secure data integrity and confidentiality.[19,51]

Emerging Technologies and Their Consequences for Cybersecurity in Healthcare

As new technologies evolve and pervade healthcare, so will their consequences for the security of that healthcare. That could be the case with telehealth, in which virtual consultations and remote patient monitoring are key examples. Telehealth provides many conveniences around accessibility, but with that convenience comes a new set of cybersecurity threats. Also, sensitive patient information must be transmitted over electronic networks that are vulnerable to interception and unauthorised access on telehealth platforms. As healthcare delivery rapidly embraces the digital frontier, from EHRs to a wide array of network-enabled medical devices, there is an ever-increasing opportunity for ill-intentioned actors to exploit vulnerabilities in these systems through cyberattacks. This means that cybercriminals have a chance to access telehealth systems and hit paydirt when they either unauthorisedly view sensitive patient data or hack the platform to manipulate virtual consultations themselves. The fine reflects a growing awareness of the dangers of identity theft and privacy breaches affecting patients.[19,52]

Conclusion

Blockchain technology in the Healthcare system has huge potential in securing data, protecting patient privacy, and making blockchain efficient for medical records. However, with blockchain innovation comes the introduction of new cybersecurity threats that target sensitive health information. Vulnerabilities in blockchain networks can spell disaster when it comes to having patient data confidentiality and integrity of systems as the highest priority, as they may lead to financial loss, reputation damage, and lapses in patient care within a healthcare organisation.

The cyberattack that blockchain technology has brought into the healthcare system results in Cybersecurity risks. Injection attacks, such as SamSam, Locky, and Netwalker ransomware that encrypt healthcare data and ask for ransom for its decryption, are just one of many types. These types of attacks can incapacitate healthcare operations, impede treatment delivery, and put lives at risk. Phishing is one form of social engineering, a tactic that preys upon human weaknesses to compromise healthcare systems and DoS attacks flood networks with traffic that interrupts the ability of networks to provide services.

These cyberattacks have widespread effects impacting both the healthcare provider, the patient, and the economy as a whole. Healthcare Providers lose downtime, trust, and fines due to a breach of regulations, while patients suffer identity theft and privacy issues all while waiting for care. Additionally, the financial toll of these attacks on the healthcare sector has been colossal, with billions lost yearly in ransom payments, recovery efforts, and legal liabilities.

Such dangers could be met with regulations, like the HIPAA, that must exist to ensure adequate protection of patient data. HITRUST, on the other hand, is a relevant framework but not a standard that requires healthcare organisations to have rigorous cybersecurity controls and protections around ePHI. However, following guidelines is insufficient to protect against advanced forms of cyber warfare.

Mitigation methods in blockchain healthcare include layered defence strategies, where different security measures are used at multiple levels to identify and prevent an attack. While handbook protection protects all devices that can access your community, intrusion detection systems examine your community site visitors to check for malign or suspicious functions. System updates and patches regularly address vulnerabilities, and training and awareness programs help ensure that the healthcare staff is well-versed in all cybersecurity best practices.

With the telehealth services growing wider in the healthcare sector, future blockchain healthcare cybersecurity will witness some changing challenges. Proactive cybersecurity: The rise of new technologies such as IT and IoT also brings in newer vulnerabilities, so it is important to invest in proactive cybersecurity heavily. The security of such systems will depend upon the mobilisation and coordination between healthcare organisations, governments, and technology providers.

References

1 Deshpande, Advait, Katherine Stewart, Louise Lepetit, and Salil Gunashekar. "Distributed Ledger Technologies/Blockchain: Challenges, opportunities and the prospects for standards." *Overview Report the British Standards Institution (BSI)* 40, no. 40 (2017): 1–34.

2 Das, Moumita, Xingyu Tao, Yuhan Liu, and Jack CP Cheng. "A blockchain-based integrated document management framework for construction applications." *Automation in Construction* 133 (2022): 104001.

3 Abraham, Ajith, Hideyasu Sasaki, Ricardo Rios, Niketa Gandhi, Umang Singh, and Kun Ma, eds. *Innovations in Bio-Inspired Computing and Applications: Proceedings of the 11th International Conference on Innovations in Bio-Inspired Computing and Applications (IBICA 2020) Held During December 16–18, 2020*. Vol. 1372. Springer Nature, 2021.

4 Køhlert-Larsen, Nicklas, and Søren Bomholtz Thomsen. "Blockchain technology in healthcare." (2023). Master's Thesis MSc in Business Administration and Innovation in Health Care Copenhagen Business School 2023.

5 Jyothilakshmi, K. B., Vandana Robins, and A. S. Mahesh. "A comparative analysis between hyper ledger fabric and Ethereum in the medical sector: A systematic review." *Sustainable Communication Networks and Application: Proceedings of ICSCN 2021*. Vol. 93 (2022): 67–86.

6 Laroiya, Chetna, Deepika Saxena, and C. Komalavalli. "Applications of blockchain technology." In *Handbook of Research on Blockchain Technology*, pp. 213–243. Academic Press, 2020.

7 Nwosu, Anthony Ugochukwu, S. B. Goyal, and Pradeep Bedi. "Blockchain transforming cyber-attacks: Healthcare industry." In. Ajith Abraham, Hideyasu Sasaki, Ricardo Rios, Niketa Gandhi, Umang Singh, Kun Ma (Eds), *Innovations in Bio-Inspired Computing and Applications: Proceedings of the 11th International Conference on Innovations in Bio-Inspired Computing and Applications (IBICA 2020) Held on December 16–18, 2020 11*, pp. 258–266. London, New York, Berlin, Shanghai, and Tokyo: Springer International Publishing, 2021.

8 Razdan, Sahshanu, and Sachin Sharma. "Internet of medical things (IoMT): Overview, emerging technologies, and case studies." *IETE Technical Review* 39, no. 4 (2022): 775–788.

9 Khatoon, Asma. "A blockchain-based smart contract system for healthcare management." *Electronics* 9, no. 1 (2020): 94.

10 Haleem, Abid, Mohd Javaid, Ravi Pratap Singh, and Rajiv Suman. "Telemedicine for healthcare: Capabilities, features, barriers, and applications." *Sensors International* 2 (2021): 100117.

11 Coventry, Lynne, and Dawn Branley. "Cybersecurity in healthcare: A narrative review of trends, threats and ways forward." *Maturitas* 113 (2018): 48–52.
12 Khari, Manju, Gulshan Shrivastava, Sana Gupta, and Rashmi Gupta. "Role of cyber security in today's scenario." In *Detecting and Mitigating Robotic Cyber Security Risks*, pp. 177–191. Hershey, PA: IGI Global, 2017.
13 Wani, Sharyar, Mohammed Imthiyas, Hamad Almohamedh, Khalid M. Alhamed, Sultan Almotairi, and Yonis Gulzar. "Distributed denial of service (DDoS) mitigation using blockchain—A comprehensive insight." *Symmetry* 13, no. 2 (2021): 227.
14 Caine, Kelly, and Rima Hanania. "Patients want granular privacy control over health information in electronic medical records." *Journal of the American Medical Informatics Association* 20, no. 1 (2013): 7–15.
15 Yang, Ji-Jiang, Jianqiang Li, Jacob Mulder, Yongcai Wang, Shi Chen, Hong Wu, Qing Wang, and Hui Pan. "Emerging information technologies for enhanced healthcare." *Computers in Industry* 69 (2015): 3–11.
16 Ramya, M., and Sudhakaran Pradeep. "A review on security issues and attack detection in Internet of Medical Things (IoMT)." In *AIP Conference Proceedings*, vol. 3075, no. 1. AIP Publishing, 2024.
17 Tetteh, Bessie Mae. "Does HIPAA provide enough protection for healthcare in the age of ransomware and current cybersecurity threats." pp. 8–110, Bessie Mae Tetteh, Medical University of South Carolina MEDICA (2019).
18 Arapi, Kreshnik. "The healthcare industry: Evolving cyber threats and risks." Master's thesis, Utica College, 2018.
19 Okafor, Chiedozie Marius, Abosede Kolade, Tochukwu Onunka, Chibuike Daraojimba, Nsisong Louis Eyo-Udo, Okeoma Onunka, and Adedolapo Omotosho. "Mitigating cybersecurity risks in the US healthcare sector." *International Journal of Research and Scientific Innovation (IJRSI)* 10, no. 9 (2023): 177–193.
20 Manap, Nazura Abdul, Anita Abdul Rahim, and Hossein Taji. "Cyberspace identity theft: The conceptual framework." *Mediterranean Journal of Social Sciences* 6, no. 4 (2015): 595.
21 Javaid, Mohd, Abid Haleem, Ravi Pratap Singh, and Rajiv Suman. "Towards insighting cybersecurity for healthcare domains: A comprehensive review of recent practices and trends." *Cyber Security and Applications* 1 (2023): 100016.
22 Luna, Raul, Emily Rhine, Matthew Myhra, Ross Sullivan, and Clemens Scott Kruse. "Cyber threats to health information systems: A systematic review." *Technology and Health Care* 24, no. 1 (2016): 1–9.
23 Dar, Usman Ali, and Arsalan Iqbal. "The silent art of reconnaissance: The other side of the hill." *International Journal of Computer Networks and Communications Security* 6, no. 12 (2018): 250–263.
24 Uma, M., and Ganapathi Padmavathi. "A survey on various cyber attacks and their classification." *International Journal of Network Security* 15, no. 5 (2013): 390–396.
25 Rid, Thomas, and Ben Buchanan. "Attributing cyber attacks." *Journal of Strategic Studies* 38, no. 1–2 (2015): 4–37.
26 Al-Qarni, Elham Abdullah. "Cybersecurity in healthcare: A review of recent attacks and mitigation strategies." *International Journal of Advanced Computer Science and Applications* 14, no. 5 (2023): 135–140.
27 Halouzka, Kamil, Aneta Coufalíková, Ladislav Buřita, and Pavel Kozak. "The impact of the Covid-19 pandemic on the evolution of cyber threats." In *2023 International Conference on Military Technologies (ICMT)*, pp. 1–8. London, New York, Berlin, Shanghai, and Tokyo: IEEE, 2023.

28 Khatkar, Monika, Kaushal Kumar, and Brijesh Kumar. "An overview of distributed denial of service and internet of things in healthcare devices." *2020 Research, Innovation, Knowledge Management and Technology Application for Business Sustainability (INBUSH)* (2020): 44–48.

29 Djenna, Amir, and Diamel Eddine Saïdouni. "Cyber attacks classification in IoT-based-healthcare infrastructure." In *2018 2nd Cyber Security in Networking Conference (CSNet)*, pp. 1–4. IEEE, 2018.

30 Ness, Stephanie, and Tushar Khinvasara. "Emerging threats in cyberspace: Implications for national security policy and healthcare sector." *Journal of Engineering Research and Reports* 26, no. 2 (2024): 107–117.

31 Gostin, Lawrence. "Health care information and the protection of personal privacy: Ethical and legal considerations." *Annals of Internal Medicine* 127, no. 8_Part_2 (1997): 683–690.

32 Porter, Gregory, Matthew Trevors, and Robert Vrtis. "Mapping of the Health Insurance Portability and Accountability Act (HIPAA) security rule to the cyber resilience review (CRR)." (2018), 1-11,

33 Burke, Taylor. "The health information technology provisions in the American Recovery and Reinvestment Act of 2009: Implications for public health policy and practice." *Public Health Reports* 125, no. 1 (2010): 141–145.

34 Sönmez, Ferda Özdemir, Chris Hankin, and Pasquale Malacaria. "Decision support for healthcare cyber security." *Computers & Security* 122 (2022): 102865.

35 Coronado, Anthony J., and Timothy L. Wong. "Healthcare cybersecurity risk management: Keys to an effective plan." *Biomedical Instrumentation & Technology* 48, no. s1 (2014): 26–30.

36 Poongodi, C., K. Lalitha, and Rajesh Kumar Dhanaraj. "The role of blockchains for medical electronics security." In Kavita Saini, Pethuru Chelliah, Deepak Saini (Eds), *Essential Enterprise Blockchain Concepts and Applications*, pp. 231–262. Boca Raton, FL: Auerbach Publications, 2021.

37 Hyman, William A., and Ami Rakshit. "Information sources for medical equipment risk management." *Journal of Clinical Engineering* 14, no. 2 (1989): 113–120.

38 Drake, Ryan, and Evan Ridder. "Healthcare cybersecurity vulnerabilities." In *International Conference on Cybersecurity and Cybercrime*, vol. 9, pp. 49–56. 2022.

39 Pande, Sagar, Aditya Khamparia, and Deepak Gupta. "An intrusion detection system for health-care system using machine and deep learning." *World Journal of Engineering* 19, no. 2 (2022): 166–174.

40 Meingast, Marci, Tanya Roosta, and Shankar Sastry. "Security and privacy issues with health care information technology." In *2006 International Conference of the IEEE Engineering in Medicine and Biology Society*, pp. 5453–5458. IEEE, 2006.

41 Iqbal, Mubashar, and Raimundas Matulevičius. "Blockchain as a countermeasure solution for security threats of healthcare applications." In *Business Process Management: Blockchain and Robotic Process Automation Forum: BPM 2021 Blockchain and RPA Forum, Rome, Italy, September 6–10, 2021, Proceedings 19*, pp. 67–84. Springer International Publishing, 2021.

42 Abraham, Chon, Dave Chatterjee, and Ronald R. Sims. "Muddling through cybersecurity: Insights from the US healthcare industry." *Business Horizons* 62, no. 4 (2019): 539–548.

43 Savanović, Nikola, Ana Toskovic, Aleksandar Petrovic, Miodrag Zivkovic, Robertas Damaševičius, Luka Jovanovic, Nebojsa Bacanin, and Bosko Nikolic. "Intrusion detection in healthcare 4.0 internet of things systems via metaheuristics optimized machine learning." *Sustainability* 15, no. 16 (2023): 12563.

44 Nifakos, Sokratis, Krishna Chandramouli, Charoula Konstantina Nikolaou, Panagiotis Papachristou, Sabine Koch, Emmanouil Panaousis, and Stefano Bonacina. "Influence of human factors on cyber security within healthcare organisations: A systematic review." *Sensors* 21, no. 15 (2021): 5119.

45 Jerry-Egemba, Nma. "Safe and sound: Strengthening cybersecurity in healthcare through robust staff educational programs." In *Healthcare Management Forum*, vol. 37, no. 1, pp. 21–25. Thousand Oaks: SAGE Publications, 2024.

46 Julie Anne Chua, PMP, CAP, CISSP: https://www.physicianleaders.org/articles/cybersecurity-in-the-healthcare-industry

47 National Academies of Sciences, Medicine Division, Board on Global Health, Committee on Global Health, and the Future of the United States. "Global health and the future role of the United States." pp. 1–384, Washington, DC: The National Academies Press, 2017.

48 Ireland, Leslie. "21st century intelligence: The need for a one-team-one-fight approach." *PRISM* 7, no. 1 (2017): 46–57.

49 Wilkinson, Ian Cornelius. *Cybersecurity Using Risk Management Strategies of US Government Health Organizations*. Minneapolis, MN: Walden University, 2020.

50 He, Ying, Aliyu Aliyu, Mark Evans, and Cunjin Luo. "Health care cybersecurity challenges and solutions under the climate of COVID-19: Scoping review." *Journal of Medical Internet Research* 23, no. 4 (2021): e21747.

51 Agarwal, Reshu, and Mukul Kumar. "Cyber security for handling threats in healthcare devices." In Pawan Singh Mehra, Lalit Mohan Goyal, Arvind Dagur, Anshu Kumar Dwivedi (Eds), *Healthcare Systems and Health Informatics*, pp. 217–233. Abingdon: CRC Press, 2022.

52 Bhuyan, Soumitra Sudip, Umar Y. Kabir, Jessica M. Escareno, Kenya Ector, Sandeep Palakodeti, David Wyant, Sajeesh Kumar, Marian Levy, Satish Kedia, Dipankar Dasgupta, and Aram Dobalian. "Transforming healthcare cybersecurity from reactive to proactive: Current status and future recommendations." *Journal of Medical Systems* 44 (2020): 1–9.

10 User Experience and Adoption Challenges in the Healthcare Industry

Shaweta Sharma, Akanksha Sharma, Ashish Verma, Sunita, Shivkanya Fuloria and Akhil Sharma

Introduction

Healthcare UX, or Healthcare user experience, is designing the customer experience of health products and services with a focus on delivering value and insights to the customer (as opposed to keeping them in the product loop). The complex environment of healthcare technology influences the communication that occurs between patients, clinicians/doctors, and software systems, affecting the quality, accuracy, and efficiency of healthcare delivery. Healthcare UX is a balance between business and profitability

Healthcare UX makes an impact, so it must be watched very specifically. Suppose there is a poorly designed product or digital interface. In that case, the consequence can be too big, and it may even lead to misreading for customers, improper judgment, and sometimes a bad impact on customer health.[1]

Importance of Healthcare UX

Figure 10.1 depicts the importance of blockchain assisted healthcare user experience.

Better Clinical Experience

Clinical experience is not only critical to the patient's overall experience with the product or organisation but also a key driver of their mental well-being. An emergency room patient or a patient waiting for their test results is already going through a lot of stress, which can be reduced substantially with a proper Healthcare UX.

Reduced Errors and Miscommunications

However, research published in 2020 shows that nearly 80% of all clinical mistakes are due to miscommunication and medical faults between patients and medical organisations. This should be alarming, and it is also the foremost reason you must improve your UX to communicate the information with results correctly.[2]

DOI: 10.4324/9781003529910-10

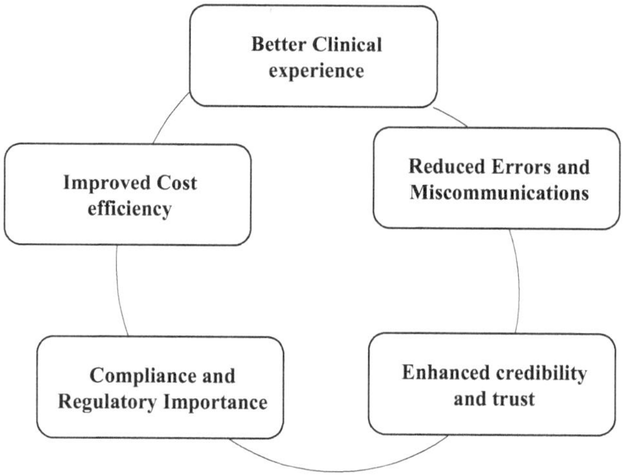

Figure 10.1 Importance of Healthcare UX.

Enhanced Credibility and Trust

When there is a proper healthcare UX, the patients will feel good, which will help the medical organisation. That eventually leads to a well-designed healthcare UX that gets more trust from the customers, and eradicating miscommunication and even medical errors increases the credibility of the organisation.

Compliance and Regulatory Importance

The importance of Healthcare UX is tremendous since it becomes obligatory for every medical organisation to comply with the regulations of HIPAA (Health Insurance Portability and Accountability Act). This is the reason why organisations can adhere to regulatory requirements regarding data privacy, patient confidentiality, etc., with a well-balanced UX.[3]

Improved Cost Efficiency

Healthcare UX is the set of good practices that enhance administrative productivity and reduce adverse health outcomes in the long run. A well-designed healthcare app also reduces the administrative overhead costs for any organisation; hence, Healthcare UX also enhances cost effectiveness.[4]

Importance of Technology Adoption in Improving Healthcare Services

The adoption of technology in healthcare is crucial for enhancing service delivery and improving patient outcomes. Highlighting its importance:

Improved Patient Care

Accurate Diagnoses

Adopting EHRs and telemedicine leads to accurate diagnoses and customised treatment plans that allow patients to manage chronic conditions effectively while making it easier to detect diseases in their early stages.

Real-Time Monitoring

From real-time monitoring of patient health to timely interventions and adjustments in treatment plans, digital tools play a critical role.[5]

Streamlined Operations

Efficiency in Processes

Technology can reduce the administrative burden of scheduling, billing, and inventories. He notes that with this, healthcare professionals can spend more time treating the patient, which leads to cost savings and better allocation of resources.

Enhanced Coordination

Better data management through digital systems can lead to enhanced communication between different healthcare units that will limit errors and further improve care coordination.

Increased Patient Engagement

Empowerment Through Technology

Digital platforms provide access to health information, appointment scheduling, and communication with providers. Such engagement results in increased satisfaction and compliance with the treatment plans.[6]

Telehealth Adoption

The COVID-19 pandemic fast-tracked the acceptance of telehealth services, which made healthcare more accessible and convenient, especially for patients in remote areas.

Enhanced Data Management

Data Security and Compliance

When it comes to patient data, however, their systems were never designed to keep them up-to-date on regulations like HIPAA that govern such things and protect sensitive records from breaches. CVD creates trust between patients and healthcare professionals.[7]

Analytics for Better Decision-Making

With AI, machine learning analyses massive amounts of health data, which assists in identifying trends and improving clinical decisions.

Economic Benefits

Cost Reduction

The adoption of technology can help healthcare organisations realise large cost savings by standardising and automating processes. Well, given the rising financial strains in the industry, it is especially relevant.[8]

Investment Growth

The increase in digital health investments signifies an expanding credit of technology's ability to revolutionise the delivery of care. Digital health investments amounted to $29 billion in 2021 alone, highlighting the economic viability of tech adoption in healthcare.[9]

Need for Addressing Adoption Challenges

Addressing adoption barriers in healthcare technology is critical for a variety of reasons, as evidenced by the search results. The points emphasising the need to tackle these challenges are

Enhancing User Engagement

Most healthcare applications are viewed as intimidating, which results in low user engagement. For example, the MyFitnessPal app saw a drastic improvement in retention rates following a UX overhaul that made the user journey much easier. Satisfying these complexities will improve the UX and motivate them to keep using it.[10]

Meeting Diverse User Needs

Inclusive Design: Healthcare systems have many users: patients from the age of 0 and above, each with a different level of experience with technology, and health specialists who are also our end-users. All demographics must be accessible and easy to use on applications. This means creating simple-to-use interfaces for patients and providers, which can improve health.

Compliance and Data Security

Medical data is extremely sensitive information requiring compliance with HIPAA and other regulations. Ignoring these legal requirements will slow down technology adoption and create distrust among users. It is important to design from the security aspect and draw early attention away from usability; this will build trust in healthcare technologies.[11]

Reducing Cognitive Load

Simplifying information means enabling seamless access to all relevant ancillary and complementary content. Interfaces that are simplified and focus on delivering clear, actionable information can enhance decision-making processes and reduce user stress. This is essential within high-stakes environments where fast delivery of pivotal data is a requirement.[12]

Facilitating Seamless Integration

As emerging technologies come on the funnel of innovation, it is really important from a user perspective that they be able to use them across all social media platforms. The technologies used to support these goals also need to be multidisciplinary and cross-platform, merging care solutions with consumer solutions. Solving interoperability problems could make transitions seamless and improve user interests.

Improving Patient Outcomes

At the end of the day, addressing adoption challenges will affect care directly. User-friendly and seamless technology implementations improve the ways we manage health, engage patients, and enhance clinical outcomes.[13]

Lack of Technology Adoption in Healthcare

Healthcare will never progress without the adoption of technologies. For example, HIPAA and PIPEDA help shield clients' health information through standard compliance by many doctors and practitioners.

If these professionals fail to use security- and privacy-compliant technologies to safeguard health information, they may risk client information, which will carry substantial penalties. This is just one example of the role that the absence of technology plays in healthcare.[14]

Even though technology adoption has become convenient over time, there are certain barriers to this endeavour. Some of them are

- Several healthcare providers are unsure about how to use the technology or how it will impact their workflow.

- The comfort and ease of use of current systems make users reluctant to change to new technology.
- The perception that new technology is costly, complicated, and unclear of how much value it could bring.
- Hospitals and clinics may be sceptical about the safety or efficacy of new technologies.

Adopting technology is a gradual process, but in the long run, it pays off. The industry is helping to shift the paradigm, realising that telemedicine and remote consultation have advantages. The remote work and revolution proceeded, and now you may need all the right workflow out of productivity software to keep in line with your organisation.

There are several reasons why the technology isn't fully utilised anyway. This involves opposition from staff, inefficient technology preparation, and a lack of process adherence. Now, let us take a look at these challenges that hinder the adoption of technologies in any healthcare sector.[15]

Challenges in the Adoption of Technology in Healthcare

Serious Digital Risk

The prevailing model of healthcare delivery is highly complex. It includes layers of processes, a network of patients and partners, insurance reimbursement models, delivery models, and regulatory requirements. Along with technological advancements, these complexities expose the industry to extreme digital risks.[16]

Cyberattack Risks

The increasing evolution of the Internet of Medical Things (IoMT), taking the form of devices and applications, has made cybersecurity concerns inevitable ever since. Some of the devices that you find in this ecosystem may not have any or only standard security. This leaves these IoMT devices susceptible to cyber-attacks and other threats related to information security. The second cause of cyberattack risks is the increase in volume and access to healthcare data. In the last two years, the healthcare data has spiked by 78%.[17]

Dynamic Workforce Risk

Devices, gadgets, and data are empowering the healthcare workforce with what they need to treat their patients better today. This, as well as the pandemic, has led from a traditional model to a more dynamic model in which healthcare workers use telemedicine services to treat patients remotely. However, this creates the risk of inaccurate workforce authentication and authorisation. It also makes it more difficult to keep tabs on what employees are doing.

Data Privacy Risk

Patient Health Information: A variety of methods can collect PHI. It remains unclear who is responsible for protecting the data and information of patients. But there would be a false equivalency here, and it is reasonable to say that, ultimately, this need should be borne by the institution. Not doing so could end up costing money and, in some instances, even pose health threats to the patient. Thus, you need a remedy that not only protects the business but also gives an integrated approach to mitigate all digital risks across an organisation to counter all this. This should include robust systems for access control, fast detection and response, and comprehensive risk management. Equipped with such a tool, the healthcare sector can flourish and evolve seamlessly to transformational change without any security concerns.[18]

Poor Training and Onboarding

In healthcare, we find many applications coming into use. Whether they are providers of equipment, manufacturers of medicines, or hospitals, they all use numerous applications daily to ensure the smooth flow of activities.

Strict Compliance Regulations and Data Integrity

Compliance rules, regulations, and laws attached to the industry are given to any organisation connected with healthcare. Healthcare adopts new technology like any other industry, but this wide array of rigid rules and regulations is holding back the overall process of Technology and Application adoption. Consequently, it leads hospitals and other healthcare organisations to shy away from advanced technology. These regulations exist because poor entry of data leads to inaccurate data, which is terrible for an organisation, either from an administrative perspective or even a medical one.[19]

Factors Affecting UX in Healthcare

Several factors influence UX in healthcare, particularly how patients, healthcare providers, and administrators interact with healthcare technologies. Some factors affecting UX in healthcare are as follows:

Accessibility

Accessibility is a core aspect of ensuring that healthcare technologies are accessible to everyone, regardless of their physical, cognitive, and technological limitations. This includes developing platforms for individuals with disabilities (e.g., vision and mobility) and older adults with limited technology experience. Resume device compatibility is another important factor, as well as the healthcare tools you need to work quickly and easily on smartphones, tablets, and desktop computers. Geographic accessibility is also important, particularly in rural or underrepresented communities where services are limited. In these contexts, providing the ability for healthcare technologies to function with little infrastructure or connectivity is critical for closing the value gap.[20]

Usability

Usability refers to the ease with which healthcare professionals and patients can interact with technology. Intuitive interfaces that are easy to understand and navigate help reduce frustration and prevent errors, which can be critical in high-stakes healthcare environments. Healthcare tools should also minimise the learning curve by being designed with the end-user in mind, whether that user is a clinician, administrative staff, or a patient. A good UX design also incorporates error-tolerant features, such as warnings before irreversible actions or confirmation prompts, reducing the likelihood of mistakes that could negatively affect patient outcomes.[21]

Workflow Integration

A tension point in healthcare is incorporating new technology simply and effectively into current clinical workflows. Healthcare providers are already opening their eyes to the complex work needed and time pressures faced, so any new tech should be built around how they already do things. Technology needs to integrate into clinical workflow without creating disruption either in documenting a patient record, retrieving data, or working with other health system partners. Technologies must connect seamlessly with EHR systems, lab reports, and billing platforms so that they form a single interface for the user that does not present an extra burden on the healthcare worker.[22]

Personalisation

The real deal of personalisation is making healthcare technology applications specific and suited for the help seekers/stakeholders, who are either patients or healthcare providers. Pick Packer User is a custom UX in the system that helps users better interact with the system in a personalised way. For patients, this could be customised health-tracking features or medication reminders; it can also be dashboards for clinicians that present pertinent patient information in a format most appropriate for their speciality. The system should also be applicable to process diverse languages, cultural backgrounds, and personal preferences so that the ordinary population can access and use this technology easily.[23]

Security and Privacy

Health information is highly sensitive, and security and privacy are critical in the healthcare domain. User trust in the technology is predicated on ensuring that breaches and unauthorised access to data are prevented. Factors like strong encryption, secure authentication methods, and regular security updates come together to shield user data. In addition, transparency regarding where data would be collected, stored, and used is very important in maintaining users' trust. Patients must be assured that their private health data is safe from being disclosed and that its use complies with healthcare regulations (for instance, HIPAA in the U.S. or GDPR in the EU).

Engagement and Feedback Mechanisms

One of the most critical factors for healthcare technologies is user engagement. Telemedicine platforms and health apps designed for patient use should be structured for regular use, while those designed for healthcare professionals should promise efficiency and value inside of clinical tasks. Integrating feedback loops into the technology so users can notify developers of problems or recommend improvements through its use and experience – gamification is another feature that can keep the patients focused on continuing their therapy during chronic conditions where they have to constantly monitor or do something, as special badges could be given for tracking progress which motivates the patients.[24]

Aesthetic Design

Actually, the graphic aspect of healthcare technology is often underestimated in UX. User satisfaction and adoption can usually be improved by having a clean, well-designed interface that is aesthetically pleasing yet functionally effective. Making sure what the user sees font, colour, and layouts are consistent gives comfort to the user when navigating around the system and enables a decrease in cognitive load along with fewer possibilities of confusion. Healthcare is an arena where sophisticated aesthetic simplicity is a necessity to help ensure that users be they clinicians or patients are able to complete high-impact tasks without distraction from overly ornate or complex user interfaces.[25]

Performance and Reliability

Trust and the effectiveness of healthcare technologies heavily rely on their performance and reliability. Low Latency Systems have a fast response time from user inputs. Slow pages or lagging responses annoy users as timely healthcare needs call for quick decision-making. Reliability is just as vital healthcare platforms should always be available with little downtime or crashing since any interruption from reliability can result in a downright dangerous lapse of patient care. Scalability is an influential criterion since hospitals and other healthcare systems would need the ability to support increasing amounts of end-users and greater volumes of data over time.[26]

Patient Empowerment and Control

Healthcare technology empowers patients by increasing their health data and care control. Self-service functionalities, like allowing the user to view their medical records, book an appointment or track health milestones (blood pressure or sugar levels), can empower a patient. In addition, decision-support tools that deliver personalised recommendations to patients or give them insights into their health data can help empower better decisions regarding their care. This enhances engagement, incentivises participation, and cultivates ownership over health management.[27]

Trust and Familiarity

Trust is fundamental for the (wider) adoption of healthcare technologies. Consistency in UXs across devices (smartphones, tablets, and desktops) makes it easy for users to identify with the platform and subsequently engage with it regularly. People easily prefer using a technology that seems familiar enough to understand and use. Furthermore, when technology is validated by social influencers such as healthcare practitioners and health systems, it does make a difference in the perception of users both patients and clinicians regarding reliability and value, which can further enhance adoption and utilisation.

Adoption Challenges in the Healthcare Industry

Adoption challenges in the healthcare industry are multifaceted, involving technical, organisational, patient-centric, and regulatory issues that make it difficult for new technologies and systems to be fully embraced.[28] The main adoption challenges in the healthcare industry of blockchain technology are described below and mentioned in Figure 10.2.

Technical Challenges

One of the biggest challenges in adopting new healthcare technologies is technical issues. Integration with existing systems, especially electronic health records (EHRs), medical devices, and hospital management, is one of the main barriers. Healthcare organisations often have legacy systems, and to fit new technologies without disrupting them can be a complicated and expensive initiative.[29]

Interoperability (the ability of different systems to communicate and exchange information) is another key technical challenge that many have noted. A lot of healthcare systems and devices are siloed, so it is challenging to transfer patient

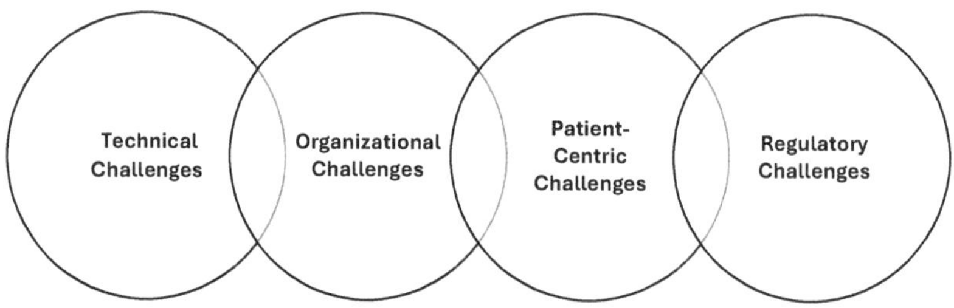

Figure 10.2 Challenges in Adoption of Blockchain Technology by Healthcare System.

information from one platform or provider to the next. Ineffective interoperability slows treatment and undermines the impact of technology.

Another key area of concern is around data security and privacy. With improvements in healthcare technologies, the risks of cyber-attacks, data breaches, and access by unauthorised users are increasing. The need for strong security combined with compliance with healthcare regulations (HIPAA in the U.S., etc.) increases the complexity of technology adoption.[30]

Organisational Challenges

One of the common challenges in embedding new healthcare technologies is resistance to change at an organisational level. Health professionals who traditionally work and are not familiar with emerging technologies will always doubt whether it would add value by complicating their workflows or need more time to learn. Such type of resistance typically comes from ignorance or unaware of the advantages it may present.

One of the most important factors, though commonly neglected, that leads to a successful adoption is training and education. If healthcare staff are not properly trained, they may not use new systems correctly, which can lead to inefficiencies or errors. Time and resources needed for training could also be a barrier, especially for healthcare organisations already burdened by time and budget constraints. Time and resources required for training could also be a barrier, especially for healthcare organisations already burdened by time and budget constraints.[31]

Another type of organisational challenge is the lack of a budget. Implementation of new technologies, infrastructure upgrades, and maintenance costs can be out of reach for many healthcare facilities (especially smaller clinics or those in resource-limited environments). Some may consider the financial investment required for new technology as too high relative to perceived benefits.

Patient-Centric Challenges

Digital literacy is one of the major adoption challenges from a patient's perspective. Not every patient is tech-savvy, which leads them to appreciate healthcare apps, telemedicine platforms, or any other such digital tool. This is especially the case for older adults or those from lower-income populations who may have less frequent access to technology or the Internet.

The other major issue is that of data privacy. If patients do not know how their health information will be used or are worried about breaches, they may be reluctant to disclose personal health information digitally. However, we know that for healthcare to work at its best level, patients must have complete trust in the system around them and feel reassured that their privacy is being properly safeguarded.[32]

Furthermore, patient engagement itself is an uneven experience. Not all digital health tools will be effective for every patient, as some patients are eager to apply the use of these tools in their care, while others can be overwhelmed or apathetic. By keeping tech simple and suitable for the patients at hand, adoption rates can dramatically improve.

Regulatory Challenges

Regulations in healthcare are strict and complicated, which sets up important barriers to the entry of new technology. Although adherence to such standards is crucial, meeting them tends to inhibit innovation rollout. For example, new medical devices or digital tools usually must undergo long certification and approval processes to guarantee their safety and effectiveness.[33]

Data governance is another issue that comes into play, especially following the accelerated use of digital tools and cloud-based systems. Providers have to make sure data is stored, managed and shared compliantly with laws such as the Health Insurance Portability and Accountability Act (HIPAA) or the General Data Protection Regulation (GDPR). The process of navigating through such regulations is tedious and tiring. It could lead organisations away from new technologies as they add a compliance burden.

Cultural and Behavioral Challenges

If we consider adoption resistance, cultural challenges are also one of the contributing factors. Particularly in healthcare, practices have remained for decades, creating an institutional culture that may be resistant to the technological innovation you desire. Certain providers may be concerned that technology would threaten the human element of patient care and see digital tools as impersonal or disconnected from the personal nature of medical interaction.

Fear of job loss is another factor behind behavioural resistance. The fear that automation and AI-driven technologies will eliminate their functions causes some to continue resisting these innovations.[34]

Infrastructural Challenges

Several health service providers, especially in third-world countries or rural places, do not have the infrastructure needed to make use of new-age health technologies. One fundamental challenge remote regions face is that of internet connectivity and network reliability, which limits the deployment of telemedicine or cloud-based health systems. Outdated hardware and software a particular challenge for areas that are urban but still lack access to modern healthcare technologies can also serve as a substantial barrier.[35]

Economic and Cost-Benefit Perception

This could also explained by the perception of the cost-benefit ratio as a barrier towards technology adoption. Although the entry of any new technology may be cautious due to a lack of clear Return on Investment (ROI), healthcare organisations, especially those under financial strain, may not be willing to take a chance with any new deployment. The ambiguity regarding ROI and the apprehension about sustaining new systems, in the long run, will cause them to stall decisions around adoption.

Impact of Poor UX on Technology Adoption

The role of UX is multifaceted when it comes to technology adoption, as all feedback – good or bad – impacts the level of satisfaction that users find from its use.

High Abandonment Rates

When the UX is poor, users tend to abandon apps at a higher rate. It has been observed that 24% of the Android apps get uninstalled within one day and 49% in a month because of poor UX. This is a stark reminder of the current state of expectations for users leaving technology that does not live up to the hype.[36]

Negative First Impressions

Users take just 500 milliseconds to pass a very sensitive, short, critical first temper about any website or application. Users will jump off immediately if an ugly or kludgy design. So it strengthens the idea that to get people back, we need to make first experiences happen as well as they can.

Reduced Customer Satisfaction

Bad UX leads to less customer content. Studies have found that 88% of users are unlikely to return to a site after a bad experience, blossoming into poor word-of-mouth and decreased loyalty.[37]

Increased Training Burden

The complexity of the user requires a huge amount of training, which discourages people from adopting new technologies. Users will always get annoyed and avoid using an application even when it offers meaningful functionality if it is not easy to learn. An established and simple-to-use design can minimise training.

Resistance to Change

If a technology is poorly designed and affects users negatively, it may lead to resistance against any new system being adopted. Such resistance is often based on some uneasiness with change; it reflects scepticism about the latest technology and its value. However, good UX design can minimise that resistance by smoothening and beautifying transitions.

Financial Implications

Companies that do not consider UX are leaving tons of revenue potential on the table. Companies can get up to $100 return for every dollar spent on UX, showing how important design is for your bottom line. On the flip side, bad UX can mean higher support costs and lost sales.[38]

Long-Term Brand Impact

A poor UX can harm a brand that the user can't recover. Companies focused on UX outperform competitors by an average of 228% in terms of shareholder return, according to studies.[39]

Overcome Adoption Challenges in Healthcare Technology

There are a few approaches available to address inherent healthcare technology and adoption challenges. By their nature, these strategies complement one another to improve UX, security, and stakeholder collaboration. Hence, the elaborated description of every point is as follows:

Enhancing UX Design

Involving End-Users in the Design Process

It is important to include end-users (e.g., patients, clinicians, and administrative staff) in the design process so that the technology is developed according to their real needs. This allows designers to observe pain points and preferences from the actual users of the system, resulting in intuitive interfaces that enable ease of use through a tailored design process. Not only does this approach improve usability, but it also creates a sense of ownership with users that increases their likelihood of embracing the technology.[40]

Simplifying Interfaces for Different User Groups

Healthcare professionals and patients have different backgrounds and levels of technology literacy. If a system is used by users who belong to other groups, it is critical to keep the interfaces simple and focused to ensure that everyone understands how to make use of the same. The UX approach can also vary widely depending on the users; for example, clinicians may need immediate access to patient data, while patients might want simpler navigation for booking appointments or viewing health information. An easygoing design reduces cognitive load and leads to a better UX.[41]

Ensuring Consistent and Intuitive Design

There are many different platforms available. Users should be able to anticipate how they will interact with the system based on everything they have done that has come before. A clear and simple design reduces the need for extensive training. It allows users to use the technology more easily, using existing design principles, which will enable you to provide a more consistent experience that the users can easily navigate.

Education and Training

Training Programs for Healthcare Staff

Training programs are essential to ensuring healthcare teams can effectively utilise new technologies. Such programs need to be conducted for various roles in the organisation, covering only those functionalities that are pertinent to them. Regular training sessions can continuously reinforce skills and allow staff to learn about new aspects and updates, which in turn improves adoption rates.[42]

Patient Education on Digital Health Tools

Patient education on digital health tools is just as vital for successful adoption. Consider implementing patient education through tutorials, workshops, or hand-outs to allow patients to use these tools properly. Patients are more likely to engage highly with their healthcare management when they know how to access their health information or communicate with providers digitally.

Improving Interoperability

Using Standardised Protocols for Data Exchange

Benefit from Interoperability challenges are frequently encountered due to difficulties in achieving seamless integration between healthcare technologies. For example, the use of standardised protocols for data exchange HL7 or Fast Healthcare Interoperability Resources (FHIR), for instance, can also allow better bidirectional communication between systems. This ensures that patient information integrates seamlessly across platforms, improving care coordination and achieving better results for the patients.[43]

Collaborating Across Organisations for Seamless Data Flow

This can only be possible through collaboration between healthcare providers, technology vendors, and regulatory bodies. It enables organisations to make a true ecosystem where the data shared is seamless and standards-based insight. This joint effort improves efficiencies and factors into better care by delivering complete information on patients exactly where it matters.

Change Management Strategies

Engaging Stakeholders Early

Engaging stakeholders early, particularly clinicians, administrators, and IT staff, is important to ensure the successful adoption of technology. However, involving all these folks in the planning and implementation stages can help alleviate resistance and offer remedies for specific concerns. Taking this collaborative approach avoids top-down decrees and fosters a sense of shared responsibility, as well as buy-in from all parties involved.[44]

Phased Adoption with Continuous Feedback

Phased adoption of technology allows organisations to onboard a new system while continuously receiving feedback from users in smaller batches. With this iterative process, you can optimise your workflows and modify problems as they get faced in the real world. Organisations can increase satisfaction and acceptance of new technology more fully across a broad set of end users by showing they are responsive to user feedback.

These strategies help alleviate some of the pain points surrounding adoption, as a result providing an improved UX that results in higher levels of patient engagement and ultimately better health outcomes for patients.[45]

Future Trends in UX and Adoption of Technology

The outlook for healthcare can change quite dramatically with Future trends in UX and technology acceptance.

Improving UX through the Help of AI and Machine Learning

AI, and ML specifically, is changing the UX landscape by providing more personalised and adaptive experiences. These technologies are used to process vast amounts of user data, seeking meaning in the patterns and preferences that those numbers reveal. As a use-case, ML algorithms are used to recommend products/media, such as Netflix or Amazon, as per the behaviour of single users and make them stay active and satisfied. In addition to this, A/B testing can also be automated with AI, which means variations of designs that work best will automatically be identified, and it makes design optimisation easy. AI will evolve to the level where it will be able to anticipate user requirements and take necessary measures for further optimisation of a UI, thus enriching the UX in health app development.[46]

Evolution of Patient-Centric Design

An aspect of patient engagement that providers are beginning to understand represents a shift towards more patient-centric design. This is more about getting a deep insight into their needs, expectations, and behaviours to solve their touchpoints with the healthcare services. New directions also include adding processes that will allow patients to share their comments and recommendations directly as part of the design process. From there, the emphasis is on usability and emotion in care as more digital health tools are pulled towards the patient's heart. So, the more patient-centred design dimension acquired by user service quality, corresponding to higher trustful and satisfied figures attained from these services, better health outcomes would have been reached.[47]

New Technologies Such as Blockchain for Safe Data

Blockchain technology is emerging as a potential solution to provide more data protection within healthcare. It is decentralised, it will protect the patient's data and access controls are transparent to everyone. This also suggests that healthcare organisations can then utilise blockchain technology to enhance the integrity of their data and deter breaches, addressing one of the first major challenges in tech adoption. Its technology also creates interoperation between circuits by offering a secure framework for data exchange. Given the importance of data security provided by organisations as part of digital health programs, it is likely that blockchain technology will facilitate user trust and consequently promote the proliferation of health technologies.[48]

Predictions on the Future of Digital Health Adoption

As technology innovation continues to change the landscape of digital health adoption, the future looks bright. Proponents say the incorporation of AI, ML, and other emerging technologies will create individualised healthcare experiences for patients. The COVID-19 pandemic has led to a dramatic rise in telehealth, which finally helped ease acceptance among patients and providers and now seems poised for even greater digital health growth. Over the next couple of years, these investments in user-centred design and well-enforced privacy mechanisms should translate into growing levels of user trust and confidence in digital health tools. These trends, combined, represent a more integrated and agile healthcare environment with technology embedded in the patient experience.[49]

Conclusion

The UX in healthcare is one of the most important ingredients for any digital health technology to obtain successful adoption. As healthcare systems evolve, the increase in simple yet effective UX becomes essential to bridge the gap between technology and actual user engagement for patients, providers, or administrators. An effective UX, in addition to the increased access and usability, may also provide patient-centred care designed to enhance patient satisfaction and achieve better health outcomes. Approval for the adoption of healthcare technologies is not as simple as integration into systems and secure data handling. There is also the need to overcome change resistance within organisations, budgetary limits, and low digital literacy among patients; hence, more than one approach is needed. Given that proper training is the largest transfer to clinics, individuals are likely to access user-friendly, safe collections with enhanced clarifications of individual privacy. The implications of poor UX are legion, from slower technology adoption, operational inefficiencies, and increased risk of error based on systems that are confusing or overly complex. This would then make the adoption pathway smoother as it places user-centred design at its core, offers interoperability, alleviates privacy concerns, and has a robust strategy for change management.

The UX in healthcare has no limits of horizons with innovations on the zenith ahead from now as growth in artificial intelligence and machine learning gives an open sky to the prospect of integrations with blockchain innovations. So that systems are intuitive, secure, and responsive for patients and providers. Increasing UX is the key that will turn healthcare technologies (as digital health solutions) from adoption to a usage story, laying the ground for all integration over time.

References

1 Fanfarelli, Joey R., Rudy McDaniel, and Carrie Crossley. "Adapting UX to the design of healthcare games and applications." *Entertainment Computing* 28 (2018): 21–31.

2 Thomas, Kathleen C., Hillary Owino, Sana Ansari, Leslie Adams, Julianne M. Cyr, Bradley N. Gaynes, and Seth W. Glickman. "Patient-centered values and experiences with emergency department and mental health crisis care." *Administration and Policy in Mental Health and Mental Health Services Research* 45 (2018): 611–622.

3 Rossi, Marco, and Giada Russo. "Regulatory compliance in medical device software development: Strategies for navigating complex requirements." *Scientific Academia Journal* 5, no. 1 (2022): 1–8.

4 Khairat, Saif, Cameron Coleman, Thomas Newlin, Victoria Rand, Paige Ottmar, Thomas Bice, and Shannon S. Carson. "A mixed-methods evaluation framework for electronic health records usability studies." *Journal of Biomedical Informatics* 94 (2019): 103175.

5 Kalid, Naser, A. A. Zaidan, B. B. Zaidan, Omar H. Salman, Mashitoh Hashim, and H. Muzammil. "Based real-time remote health monitoring systems: A review on patients prioritisation and related "big data" using body sensors information and communication technology." *Journal of Medical Systems* 42 (2018): 1–30.

6 Tanniru, Mohan. "Engagement leading to empowerment—Digital innovation strategies for patient care continuity." *Journal of Hospital Management and Health Policy* 3 (2019): 1–12.

7 Luxton, David D., Robert A. Kayl, and Matthew C. Mishkind. "mHealth data security: The need for HIPAA-compliant standardisation." *Telemedicine and e-Health* 18, no. 4 (2012): 284–288.

8 Thomas, Ranjeeta, and Kalipso Chalkidou. "Cost-effectiveness analysis." In *Health System Efficiency: How to Make Measurement Matter for Policy and Management [Internet]*. European Observatory on Health Systems and Policies, 2016.

9 Jadad-Garcia, Tamen, and Alejandro R. Jadad. "Cracking the code: Lessons from 15 years of digital health IPOs for the era of AI." arXiv preprint arXiv:2410.02709 (2024).

10 Mustafa, Abdulsalam Salihu, Nor'ashikin Ali, Jaspaljeet Singh Dhillon, Gamal Alkawsi, and Yahia Baashar. "User engagement and abandonment of mHealth: A cross-sectional survey." In Daniele Giansanti (ed), *Healthcare*, vol. 10, no. 2, p. 221. Basel, Switzerland: MDPI, 2022.

11 Alraja, Mansour Naser, Usman Javed Butt, and Maysam Abbod. "Information security policies compliance in a global setting: An employee's perspective." *Computers & Security* 129 (2023): 103208.

12 Lindblom, Jessica, and Peter Thorvald. "Towards a framework for reducing cognitive load in manufacturing personnel." *Advances in Cognitive Engineering and Neuroergonomics* 11 (2014): 233–244.

13 Smith, Abi, Dimitrios Siassakos, Joanna Crofts, and Tim Draycott. "Simulation: Improving patient outcomes." In Dena Goffman (ed), *Seminars in Perinatology*, vol. 37, no. 3, pp. 151–156. Amsterdam, Netherlands: WB Saunders, 2013.
14 Anwar, Fozia, and Azra Shamim. "Barriers in adoption of health information technology in developing societies." *International Journal of Advanced Computer Science and Applications* 2, no. 8 (2011): 40–45.
15 Bertolazzi, Alessia, Valeria Quaglia, and Ramona Bongelli. "Barriers and facilitators to health technology adoption by older adults with chronic diseases: An integrative systematic review." *BMC Public Health* 24, no. 1 (2024): 506.
16 Renukappa, Suresh, Primrose Mudiyi, Subashini Suresh, Wala Abdalla, and Chandrashekar Subbarao. "Evaluation of challenges for adoption of smart healthcare strategies." *Smart Health* 26 (2022): 100330.
17 Dhingra, Sarthak, Rakesh Raut, Angappa Gunasekaran, B. Koteswara Rao Naik, and Venkateshwarlu Masuna. "Analysis of the challenges for blockchain technology adoption in the Indian health-care sector." *Journal of Modelling in Management* 19, no. 2 (2024): 375–406.
18 Rodwin, Marc A. "Patient data: Property, privacy & the public interest." *American Journal of Law & Medicine* 36, no. 4 (2010): 586–618.
19 Ronolo, Shyne Cindy. "Assuring data integrity towards regulatory compliance: A study on process improvement in data integrity compliance of computerized systems." Metropolia University of Applied Sciences, Helsinki, Finland (2023): 1–86.
20 Li, Yan, and Abdulaziz Saad Albarrak. "An informatics-driven intelligent system to improve healthcare accessibility for vulnerable populations." *Journal of Biomedical Informatics* 134 (2022): 104196.
21 Abdelwahab, Marwan Sameh, Dina Gamal Abboud, and Nagwa Yehia El-Adawy. "User experience and user interface (UX & UI) of medical device displays: Systematic review of literature & outline of missing opportunities." *Journal of Art, Design and Music* 3, no. 2 (2024): 4.
22 Zayas-Cabán, Teresa, Tracy H. Okubo, and Steven Posnack. "Priorities to accelerate workflow automation in health care." *Journal of the American Medical Informatics Association* 30, no. 1 (2023): 195–201.
23 Rivera-Romero, Octavio, Elia Gabarron, Jorge Ropero, and Kerstin Denecke. "Designing personalised mHealth solutions: An overview." *Journal of Biomedical Informatics* 146 (2023): 104500.
24 Domecq, Juan Pablo, Gabriela Prutsky, Tarig Elraiyah, Zhen Wang, Mohammed Nabhan, Nathan Shippee, Juan Pablo Brito, Kasey Boehmer, Rim Hasan, Belal Firwana, Patricia Erwin, David Eton, Jeff Sloan, Victor Montori, Noor Asi, Abd Moain Abu Dabrh & Mohammad Hassan Murad. "Patient engagement in research: A systematic review." *BMC Health Services Research* 14 (2014): 1–9.
25 Oyibo, Kiemute, and Julita Vassileva. "The interplay of aesthetics, usability and credibility in mobile website design and the effect of gender." *Journal on Interactive Systems* 8, no. 2 (2017): 4–19.
26 Gawanmeh, Amjad, Hussam Al-Hamadi, Mahmoud Al-Qutayri, Shiu-Kai Chin, and Kashif Saleem. "Reliability analysis of healthcare information systems: State of the art and future directions." In *2015 17th International Conference on E-Health Networking, Application & Services (HealthCom)*, pp. 68–74. IEEE, 2015.
27 Akeel, Aisha Umar, and Darren Mundy. "Re-thinking technology and its growing role in enabling patient empowerment." *Health Informatics Journal* 25, no. 4 (2019): 1278–1289.

28 Chen, Peng-Ting, Chia-Li Lin, and Wan-Ning Wu. "Big data management in healthcare: Adoption challenges and implications." *International Journal of Information Management* 53 (2020): 102078.
29 Al Meslamani, Ahmad Z. "Technical and regulatory challenges of digital health implementation in developing countries." *Journal of Medical Economics* 26, no. 1 (2023): 1057–1060.
30 Huang, Chunya, Ross Koppel, John D. McGreevey III, Catherine K. Craven, and Richard Schreiber. "Transitions from one electronic health record to another: Challenges, pitfalls, and recommendations." *Applied Clinical Informatics* 11, no. 05 (2020): 742–754.
31 Jacob, Christine, Antonio Sanchez-Vazquez, and Chris Ivory. "Social, organizational, and technological factors impacting clinicians' adoption of mobile health tools: Systematic literature review." *JMIR mHealth and uHealth* 8, no. 2 (2020): e15935.
32 Stergiopoulos, Stella, Debra L. Michaels, Barbara Lopez Kunz, and Kenneth A. Getz. "Measuring the impact of patient engagement and patient centricity in clinical research and development." *Therapeutic Innovation & Regulatory Science* 54 (2020): 103–116.
33 Mennella, Ciro, Umberto Maniscalco, Giuseppe De Pietro, and Massimo Esposito. "Ethical and regulatory challenges of AI technologies in healthcare: A narrative review." *Heliyon* 10 (2024): 1–20.
34 Galsanjigmed, Enkhzul, and Tomoki Sekiguchi. "Challenges women experience in leadership careers: An integrative review." *Merits* 3, no. 2 (2023): 366–389.
35 Li, Jane, and Laurence S. Wilson. "Telehealth trends and the challenge for infrastructure." *Telemedicine and E-Health* 19, no. 10 (2013): 772–779.
36 Mondal, Jalaluddin, and Somnath Chakrabarti. "The abandonment behaviour of the branded app consumer: A study using interpretive structural modelling approach." *Journal of Retailing and Consumer Services* 63 (2021): 102695.
37 Jimenez, Laura M., and Carla K. Meyer. "First impressions matter: Navigating graphic novels utilizing linguistic, visual, and spatial resources." *Journal of Literacy Research* 48, no. 4 (2016): 423–447.
38 Rosenzweig, Elizabeth. *Successful User Experience: Strategies and Roadmaps*. San Francisco, CA: Morgan Kaufmann, 2015: 1–52.
39 Kumar, Navaneethakrishnan, and Arumbi Saravanan Sathish. "Understanding the influence of brand reputation and trust on loyalty: A mediated role of relationship." *PalArch's Journal of Archaeology of Egypt/Egyptology* 17 (2021): 8441–8457.
40 Korte, Brenda J., Anne Rompalo, Yukari C. Manabe, and Charlotte A. Gaydos. "Overcoming challenges with the adoption of point-of-care testing: From technology push and clinical needs to value propositions." *Point of Care* 19, no. 3 (2020): 77–83.
41 Alhur, Anas. "Overcoming electronic medical records adoption challenges in Saudi Arabia." *Cureus* 16, no. 2 (2024): 1–7.
42 Greenhalgh, Trisha, Rebecca Payne, Nina Hemmings, Helen Leach, Isabel Hanson, Anwar Khan, Lisa Miller, Emma Ladds, Aileen Clarke, Sara E Shaw, Francesca Dakin, Sietse Wieringa, Sarah Rybczynska-Bunt, Stuart D Faulkner, Richard Byng, Asli Kalin, Lucy Moore, Joseph Wherton, Laiba Husain, Rebecca Rosen. "Training needs for staff providing remote services in general practice: A mixed-methods study." *British Journal of General Practice* 74, no. 738 (2024): e17–e26.
43 Torab-Miandoab, Amir, Taha Samad-Soltani, Ahmadreza Jodati, and Peyman Rezaei-Hachesu. "Interoperability of heterogeneous health information systems: A systematic literature review." *BMC Medical Informatics and Decision Making* 23, no. 1 (2023): 18.

44 Kash, Bita Arbab, Aaron Spaulding, Christopher E. Johnson, and Larry Gamm. "Success factors for strategic change initiatives: A qualitative study of healthcare administrators' perspectives." *Journal of Healthcare Management* 59, no. 1 (2014): 65–81.
45 Jackson, C., and Caroline Nicholson. "Making integrated healthcare delivery happen-a framework for success." *Asia Pacific Journal of Health Management* 3, no. 2 (2008): 19–24.
46 Kim, Ambrose, and Kyoung-jae Kim. "User experience and the multi-stage adoption of mobile apps." *Journal of Information Technology Applications and Management* 21, no. 2 (2014): 49–79.
47 Burke, Matthew D., Melissa Keeney, Rochelle Kleinberg, and Rubi Burlage. "Challenges and opportunities for patient centric drug product design: Industry perspectives." *Pharmaceutical Research* 36 (2019): 1–7.
48 Abernethy, Amy, Laura Adams, Meredith Barrett, Christine Bechtel, Patricia Brennan, Atul Butte, Judith Faulkner et al. "The promise of digital health: Then, now, and the future." *NAM Perspectives* 2022 (2022): 1–24.
49 Bell, Sarah, Calvin D. Lawrence, Seth Dobrin, William Cherniak, Fernando De La Peña Llaca, Jefferson G. Fernandes, Aditi U. Joshi, and Geoffrey Rutledge. "Near-term digital health predictions: A glimpse into tomorrow's AI-driven healthcare." *Telehealth and Medicine Today* 8, no. 5 (2023): 1–6.

11 Blockchain for Clinical Trials and Research Data Integrity

Akhil Sharma, Sunita, Akanksha Sharma, Ashish Verma, Shaweta Sharma and Neeraj Kumar Fuloria

Introduction

Blockchain technology has revealed never-before-mentioned opportunities in the healthcare sector that are opening up the true value of interoperability. By harnessing various compelling attributes of blockchain technology like data provenance, transparency, decentralised transaction verification, and immutable data registry, stringent Clinical Trials (CTs) management challenges (e.g., subject recruitment, long-term follow-up and monitoring, clinical trial maintenance, and operational issues related to data analytics and reliable reporting) can efficiently be addressed. While multiple previous research studies have demonstrated the potential of blockchain solutions in enhancing patient retention, data integrity, and privacy and ensuring compliance of CTs with regulatory policy, a holistic review of this theme is missing. In this survey, we highlight the recent trends towards blockchain technology adoption in CTs. Using certain parameters, we establish a thorough taxonomy of the decentralised CT tasks and practices in order to help us organise and classify the literature.[1,2]

Clinical data management (CDM), a crucial step in clinical research, brings out good quality, reliable, and statistically valid data from clinical trials. Thus, it assists in saving the period from drug development to marketing to an extreme extent. CDM team members participated in every aspect of a clinical trial from beginning to end. They must possess sufficient process knowledge that aids in upholding the quality standards of CDM processes. During a trial, different activities such as designing of case report form (CRF), CRF annotation, database designing, data entry, data validation, discrepancy management and medical coding, data extraction, and locking of the clinical trial database are amply checked for quality abound. Under the current scenario, there has been increased pressure to raise CDM standards, as the regulatory need while competing in the market is faster commercialisation of the products. Regulatory-compliant data management tools will meet these demands of the CDM Team. It is also compulsory for corporations to furnish the data electronically. CDM professionals expected appropriate setting up data quality benchmarks and an urge to respond to the fast-paced technology transition. Inherent data storage space will be obtained from the blockchain

DOI: 10.4324/9781003529910-11

during the application process to guarantee that existing transaction data will not be modified or deleted.[3,4]

Blockchain technology for transaction verification can be used to analyse and confirm that information data is real and reliable without any third-party authentication. Historical transactions are untamperable, which guarantees the authenticity and effectiveness of the data stored. For those applications of blockchain technology, the application of the cryptographic algorithm and digital signature identity authentication and authenticity technology is more common; it can highlight the advantages that blockchain architecture encapsulated access control at both read-write levels with many data types, simply as one sub-method to enhance security for specific blockchain technologies during real-life applications. Nowadays, accompanied by the development of information technology, the application of blockchain technology is gradually becoming more mature and perfect. The non-tamper and decentralisation of its data quality are the key foundations that enable the exertion of blockchain technology advantages. One of the important means to improve data security technology and management level is through effective prevention of security risks, especially in the Internet of Things (IoT) environment, which collects large amounts of sensitive private information and restricts its mass transmission and secure storage process. The process of data processing and application without effective security measures may lead to the loss, leakage, or expiration of data. Such issues will all have some degree of influence on data integrity and damage the application value of data in the IoT environment. Hence, the successful implementation of blockchain technology in clinical research provide benefit for storing and managing of data. The inherent decentralised and anonymous nature of blockchain technology, which can verify the integrity of data without transferring the entire data to the network server, makes it potential to address the problem that privacy-preserving is needed in data integrity verification.[5,6]

Importance of Data Integrity in Clinical Research

Data integrity is important to ensure the collected raw data, after processing, is valid, complete, and well documented. The objective of data integrity is to ensure that all the data, which include original records and observations such as any other documented activity that is necessary to reconstruct the clinical trial along with the assurance of the safety, efficacy, and quality of the product, should be accessible, intact, valid and genuine.[7] Reasons why data integrity is essential in clinical research are shown in Figure 11.1.

Ensures Patient Safety

Data integrity ensures that the clinical trial outcomes, and by extension, patient safety, remain protected since the data itself would be real and constant. Data misrepresentation, tampering, or unintentional errors can lead to false conclusions regarding treatment safety and efficacy resulting in patients being put at risk.

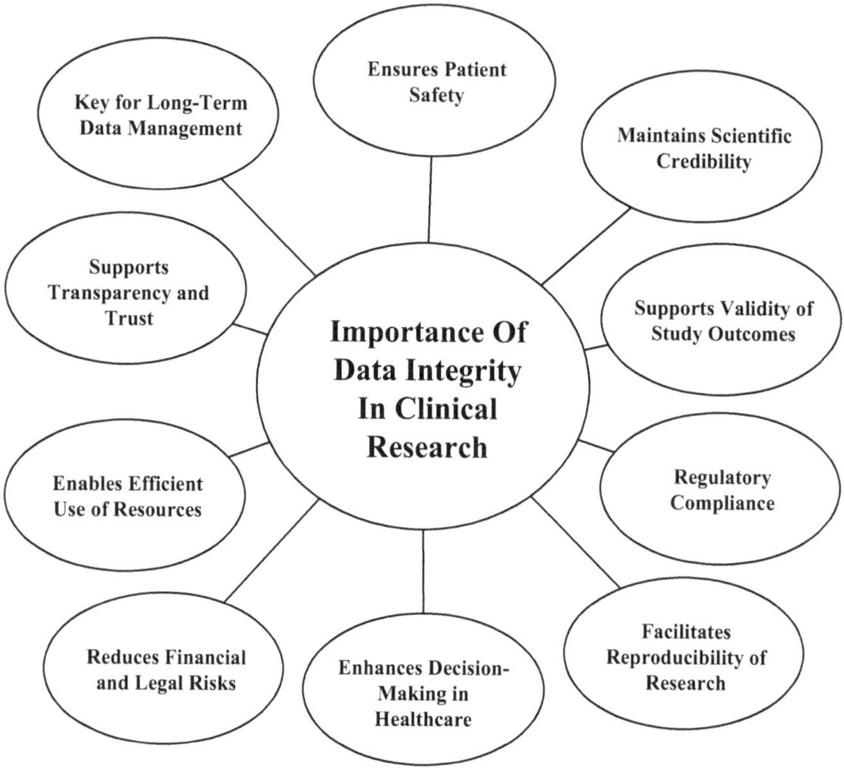

Figure 11.1 Importance of Data Integrity in Clinical Research.

Regulatory Compliance

It is already heavily regulated by guidelines and standards set forth by the U.S. Food and Drug Administration (FDA), European Medicines Agency (EMA), and other regulatory agencies that govern clinical research. Data integrity standards are extremely rigid with these agencies. If not followed, penalties can be imposed, the trial may be suspended, and even drug acceptance or appropriation by authorities may be denied.[8]

Maintains Scientific Credibility

Data integrity is important for any study hoping to be scientifically valid. If the data is accurate and consistent, and therefore, the results are trustworthy, it can add value to scientific knowledge. Sound data integrity, on the other hand, enhances the quality of research as important by way of credibility and recognition to researchers.

Supports Validity of Study Outcomes

Data integrity ensures that the conclusions drawn from a study are based on genuine and unaltered data. This is crucial for the validity of the study's outcomes, which inform clinical decision-making and policy development.[9]

Facilitates Reproducibility of Research

Reproducibility is a cornerstone of scientific research. Maintaining data integrity enables other researchers to reproduce the study and verify the results, reinforcing the study's findings and building a foundation for future research.

Enhances Decision-Making in Healthcare

Data from clinical trials influence medical practices and treatment guidelines. Reliable data ensure that healthcare professionals make informed decisions based on sound evidence, leading to better patient outcomes.[10]

Reduces Financial and Legal Risks

Inaccurate or falsified data can lead to significant financial losses, including costly delays in drug development and potential legal liabilities. Ensuring data integrity helps prevent these risks by providing a solid foundation for clinical research.

Enables Efficient Use of Resources

Good quality data is also essential to ensure that resources, like time and money, are not spent on extraneous efforts. When data quality is poor, studies (or indeed re-analysis) will often need to be repeated, resulting in a misallocation of resources.[11]

Supports Transparency and Trust

Control over data integrity establishes transparency and trust among stakeholders such as regulatory authorities, funding bodies, researchers, healthcare providers, and patients. This trust is critical for accepting new treatments and continuous support of clinical research projects.[12]

Key for Long-Term Data Management

Clinical research can often require revisiting data for longitudinal analysis or other follow-up studies. Starting with intact data helps streamline the process of handling, analysing, and verifying future data especially. It follows that data integrity is critical, which represents the core of ethical clinical research, regulatory compliance, and advancement of science.

Need of Blockchain in Clinical Trials and Research Data

Blockchain technology, which is involved in clinical trials and managing research data, is a solution for some challenges like data integrity, transparency, and patient empowerment. Blockchain, as an immutable decentralised framework, increases the traceability of clinical trial processes and consequently reduces the opportunity for misconduct and fraud. With implementations such as time-stamping and smart contracts, a blockchain can record every interaction with very clear evidence of the previous chain of events. Such a tool would not just strengthen trust between stakeholders but also wire up-the-spot monitoring and spirit of regulatory compliance. In addition, blockchain enables patients to ownership their data and see how it is used in trials. Better access increases participation in clinical research and improves the data itself. While there is no shortage of information surrounding blockchain technology in healthcare, the article provides an overview of its potential to retain the efficiency and integrity of clinical trials due to high levels of security and reliance on decentralised databases.[13]

Challenges in Clinical Trials and Research Data

The challenges associated in clinical trials and research data are discussed in Figure 11.2.

Data Integrity and Reliability

Data integrity, on the other hand, means preserving the accuracy and consistency of data over its entire lifecycle. The data is guaranteed to be original, unchanged, and valid as it was at the time of collection until it is retained or deleted. This means safeguarding data from corruption, unauthorised access, or unwanted changes, whether it is original raw data from malfunctions, human error, or a cyber-attack. Data integrity focuses on accuracy (correct representation of information), consistency (the same character across the systems), and completeness. Data integrity is essential to making sure that the data used for decision-making processes are sound and reproducible.[14]

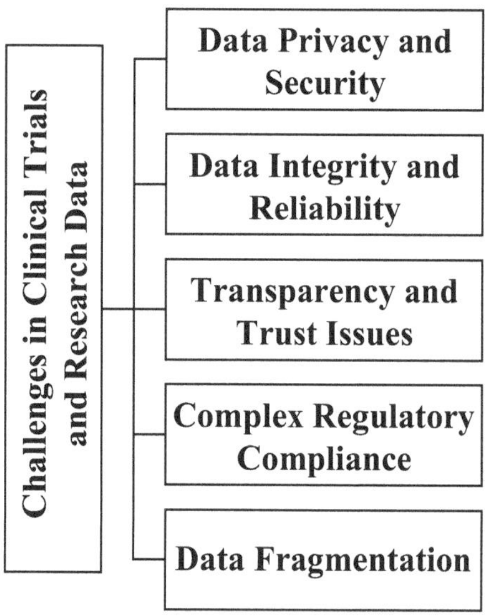

Figure 11.2 Challenges in Clinical Trials and Research Data.

Data reliability is the ability of data to be good and valuable over time. So, it refers to the degree of repeatability and variation in data that may provide similar results through measurements or analysis under different conditions. Standardised, repeatable methods produce reliable data; the information will be constant and trustworthy for decision-making. It is important for mitigating variability and uncertainty in any data-driven processes and boosting confidence in analysis results. In scientific research, healthcare, finance, and diverse other industries where reliable and repeatable results are crucial for reaching valid conclusions and making sound decisions, data efficiency is an essential element.[15]

Data Privacy and Security

Digital health technology presents challenges to bringing standards up to date concerning privacy, safety, ethics, and regulation. The use of digital technology and remote monitoring increases the risk of security breaches involving the improper collection, dissemination, or storage of data. Some of these data, namely global positioning system (GPS)/location data, may place trial participants in greater jeopardy than anticipated at a great personal and economic cost of stigma (e.g. litigation). In pursuit of this, the FDA has incorporated cybersecurity into finding ways to certify such medical devices. While we are working on increasing the patient's access, the risks and benefits of sharing patient data either individually or assembled have to be communicated with all stakeholders. Confidential databases will still be at risk of breaches but dispersed ledgers like blockchain or decentralised databases will lower the risk. The need for guidance for digital trials, especially related to consent requirements, reporting, and oversight, will be addressed through further work with IRBs. For instance, a site-less study may include virtual visits crossing state lines or international boundaries instead of at an actual physical study site and the variable state regulations around investigator oversight must be accounted for trials to zone function appropriately. While the Interstate Medical Licensure Compact may resolve this uniformity issue by enabling multiple states to join an agreement, all states and territories must be encouraged to participate under cross-state telehealth licensing agreements. Moreover, documentation of informed consent will need to include remote consent technologies but remains critical to ensure the coverage of individuals' consent on data collection, transmission, sharing, and security.[16]

Transparency and Trust Issues

Data handling transparency is when you do not disclose the processes involved in data collection, storage and analysis and share of all such information. In clinical research, this may mean undisclosed data modifications, selective result reporting, or withholding raw data from regulators and other scientists. Stakeholders, both internal and external, may not be able to confirm the accuracy of results if they cannot access reliable data or information on how it is managed. In such cases, it impedes the replication of study findings and compromises research credibility while leading to a general erosion of public confidence in the results. Transparency of data handling is therefore essential for independent verification; it ensures that the data relied upon to make decisions follows sound methodologies.[17]

Trusting the authenticity of trial results is paramount, as clinical research provides the basis for healthcare practices, drug approvals, and policy decisions. If the practices for handling data are not clear or there is potential for manifest manipulation of data, this casts doubt on the integrity of the results. As a result, it makes people doubt that the results reflect true intervention benefits and instead are affected by biases, i.e. commercial interests or pressure to publish positive findings. In addition, we have seen a loss of trust in clinical trials and the organisations that conduct them due to the discovery of data fabrication/falsification/withholding of relevant data. Put simply, rigorous adherence to the highest ethical standards, transparent reporting of results, and third-party validation are essential for building trust in the integrity of trial results.[18]

Complex Regulatory Compliance

Difficulty in Meeting Requirements

Clinical research organisations routinely struggle to meet the requirements of the regulatory standards set forth by bodies like the FDA and the EMA due to their complexity and strictness. These agencies govern specific rules of data collection, storage, monitoring, and reporting to guarantee that new treatments are safe and effective. Compliance is primarily about GCP, but as regulations change over time or from region to region, compliance must also provide the flexibility needed. Dealing with these requirements is not only time-consuming but also resource-intensive and requires expertise to interpret the regulations correctly and implement them on the right side. This can make compliance a challenge and lead to delayed timelines, higher costs, and sometimes rejection of the trial data or approval application.[18]

Managing Regulatory Documents and Audit Trails

Handling regulatory documents and audit trails is an integral part of compliance in clinical research, yet it is a challenging endeavour. There is no shortage of paperwork in clinical trials, with protocols, informed consent forms, CRFs, and safety reports needing to be carefully filed, updated, and made available for inspection. A relevant audit trail will also ensure that any changes made to the data during a study are recorded along with an appropriate justification (traceability and data integrity). Handling such records, maintaining version control, and accessing and securing data must all be very well documented. The risk here is that if regulatory documents and audit trails are not properly managed, it results in noncompliance, a fine, or even worse, invalidation of trial result.[19]

Data Fragmentation

Information management is plagued by data fragmentation. This means that data is distributed across multiple storages, and little analysis can be done from it, or accessing the required data becomes a hassle. For starters, data fragmentation refers to both physical and logical fragments. Fragmentation in physical terms means that files are far apart on different servers, maybe even in other countries or hosted devices through data clouds as a model. At the same time, logical fragmentation occurs due to having multiple versions of the same data on various platforms. Fragmented data is inconsistent, difficult to aggregate together, and takes longer to retrieve. This type of mess is hard to control with data. This complicates maintaining a single source of truth. This problem is about who knows what about the customer and running things inside the organisation. It undermines the ambition of creating a strong data-organisational culture. Companies find it difficult to utilise their data fully due to fragmentation that occurs for various reasons.[20] These problems arise primarily from the following causes:

Data Silos

Data silos develop when different departments in an organisation deploy their systems without collaboration. Having these systems apart makes it difficult to integrate data. This means that without talking through important concepts, teams will duplicate work upon work and share data in various locations. This prevents it from getting a complete view of what data the company holds.

Duplicate Data

Duplicate data emerges when a company creates multiple copies of the same information for various purposes. It causes the data to become unmanageable. Often, not having one single source of truth means that it can be difficult to know which data is correct and keep track of all the disparate datasets.[21]

File Sharing Practices

The fragmentation of data can worsen this problem due to inefficiency in sharing files. When data travels between teams or places, it spreads out even more. This adds more copies and conceals the nature of the data mutations. Following all the versions and updates is a huge work.[22]

Blockchain Solutions for Clinical Trials

Decentralised Data Management

Immutable and Transparent Records for Clinical Data

The use of decentralised data management in clinical research allows for the establishment of immutable and transparent records for optional clinical data. For example, blockchain – using this technology, data entries can be permanently recorded so that no tampering is done on the register. Every data entry or transaction is timestamped and secured via a cryptographic hash, resulting in a verifiable record of every action performed in the clinical trial. This immutable nature addresses problems like data manipulation, fraud, or selective reporting because all players have the same unchangeable version of the data. The process of conducting clinical research becomes a step-by-step, transparent, and immutable record; this goes a long way to demonstrate trust in the process, including real-time monitoring and verification of data integrity (which cannot be altered even by the sponsors) at every level throughout an entire trial.[23]

Consensus Mechanisms for Data Validation

In decentralised data management, consensus mechanisms are essential to guaranteeing data integrity and reliability through a distributed agreement between multiple participants. These mechanisms can be applied to clinical research by demanding that data entries acquire validation from a distributed network of nodes (participants) before being entered into the blockchain. The data itself cannot be changed by one party in a way that may lead to bias or manipulation. Examples include consensus protocols (i.e., Proof of Work, Proof of Stake, or Practical Byzantine Fault Tolerance) that create a majority agreement to confirm the truthfulness of the data. Decentralised systems can improve data quality, foster transparency, and make sure that clinical trial results are verifiable and accurate by using consensus mechanisms for data validation.[24]

Smart Contracts

Automating Trial Processes (e.g., Informed Consent)

In clinical research, smart contracts can automate different trial processes, including but not limited to informed consent management. These blockchain-based agreements execute themselves and trigger automatic actions when certain criteria are met. One example is informed consent, through which smart contract technology can automatically verify study participants with all the necessary information needed to enter the experiment, as well as ensure that they comprehend this knowledge while tracking their consent via a secure and encrypted record on the blockchain. Automating these steps reduces administrative burden, human error, and regulatory compliance. Similarly, smart contracts could also trigger notifications or follow-up tasks (e.g., reminding participants that their consent may need to be renewed), and in both cases, updating records where appropriate. Automation of these trial processes brings efficiency along with the fact that all activities are performed safely and transparently.[25]

Facilitating Real-Time Updates to Protocol Changes

Moreover, smart contracts can allow clinical trial protocols to be updated during the trial in near real-time, providing flexibility to trial management. Any time a protocol changes, such as a change to dosing schedules, eligibility criteria, or monitoring requirements, smart contracts can automatically enforce new rules throughout the system and update relevant parties in real time. Additionally, since protocol conditions are embedded within the smart contract code, all network participants (including investigators and regulators) can reference updated versions instantly through a decentralised network. Minimising time lag in rolling out changes enhances compliance with the new processes and achieves consistency in how trials are done.[26]

Secure Data Sharing and Access Control

Cryptography for Secure and Selective Data Sharing

Cryptography is key for secure and selective data sharing in clinical research. Encryption and digital signature techniques restrict sensitive clinical data so that access is only possible to authorised individuals. Encryption renders data only readable to those with the proper decryption keys, therefore protecting patient privacy and keeping it away from unauthorised users. There also exist cryptographic methods to selectively share data among individuals, where researchers can allow limited access to certain parties, like regulators, research partners, or service providers, on a case-by-case basis. By managing the access through it, sensitive information only gets shared on a need-to-know basis, which mitigates the data breach risk as well as ensures compliance with privacy regulations.[27]

Permissioned Blockchains for Controlled Data Access

In clinical research, permissioned blockchains enable a model for decentralised but controlled data access. When it comes to types of blockchain, permissioned blockchains differ from public ones that anyone can use; only a specific group of trusted participants (e.g. clinical researchers, regulators, and healthcare institutions) have access to permissioned ones. These types of blockchains employ access control mechanisms to define the capabilities of various parties with respect to reading, writing, or validating data on these ledgers, ensuring that only authorised entities can interact with the data. Such a controlled ecosystem helps maintain data privacy, assists with regulations such as GDPR or HIPAA, and facilitates the safe sharing of clinical data between institutions. With permissioned blockchains, information can be accessed and collaborated, much like other databases, but with rules and frameworks that ensure the security and integrity of the data.[28]

Tokenisation and Incentive Systems

Reward Mechanisms for Data Sharing and Participation

The process of tokenisation applied in clinical research can also establish reward-based schemes for incentivising data sharing and participation. Digital tokens can then be given in a way similar to many other areas where individuals, researchers, or institutions contribute valuable data or actually engage in the study. Patients can be rewarded tokens when they provide their health information or follow up for a survey, which is routed back to them as discounts on healthcare or benefits services and might also come in the form of cash. This incentivisation drives deeper engagement and better data capture along with patient involvement through the trial. Researchers are incentivised to share their datasets or work together, establishing an openness and data exchange ecosystem in the scientific community, thanks to token-based reward systems.[29]

Tokenised Access to Data for Research Collaborators

Tokenisation can also help manage access to clinical data, whereby research collaborators use tokens as a means of restricting access rights. In a token system, access to the data can be given to collaborators who hold a defined number of tokens (which equate to permission to view or analyse specific datasets). Here, we can make access precise by just explaining how much or what type of tokens should be owned by the researcher, and we can update the change so that a researcher gets access. It would make data-sharing contracts visible and traceable, helping to ensure that they use data in ways that are ethical and comply with legal norms. Tokenised access offers a controllable and collaborative solution by allowing the ability to set specific permissions for data in order to separate sensitive clinical data from less secure information.[30]

Ensuring Data Integrity with Blockchain

Blockchain technology offers a solid structure for maintaining data integrity at numerous layers of application. The decentralised, immutable, and cryptographically secure nature of blockchain makes it a great service for storing and protecting data. An in-depth discussion on how blockchain delivers data integrity using a number of mechanisms.

Data Timestamping

Creating Verifiable Records with Timestamps

All transactions are time-stamped on a blockchain, and this gives an order of events. Not only can the data verification be done, but it also provides a definitive audit and compliance trail of actions taken.

Tracking the Provenance of Data

The immutable and traceable nature of blockchain allows tracking the provenance of data as well. Every modification or addition to the data is logged in an immutable way, maintaining the source and history of the data.[31]

Version Control

Managing Data Changes and Updates across Trial Sites

When running multi-centre trials, keeping the same data across different sites is paramount. This is made possible because blockchain creates a single source of truth that everyone in the network can refer to. All sites have access to the same information, and any changes or updates are made in real time.

Ensuring Consistency in Multi-Centre Trials

The decentralised ledger of blockchain can minimise inconsistencies in data. It gives every trial site the ability to independently verify the data integrity of what they receive, and so trust and uniformity across all key stakeholders.[32]

Preventing Data Tampering

Cryptographic Techniques to Secure Data against Alterations

Blockchain uses cutting-edge cryptographic technologies to protect data records. Each block includes a unique hash connecting it to the previous one; should any data be altered, its corresponding hash would revert to another value, thus signalling distortion.

Using Consensus Protocols to Validate Data Entries

The consensus mechanisms (proof of work and proof of stake, etc.) will be checked, and only valid transactions will be added to the blockchain. This collective decision by the participants in the network ensures that no one can guarantee locking or changing anything and ensures preventative security.[33]

Auditable Data Trails

Maintaining a Traceable History of All Data Interactions

Blockchain does not own the data, so it has a full audit trail of every transaction or interaction with it. For regulatory compliance, this traceability is priceless as it will allow organisations to showcase their adherence through transparent records.

Enabling Efficient Regulatory Audits and Inspections

This unchanging nature of records on the blockchain makes audits very easy as they give auditors an indisputable history of transactions. Such transparency ensures that the audit does not take much time and also instils confidence in the auditors regarding the correctness of the data they are auditing.[34]

Integration with Existing Clinical Trial Systems

Interoperability with Electronic Health Records

The ability to interface with electronic health records (EHR as integration of clinical trial information into patient health records is indispensable. Connecting trial data with EHRs can provide researchers with a wealth of information regarding each patient, such as their medical history, demographics, and concurrent treatments. Linking trial results with records of care providers helps improve the context of what is gained from trials. It enables improved patient selection and management during a trial, compared to ordinary clinical practice. It allows patient records to be updated in real-time, meaning that what is learned from clinical trials can help guide care being provided for patients at that very moment and the other way around. For this integration, it is important to set up secure data exchange protocols from EHRs to blockchain systems that allow for the efficient communication and sharing of data while ensuring patient privacy and compliance with health regulations.[35]

Data Standards and Protocols

The standardisation of protocols like Fast Healthcare Interoperability Resources (FHIR) is a must for clinical trials to ensure that data sharing and integration can happen seamlessly. It enables systems (including blockchain platforms) and EHRs to communicate with each other in a standard way using FHIR. In this way, researchers will be able to make sure that the compliance of the clinical trial data, along with blockchain data matching foreseeable regulatory requirements, has a good degree of interoperability. Such standardisation improves data quality and explains how stakeholders across the clinical research ecosystem work together, leading to faster and better clinical trials. Using data standards guarantees that everyone involved in a clinical trial will talk about the same thing, and every dataset will be interpreted correctly without ambiguity. The data standards protocol are described in Table 11.1.[36]

Future Opportunities and Trends

Decentralised clinical trials will vastly change the future of clinical research by making patient recruitment and engagement easier while decreasing costs and logistical hurdles. These trials harness digital tools and remote monitoring, providing wider access to patients across demographic backgrounds with the ability for participants to join their trials from home and interact more flexibly. As a result, in addition to enhancing recruitment rates, this method improves participant retention and satisfaction while also making clinical research more inclusive and streamlined.[37]

Moreover, the incorporation of new-age technologies like Artificial Intelligence, IoT and big data analytics offer promising innovations for clinical trials. Integrating blockchain with these technologies can ensure security and trust in the data collected from IoT devices, enabling fast and accurate results as well as a large ecosystem of data for researchers to leverage. By monitoring patient data in real-time, adaptive trial protocols permit rapid response to safety issues and the

Table 11.1 Data Standards Protocols

Topic	*Description*
Compliance with data protection regulations	Compliance with regulations such as GDPR and HIPAA means protecting personal data, employing reasonable safeguards, and providing access to individuals. Researchers must play Pudding direction behaviour up to points of settlement funds and requisition their systems with relation action. The immutable and transparent record helps regulatory compliance, which is really important for them. Its distributed nature can aid in preserving the integrity of the data and compliance with data protection rules.[38]
Patient consent and data ownership	Every patient will be able to own their health data using blockchain, which will provide access and set conditions on who can access the data. It encourages patient participation and autonomy in clinical research. Consent, in particular, raises problems of ethically valid management regarding its information content, voluntariness, and possibility of revocation. This means that researchers may need to create systems that show what data is used and respect patients' wishes regarding their information.[39]
Blockchain governance models	Blockchain governance models describe rules, protocols, and decision-making processes to operate the blockchain networks with data sharing. Good governance allows the network to operate transparently and fairly. For good governance, precise delineation of the roles and responsibilities of stakeholders patients, researchers, data managers, and regulators—is very important. Such transparency encourages responsibility and reduces potential conflicts of interest in the blockchain environment.[40]

opportunity for personalised treatment strategies, which may enhance both trial efficacy and, subsequently, patient outcomes. The momentum instead is towards the patient more user-driven models in which individuals own and control their health data. This enhances patient autonomy over data access, which minimises the complication of transparency and helps to gain trust within data practice. Tokenised Data Marketplaces Tokenised data marketplaces are a new way to approach research collaboration through direct token sales for patient data with an emphasis on patient safety. This not only helps with data availability to drive research but also creates a culture of using such data while upholding patient privacy and consent, leading the way for the future of clinical innovations.[41,42]

Challenges and Limitations

Technical Barriers

While blockchain has significant potential to improve clinical research, its use is limited by various technical challenges. From the scalability of current blockchain networks, most of which cannot accommodate the large data volume generated during clinical trials. Since healthcare apps require high transaction throughput and fast processing time, existing blockchain solutions may come short of providing sufficient or satisfactory performance. Moreover, there are significant challenges associated with the complexity of integrating blockchain into existing healthcare systems. Most of the organisations are running on legacy systems, which will not talk to new technologies without programming this will take significant engineering capabilities and resources to create natural interoperability.[43]

Adoption and Awareness

There are also barriers to the adoption and awareness of blockchain technology in healthcare, including a reluctance to change within the industry. There may be resistance to adopting new technology among many stakeholders, including healthcare providers, researchers, and regulatory bodies, who worry about data security, regulatory compliance, and the general disruption of well-established workflows. In other words, to overcome this resistance, we will need to not only show the impact of blockchain but also understand the cultural and organisational challenges that will help us come up with new solutions. In addition, there is an urgent necessity for education and training about blockchain technology because numerous professionals in the healthcare sector are not familiar with its concepts and applications. Adequate training to help develop the know-how and expertise required for successful implementation and integration.[44]

Cost and Resource Considerations

Two more reasons standing in the way of blockchain adoption in clinical research are those related to cost and resource management. The steep upfront costs of implementing blockchain systems can be off-putting for organisations, especially smaller institutions or startups with limited budgets. These costs are not just the hardware and software but also training staff and reengineering processes to fit new systems. Furthermore, it does create challenges with long-term maintenance and sustainability problems because organisations subsequently have to look at continual operational costs of running the apps, updating them, and possible scalability requirements as their data and usage increase. Financial implications must be assessed by organisations considering the deployment of blockchain technology in the world of clinical research, and collaborative models or sources of funds to support this agenda should be regarded as success.[45,46]

Conclusion

Blockchain technology offers a transformative opportunity to advance the integrity and efficiency of research data and stakeholders in healthcare clinical trials. Blockchain helps to combat serious issues like data manipulation, transparency, and adherence to regulatory guidelines by adding a secure, transparent, and permanent foundation for managing data exposure. Decentralised clinical trials enable more patient-centric approaches and recruitment by reducing logistical hurdles, making it possible to conduct research in a wider range of real-world environments and leading the way towards more scalable and convenient sexual health research methods. However, to gain the most from the potential of blockchain technology in clinical trials, strategic partnerships involving stakeholders such as researchers, healthcare providers, regulatory bodies, and technology partners need to be created. Organisations will need to overcome various technical and cultural barriers and additionally commit time and resources to education, training, and awareness. Establishing data integrity best practices and taking steps to align initiatives with the relevant regulatory framework is a major part of building trust and compliance. Moving ahead, the road ahead for further research and development will be key to opening up postulations for blockchain in clinical research. Stakeholders can build on and expand the use of blockchain with increased interoperability, scalability, and incorporation of new technologies to further enhance patient care and medical research. As the landscape of clinical trials evolves, the adoption of blockchain technology will serve to improve data integrity while also driving a more patient-centric and collaborative healthcare innovation process.

References

1 Omar, Ilhaam A., Raja Jayaraman, Khaled Salah, Ibrar Yaqoob, and Samer Ellahham. "Applications of blockchain technology in clinical trials: Review and open challenges." *Arabian Journal for Science and Engineering* 46, no. 4 (2021): 3001–3015.

2 Mohammed Abdul, Shezon Saleem. "Navigating blockchain's twin challenges: Scalability and regulatory compliance." *Blockchains* 2, no. 3 (2024): 265–298.

3 El Fadly, AbdenNaji, Bastien Rance, Noël Lucas, Charles Mead, Gilles Chatellier, Pierre-Yves Lastic, Marie-Christine Jaulent, and Christel Daniel. "Integrating clinical research with the Healthcare Enterprise: From the RE-USE project to the EHR4CR platform." *Journal of Biomedical Informatics* 44 (2011): S94–S102.

4 Chilukuri, Harihar, Narasimha Pothula Reddy, Ram Mohan Pathapati, Arkalgud Nagesha Manu, Sharada Jollu, and Ahammed Basha Shaik. "Acute antidepressant effects of intramuscular versus intravenous ketamine." *Indian Journal of Psychological Medicine* 36, no. 1 (2014): 71–76.

5 Hayes, Adam. "Blockchain facts: What is it, how it works, and how it can be used." *Investopedia* (2022). https://www.investopedia.com/terms/b/blockchain.asp

6 Habib, Gousia, Sparsh Sharma, Sara Ibrahim, Imtiaz Ahmad, Shaima Qureshi, and Malik Ishfaq. "Blockchain technology: Benefits, challenges, applications, and integration of blockchain technology with cloud computing." *Future Internet* 14, no. 11 (2022): 341.

7 Wallach, Joshua D., Gregg S. Gonsalves, and Joseph S. Ross. "Research, regulatory, and clinical decision-making: The importance of scientific integrity." *Journal of Clinical Epidemiology* 93 (2018): 88–93.

8 Gogtay, Nithya J., Renju Ravi, and Urmila M. Thatte. "Regulatory requirements for clinical trials in India: What academicians need to know." *Indian Journal of Anaesthesia* 61, no. 3 (2017): 192–199.

9 Hawkins, Melanie, Gerald R. Elsworth, Sandra Nolte, and Richard H. Osborne. "Validity arguments for patient-reported outcomes: Justifying the intended interpretation and use of data." *Journal of Patient-Reported Outcomes* 5 (2021): 1–14.

10 Titler, Marita G. "The evidence for evidence-based practice implementation." *Patient Safety and Quality: An Evidence-Based Handbook for Nurses* 1 (2008): 113–160.

11 Botha, Marna, Adele Botha, and Marlien Herselman. "Data quality challenges: A content analysis in the e-health domain." In *2014 4th World Congress on Information and Communication Technologies (*WICT 2014), pp. 107–112. IEEE, 2014.

12 Maki, Kevin C., Joshua W. Miller, George P. McCabe, Gowri Raman, and Penny M. Kris-Etherton. "Perspective: Laboratory considerations and clinical data management for human nutrition randomised controlled trials: Guidance for ensuring quality and integrity." *Advances in Nutrition* 12, no. 1 (2021): 46–58.

13 Zhuang, Yan, Lincoln R. Sheets, Zonyin Shae, Yin-Wu Chen, Jeffrey JP Tsai, and Chi-Ren Shyu. "Applying blockchain technology to enhance clinical trial recruitment." In *AMIA Annual Symposium Proceedings*, vol. 2019, p. 1276. American Medical Informatics Association, 2019.

14 Ildstad, Suzanne T., and Charles H. Evans Jr, eds. *Small clinical trials: Issues and challenges*. Washington DC: National Academy Press (2001).

15 Sabale, Mrunal M., Varun A. Pande, Amol A. Tagalpallewar, Arti G. Swami, Anil T. Pawar, and Akshay M. Baheti. "Maintaining data safety and accuracy through data integrity (DI): A comprehensive review." *Research Journal of Pharmacy and Technology* 17, no. 5 (2024): 2431–2440.

16 Choudhary, Puneetha. "Digital information security and privacy protection in healthcare sector in India." *Indian Journal of Law & Legal Research* 4, no. 2 (2022): 1.

17 Morey, Timothy, Theodore Forbath, and Allison Schoop. "Customer data: Designing for transparency and trust." *Harvard Business Review* 93, no. 5 (2015): 96–105.

18 Institute of Medicine (US) Committee on Health Research and the Privacy of Health Information. "The value, importance, and oversight of health research." *Beyond the HIPAA Privacy Rule: Enhancing Privacy, Improving Health Through Research* (2009): 111–152.

19 Raja Rajeswari, K., C. H. Sri Durga, and V. Rama Mohan Gupta. "Regulatory challenges in clinical trials: Strategies to overcome commonly observed deficiencies." *Journal of Intellectual Property Rights* 24 (2019): 140–148.

20 Castro-Medina, Felipe, Lisbeth Rodríguez-Mazahua, María Antonieta Abud-Figueroa, Celia Romero-Torres, Luis Ángel Reyes-Hernández, and Giner Alor-Hernández. "Application of data fragmentation and replication methods in the cloud: A review." In *2019 International Conference on Electronics, Communications and Computers (CONIELECOMP)*, pp. 47–54. IEEE, 2019.

21 Xia, Wen, Hong Jiang, Dan Feng, Fred Douglis, Philip Shilane, Yu Hua, Min Fu, Yucheng Zhang, and Yukun Zhou. "A comprehensive study of the past, present, and future of data deduplication." *Proceedings of the IEEE* 104, no. 9 (2016): 1681–1710.

22 Maslove, David M., Jacob Klein, Kathryn Brohman, and Patrick Martin. "Using blockchain technology to manage clinical trials data: A proof-of-concept study." *JMIR Medical Informatics* 6, no. 4 (2018): e11949.

23 Hang, Lei, Chun Chen, Linchao Zhang, and Jun Yang. "Blockchain for applications of clinical trials: Taxonomy, challenges, and future directions." *IET Communications* 16, no. 20 (2022): 2371–2393.
24 Nguyen, Cong T., Dinh Thai Hoang, Diep N. Nguyen, Dusit Niyato, Huynh Tuong Nguyen, and Eryk Dutkiewicz. "Proof-of-stake consensus mechanisms for future blockchain networks: Fundamentals, applications and opportunities." *IEEE Access* 7 (2019): 85727–85745.
25 Abdelhamid, Manar, and Ghada Hassan. "Blockchain and smart contracts." In *Proceedings of the 8th International Conference on Software and Information Engineering*, pp. 91–95, 2019.
26 Park, Yu Rang, Young Jo Yoon, HaYeong Koo, Soyoung Yoo, Chang-Min Choi, Sung-Ho Beck, and Tae Won Kim. "Utilization of a clinical trial management system for the whole clinical trial process as an integrated database: System development." *Journal of Medical Internet Research* 20, no. 4 (2018): e9312.
27 Wang, Zhiqiang, Wenjing Gao, Ming Yang, and Rong Hao. "Enabling secure data sharing with data deduplication and sensitive information hiding in cloud-assisted electronic medical systems." *Cluster Computing* 26, no. 6 (2023): 3839–3854.
28 Helliar, Christine V., Louise Crawford, Laura Rocca, Claudio Teodori, and Monica Veneziani. "Permissionless and permissioned blockchain diffusion." *International Journal of Information Management* 54 (2020): 102136.
29 Janowski, Andrzej. "Natural language processing techniques for clinical text analysis in healthcare." *Journal of Advanced Analytics in Healthcare Management* 7, no. 1 (2023): 51–76.
30 Kondra, Sarika, Wu Xu, and Vijay V. Raghavan. "Unlocking the power of clinical notes: Natural language processing in healthcare." *Acta Scientific Medical Sciences* (ISSN: 2582-0931) 8, no. 6 (2024): 37–44.
31 Javaid, Uzair, Muhammad Naveed Aman, and Biplab Sikdar. "Blockpro: Blockchain based data provenance and integrity for secure IoT environments." In *Proceedings of the 1st Workshop on Blockchain-Enabled Networked Sensor Systems*, pp. 13–18, 2018.
32 Treiblmaier, Horst, Abderahman Rejeb, Mike Gault, Anjum Khurshid, Alex Norta, Jim Poteet, and Suresh Sivagnanam. "Harnessing blockchain to transform healthcare data management: A comprehensive research agenda." *Blockchain in Healthcare Today* 7 (2024): 10–30.
33 Sriman, B., S. Ganesh Kumar, and Prabakaran Shamili. "Blockchain technology: Consensus protocol proof of work and proof of stake." In *Intelligent Computing and Applications: Proceedings of ICICA 2019*, pp. 395–406. Springer Singapore, 2021.
34 Singh, Manpreet, Mahesh Joshi, Sharad Sharma, and Tarek Rana. "How blockchain is transforming accounting, auditing and finance: A systematic review." *Handbook of Big Data and Analytics in Accounting and Auditing* (2023): 535–560.
35 Tiase, Victoria L., William Hull, Mary M. McFarland, Katherine A. Sward, Guilherme Del Fiol, Catherine Staes, Charlene Weir, and Mollie R. Cummins. "Patient-generated health data and electronic health record integration: A scoping review." *JAMIA Open* 3, no. 4 (2020): 619–627.
36 Ayaz, Muhammad, Muhammad F. Pasha, Mohammed Y. Alzahrani, Rahmat Budiarto, and Deris Stiawan. "The Fast Health Interoperability Resources (FHIR) standard: A systematic literature review of implementations, applications, challenges and opportunities." *JMIR Medical Informatics* 9, no. 7 (2021): e21929.
37 Ng, Cho Ee, Sarah Bowman, Jonathan Ling, Rachael Bagshaw, Angela Birt, and Yan Yiannakou. "The future of clinical trials—Is it virtual?" *British Medical Bulletin* 148, no. 1 (2023): 42–57.

38 Kabanov, Ilya. "Effective frameworks for delivering compliance with personal data privacy regulatory requirements." In *2016 14th Annual Conference on Privacy, Security and Trust (PST)*, pp. 551–554. IEEE, 2016.
39 Wu, Hongjiao, Ashutosh Dhar Dwivedi, and Gautam Srivastava. "Security and privacy of patient information in medical systems based on blockchain technology." *ACM Transactions on Multimedia Computing, Communications, and Applications (TOMM)* 17, no. 2s (2021): 1–17.
40 Laatikainen, Gabriella, Mengcheng Li, and Pekka Abrahamsson. "Blockchain governance: A dynamic view." In *Software Business: 12th International Conference, ICSOB 2021, Drammen, Norway, December 2–3, 2021, Proceedings 12*, pp. 66–80. Springer International Publishing, 2021.
41 Alharbi, Shatha, Afraa Attiah, and Daniyal Alghazzawi. "Integrating blockchain with artificial intelligence to secure IoT networks: Future trends." *Sustainability* 14, no. 23 (2022): 16002.
42 Charles, Vincent, Ali Emrouznejad, and Tatiana Gherman. "A critical analysis of the integration of blockchain and artificial intelligence for supply chain." *Annals of Operations Research* 327, no. 1 (2023): 7–47.
43 Holotescu, Carmen. "Understanding blockchain opportunities and challenges." In *Conference Proceedings of» eLearning and Software for Education «(eLSE)*, vol. 14, no. 04, pp. 275–283. Carol I National Defence University Publishing House, 2018.
44 Upadhyay, Nitin. "Demystifying blockchain: A critical analysis of challenges, applications and opportunities." *International Journal of Information Management* 54 (2020): 102120.
45 Sestrem Ochôa, Iago, Luis Augusto Silva, Gabriel De Mello, Nuno M. Garcia, Juan Francisco de Paz Santana, and Valderi Reis Quietinho Leithardt. "A cost analysis of implementing a blockchain architecture in a smart grid scenario using sidechains." *Sensors* 20, no. 3 (2020): 843.
46 Alam, Shadab, Mohammed Shuaib, Wazir Zada Khan, Sahil Garg, Georges Kaddoum, M. Shamim Hossain, and Yousaf Bin Zikria. "Blockchain-based initiatives: Current state and challenges." *Computer Networks* 198 (2021): 108395

12 Blockchain-Based Supply Chain Management in Healthcare

Ashish Verma, Sunita, Akhil Sharma, Akanksha Sharma, Shilpa Thukral and Shaweta Sharma

Introduction

Supply Chain Management (SCM) is an ongoing process where the products, services, information, and money flow among the different supply chain (SC) members. To make sure that the right quantity of materials/products/services is available at the right time, at the desired place, and at the optimum cost expected by the customer, a set of decisions and activities must be made.

Effective and efficient supply logistics can enhance overall productivity, leading to better responsiveness towards customers. This can be done by controlling the flow of all resources, products, money, and information.[1] A successful SC would be one in which the different stakeholders of the chain share and flow all information required efficiently. Thus, making logistics more efficient and managing all the SC operations effectively in a network will lead to quicker responsiveness in the chain and value generation for customers.[2]

It enhances the cost and value addition of the product or services extensively while effective capital resource utilisation. While building responsiveness is the objective, organisations have attempted to integrate all the processes across the SC. Further, with the help of the tools of the Internet of Things (IoT), radio frequency identification (RFID), and e-commerce, response in a SC has also improved.

Blockchain is a technology that has been growing relatively fast over the years, and it is fundamentally based on a distributed ledger where the data is stored in a series of blocks. These features make blockchain technology (BT) non-editable, distributed, entirely anonymous, immutable, and secure; therefore, it has scopes other than cryptocurrencies, such as insurance, SCM, healthcare, etc.[3] There is not a single owner/organiser of a blockchain network. It is the distributed network with nodes existing in a peer-to-peer topology that represents the primary executors to run all transactions required on top of some blockchain. Consensus algorithms in a blockchain network help maintain the consistency of the blockchain ledger.[4]

BT in the field of healthcare is considered in such areas as storage of electronic medical records data, medicine movement passing control over the spending of budgetary funds, clinical trials data collection, and ensuring the reliability of results of clinical trials fundraising (crowdfunding) for innovative developments.

DOI: 10.4324/9781003529910-12

Reliability and correct storage of patients' medical data and problems of confidence are relevant for the electronic systems used in healthcare at present. Blockchain systems, some of them even for the registration of medical data, are used in many countries to prevent unauthorised access and modification of patient information. Hence, the development of a patient clinical summary (health history) such as lab test results, diagnosis, and treatment. In addition, such information is only accessible when using a specific list of trusted digital signatures from the doctor and patient. The information will be available not only to the doctor but also to insurance-based representatives (but this can only happen with direct patient consent and only on the condition that they receive the necessary certificate through a smart contract).[1]

The blockchain technology plays crucial role in controlling of transfer of medicines and medical devices throughout the SC. Pharmaceutical companies (Pfizer and Genentech, which have a combined market cap of more than USD 300 billion) revealed their blockchain initiative, MediLedger, built on the Ethereum platform using Quorum. The role of the blockchain is to prevent counterfeit goods from entering the supply system. Additionally, under the new Ethereum system, pharmaceutical manufacturers will be able to detect substandard medicines before they even reach the SC.[5]

SCM and related activities form the second largest bucket of healthcare expenditure. The large scale of healthcare SCM by operations encompasses on-time delivery and tracking of items along the SC right to their end application with patients. Although prior studies have assessed the strategic and competitive advantages of efficient SCM in retail and manufacturing, healthcare provider organisations have faced challenges in realising its potential benefits. A study identified significant barriers to the implementation of integrated SCM solutions in healthcare, including misaligned or conflicting incentives, insufficient data collection, and performance metrics, educational deficiencies regarding SC issues, and potential friction within and between group purchasing organisations and other SC partners. Furthermore, the challenges in HSCs are exacerbated by the utilisation of disparate information systems and software that exhibit minimal interoperability.

Healthcare SCM involves several operations, including monitoring products along the SC till their utilisation by patients. Previous studies in manufacturing and retail have assessed the competitive and strategic benefits of an efficient SCM system; however, healthcare provider organisations have not yet completely harnessed these benefits. A study identifies several significant barriers to the implementation of effective SCM solutions in the healthcare sector, including misaligned or conflicting incentives, the necessity for enhanced data collection and performance metrics, insufficient knowledge regarding SC issues, and potential conflicts between group purchasing organisations and other SC partners. SC is apprehensive about the utilisation of various information systems (IS) and software lacking adequate interoperability, which intensifies the challenges in healthcare.[3]

Blockchain in Healthcare

Blockchain characteristics (decentralised, open, and permissionless) may grant a proper layered solution for healthcare. Broader usability will enable the technology itself to break into other aspects of healthcare, though, such as wearables and medical research. The demand for blockchain innovations in the healthcare sector is escalating. A recent Deloitte survey indicates that the sector is actively seeking novel methods to utilise the blockchain to fulfil its fundamental needs.[3,7]

The second critical feature for healthcare data is the immutability of blockchain. It can safeguard clinical trial results, medical data, and regulatory adherence. An example of how blockchain facilitates real-time patient monitoring and medical intervention within hospitals is the implementation of smart contracts. They adhere to the Health Insurance Portability and Accountability Act (HIPAA) by safeguarding records for access by patients and healthcare professionals.

BT can be utilised to establish a pharmaceutical SC and to create safeguards against counterfeit pharmaceuticals. Smart contracts are employed to ensure informed consent for data utilisation, including improved identity management and data integrity, despite the high costs associated with medication development stemming from studies assessing safety and efficacy. Enabling patients to control their own identities facilitates the implementation of the informed consent process while preserving the confidentiality of personal health information.[3,8]

Overview of Healthcare Supply Chain

The Healthcare Industry is the most emerging industry in every developing nation. SCM is one of the most challenging accomplishments in the world because this industry has its uniqueness, which makes it different from other industries. Also, every patient has their requirement, so the best quality of patient care at an affordable cost cannot be achieved easily; therefore, SCM for healthcare is crucial. It is a systematic approach to procurement, management of medical supplies, and integration of supplier and hospital services by optimising the use of available resources. The advantages of responsive healthcare SCM include but are not limited to enhancing the quality of care, enhancing response time, boosting productivity, optimally utilising resources, and smoothing patient staffing.[9]

However, the healthcare sector has yet to garner optimum results from targeted SCM practices. Due to the slow rate of adoption, it is known as a disordered and inefficient sector relative to the manufacturing market. They exhibit a deficiency in coordination with other departments and members of the SC. Hospital-based programs are generally focused on reducing resource consumption and improving the quality of care, but these programs will never provide permanent outcomes. Despite recent advancements in balancing supply and demand, the domestic health SC remains its weakest link. Internally-focused medical workers are typically interested in the internal logistics performance, often in order to shorten patient care time. With the practice of health care shifting from a simple environment with few stakeholders to an advanced context characterised by multiple stakeholders and complex technology, effective implementation of best SC practices in hospitals becomes even more problematic. Selecting purchasing activities, inventory control techniques and distribution activities can help reduce the cost per service unit with good quality patient care.[10]

In short, healthcare SCM is managing various medical instruments/medical tools (like syringes, gloves, etc.) and the workforce (doctors, nurses, and supporting staff). We all know that the principal objective of any healthcare provider is to effectively cure the patient with minimum cost, in the least amount of time possible, without compromising on the quality and his overall satisfaction. Thus, at its very core, healthcare SCM aims for a hospital to be the place that performs a crucial function in fulfilling the needs of the patients, and any healthcare SCM mainly seeks to serve this purpose.[11]

The Objective of Healthcare Supply Chain Management

Responsive healthcare SCM comes with a high-quality patient care at the lowest cost. The cost of care in the healthcare system is extremely high growing, and it is not feasible in many settings in the developing world, such as India. The primary objectives of SCM are discussed in Figure 12.1.

All the trading partners will work towards the same goal, so the streamlined workflow covers all new cooperation, which in turn provides quality patient care at minimum waste and thus lowers the cost of care. Inventory management is one of the important parts of healthcare SCM, as excess inventory imposes a big cost burden on the patient. At the same time, a shortage of medical equipment, medicine, and services can harmfully affect human well-being. SCM responsiveness will directly affect materials management in healthcare. The responsiveness comes

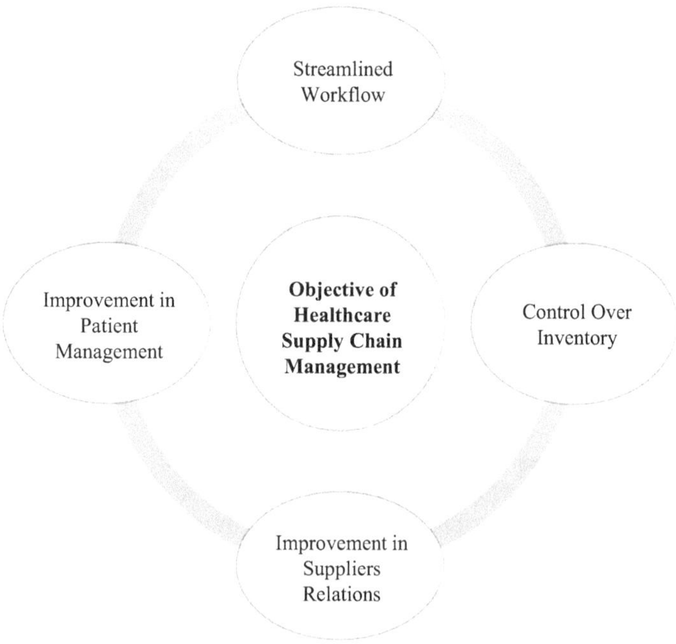

Figure 12.1 Objective of Healthcare Supply Chain Management.

from the strong and healthy relationship between the service providers/hospitals or nursing homes in relation to the suppliers. A healthier organisation with a good culture will be developed where the trading partners of the SC have a good dynamic because of responsive healthcare SCM, and each player would know who is accountable for what. The managed care segment of healthcare is useless when the patients do not get value for their money and the quality-driven care hospitals provide.[12]

Challenges in Healthcare Supply Chain

In healthcare SCM, data fragmentation degrading meaningful information and product flow highly threatens critical SC processes. For example, in healthcare and SC, non-standard product identifiers are pervasive, leading to ambiguity in the identification of products or the validation of procurement transactions. Furthermore, the fact that different SC stakeholders use multiple product identifiers in healthcare induces complexity when it comes to establishing a soundtrack-and-trace solution, considering that medicines and medical devices may pass through numerous hands while being sourced, transported, stored, and eventually consumed all over the world.[13] Manufacturers, distributors, and third-party logistics (3PL) entities are unable to reach a consensus on product identification within existing systems and transactions, as each employs its internal numbering system, which is subsequently converted to a transacting party identifier in SC transactions such as purchase orders, invoices, or advance shipping notices. Distributors and 3PL companies employ warehouse identifiers or bespoke stock-keeping units (SKUs) tailored to their operations for inventory management.[3]

Moreover, hospitals, pharmacies, and merchants are required to associate a unique identity (hospital ID) with a manufacturer identifier, which may be a Universal Product Code (UPC) or National Drug Code (NDC), whenever they procure or receive items directly from manufacturers. Moreover, few organisations document and preserve secondary product features such as batch, lot, or serial numbers and expiration dates due to IS/IT limitations, volume, and the varied nature of commodities procured in healthcare facilities. The SC monitoring issue was intensified in instances when surgical kits or pharmaceutical compounding had previously taken place, and other involved organisations could not distinctly identify each component within the kit.[3,14]

The delivery of mixed products is another element leading to information disaggregation and fragmented data inside the HSC. An illustrative example of a three-tier supply chain comprising suppliers, manufacturers, and distributors. The product flow commences when manufacturers create a batch of items, thereafter distributing them in smaller numbers to enhance quality control and inspection or for alternate packaging. Each lot is now repackaged into many cartons, which are subsequently consolidated onto one or more shipping pallets for transportation to the distributor or another location in the supply chain.[3,15]

Each individual medical device unit is often granted a unique serial number, with the lot number, batch number, and expiration dates designated by the manufacturer.

For example, if a carton contains 12 of these specific products, each is individually identified and registered by the maker with a serial number. When pallets are transferred to a third party, such as a distributor's warehouse or a 3PL provider, it is feasible for a pallet from the manufacturer to contain cartons from the same lot. Moreover, while 3PL providers are restricted from retaining extensive data (save for specialised items such as immunisations and medical equipment), they are still required to authenticate the quantities that are dispatched and received.[16]

Initially, products are not tracked individually beyond the manufacturer; just the specific carton barcodes are utilised for internal inventory control. The distributor, serving as an intermediate in the supply chain, disassembles the pallet into smaller units and retains the cartons until receiving a purchase order from a healthcare provider or wholesaler. At this juncture, the distributor will ascertain the requisite number of cartons and arrange them on a pallet or in a box according to the order's size and quantity, rather than adhering to a first-in-first-out (FIFO) methodology, thereby indicating that the shipment can no longer incorporate cartons from the same lot. Each supplied carton packed by the distributor is scanned and dispatched through a 3PL provider, without preserving batch, lot, or expiration date information. Third, when a healthcare provider receives a mixed lot shipment, the cartons are often monitored to confirm the arrival of the correct purchase order, although they are occasionally scanned individually. The supplier retains the consignment in their central storage until a clinical unit requests the item or regularly delivers it as part of replenishment.[3] On some occasions, instead of keeping the goods in the carton boxes, they are removed from their boxes and placed together with products that already exist. Last but not least, internal distribution is also done on a FIFO basis, meaning cartons are emptied regardless of the real batch and lot identifier. Consequently, items coming to the clinical unit can be from different lots and batches.[17]

Information disconnects and intractability happens inside with the providers as well as outside among SC stakeholders. Documenting usage at the patient level is essential for establishing an effective and verifiable solution, such as a product pedigree. Re-barcoding the individual item with a provider's unique identifier and other variable attributes will be necessary for providers that must monitor the batch, lot, expiration, and other relevant product characteristics. Aside from conducting human inventory counts or establishing a unique identifier for each provider, there is virtually no method for a provider to monitor its stock levels. Product management in HSCs is complicated by the utilisation of custom numbers and mixed lot deliveries, lacking associated systems for the storage of secondary identifiers.[18]

Automatically generated product labels containing identifiers such as UPC or NDC present challenges. Despite the presence of lot, batch, and expiration dates on a product, no supply chain transacting entity retains a record of these details, resulting in the product possessing dynamic qualities. A shipment may have both batch and mixed lot items. At each phase of the supply chain, stakeholders, including clinical units of healthcare providers, may receive deliveries including items from multiple lots. Counterfeiting has emerged as a significant global issue for healthcare practitioners and other supply chain members within the healthcare business. The increasing volume and diversity of healthcare products complicates the assessment of the financial and other repercussions of healthcare counterfeiting. Identifying counterfeit products is challenging due to the global production and distribution of care-related items.[3] One main reason for the practice of counterfeiting is that there are weak regulations in place, such as unregulated online pharmacies, which allow counterfeit products to enter the market easily.[19]

Application of Blockchain Technology for Supply Chain and Counterfeit Drugs Detection

The supply chain is one of the most important things for the medical industry, from raw materials and manufacturing to various levels of storage and distribution, to ensure proper monitoring from scratch so that it ends up being used in optimal numbers and in the intended manner. The problem of counterfeit drugs has gained traction over the last couple of years. This means there will have to be a mechanism whereby the end users and all other stakeholders of the supply chain can authenticate any drug's ingredients.

There are many such weak links in the supply chain where the drug can be compromised, or a fake drug can be injected into the system if there is no effective tracking mechanism. In response to these rising issues, fresh regulations have been introduced for all stakeholders of the medicine supply chain to provide a solid mechanism for tracking and tracing through which pharmaceutical supplies they pass. Here is where the requirement for tracing and monitoring could not be more perfectly met by blockchain; this data needs to be maintained in a transparent but, at the same time, secure, immutable system that has to be accessible to multiple stakeholders.[20]

As a result, several blockchain-based solutions have been proposed to monitor the pharmaceutical supply chain (PSC). The entire straight project by this pharmacy division is designated MediLedger. The network is a permissioned blockchain for partners in the PSC. The idea is consistent with the track and trace laws. One of the aims is maintaining an interoperable system that can track prescription drugs from factory to pharmacy (which is what a project called MediLedger) started with big Pharma companies, including Pfizer and Genentech, wanting to tackle using blockchain tech. AMB-net, the flagship product of Ambrosus, is one of the most ambitious products at this new frontier; it is a blockchain-based IoT network tailored for supply chains situated in the food and pharmaceutical industries. With AMB-net, companies today can build their custom supply chain solutions.[21]

Modum-MODsense T1 is a temperature sensor that ensures compliance with conditions in the supply chain of pharmaceuticals with Good Distribution Practices (GDP) of medicinal products for human use. A blockchain is used to maintain the sensor data and other digital records. Several other blockchain-based solutions within the supply chain domain have one or more application areas in the pharmaceutical industry. An example would be BlockVerify, which lists pharmaceuticals as a primary application area in its supply chain solution that doesn't permit counterfeiting.

At present, BT in healthcare is being progressively regarded as a disruptive technology, and its high popularity among a number of researchers and practitioner communities has been accompanied by an almost exclusionary use. Examples of frequently envisioned solutions include blockchain-based contract administration, electronic health records, and shared clinical trial data. BT offers essential advantages such as decentralised, secure data repositories, distributed and auditable validation capabilities in real time, and stringent access limitations across multiple stakeholders.[22]

Each time a product manufacturer presents a product for sale in the supply chain, a block is created for that transaction. This information block encompasses intra-product dynamic features, including serial numbers, batch/lot numbers, unit and quantity of measure, expiration dates, and the universal product ID (e.g., UPC). Business associates acting as transitory nodes can readily access and authenticate transaction blocks.[23]

Upon publication to the blockchain, each product transaction is instantly available to all nodes within the participating network.6 Each SC partner can oversee and verify product sales transactions occurring between distributors and care providers. Furthermore, all transaction records are documented to ensure an immutable record. This action preserves an audit trail that can verify prior transactions. This ensures essential confidence among transacting parties and guarantees that the data within this block remains unalterable if modified, removed, or relocated to another branch. With blockchain data inventory and healthcare transaction information now timestamped and readily traceable, blockchain data exhibits a high level of integrity, accuracy, and fidelity. The blockchain-enabled supply chain may assist in verifying the actual inventory observable at various stages to prevent product diversion, counterfeiting, shortages, and expiration.[24]

Utilising blockchain-based HSC can additionally facilitate stakeholders' sharing of inventory, giving up greater flexibility through resource sharing and pooling. When a product is recalled, blockchain-based SC helps the manufacturer know which trading partners should be alerted and recalled rather than triggering an unnecessary panic throughout the SC. BT essentially provides an effective method to close a recall faster, making proactive product management that also saves money. The other major advantage of blockchain is that it ensures the legitimacy of the items being transacted across the HSC.

At present, without a tangible database, it is effortless for stakeholders to extract counterfeit products, as no one knows what products and quantities are available for sale. It is feasible to improve existing blockchain-enabled smart contracts to assess and validate the pricing eligibility of suppliers across the several tiers negotiated by group buying organisations.[25]

BT could be enhanced to verify organ donor registries and medical devices. Care providers and other stakeholders exemplify entities that may accumulate resources to conceal their purchasing patterns from other participating nodes. BT ought to be employed to connect actual consumption data from patient records to enhance the end-to-end transparency of diverse HSC activities. Integrating procurement data, such as invoices or purchase orders (PO), with a patient records system represents a prospective application of BT in healthcare SCM. This type of blockchain-distributed ledger may serve as a far more potent and efficient instrument than existing solutions for facilitating the integration of diverse clinical, financial, and procurement systems along the HSC informatics and management continuum.[3,26]

Pharmaceutical Supply Chains in Healthcare Using Blockchain

PSC deliver medications to pipeline stakeholders, including biotechnology firms, health regulatory agencies, pharmacies, hospitals, and end-users (patients). The Food and Drug Agency (FDA), USA, is one of the most stringent regulators monitoring safety, quality, and efficacy in PSC.[27]

The low performance of PSCs comes from a lack of coherence within a supply chain and among stakeholders. These constitute critical factors within PSC that contribute to accelerated disease progression, drug resistance, and mortality due to a lack of transparency and visibility of drug supply. Although global sourcing and online markets facilitate access to medicines in various countries, these drugs incur a new health risk without tracking their origin. Despite extremely high standards and newer technologies (such as holograms, barcodes, and RFID tags) that help to preserve pharmaceutical integrity, counterfeiting continues to be a significant global challenge for PSC.[27]

Implementation Stages of Supply Chain Management Using Blockchain

Organisations utilise the user acceptability and technology acquisition paradigm, encompassing the adoption, pre-adoption, and post-adoption phases, to comprehend and implement IT. Numerous influential factors, including organisational and environmental components, along with user acceptance, impacted the project during the adoption phase. The protocols for incorporating or embedding new technologies into supply chain/business models, along with associated activities, appear to remain largely unaltered. It can divide blockchain implementation in terms of SCM into three stages: Initiation, Adoption decision, and Implementation which are described in Table 12.1.[28]

Initiation Stage

The objective of the blockchain initiation phase is to comprehend the advantages of BT, including the justification for its use. The adoption of blockchain is necessitated by technology advancements and external conditions. According to most conceptual studies on blockchain in the pharmaceutical sector, a transparent, efficient, and tamper-proof PSC network can be formed by using the decentralised and immutable characteristics of a distributed ledger. In the lack of universal technological standards and relevant regulations, stakeholders will be disinclined to adopt the Blockchain-based SCM solution due to associated risks. A transparent governmental oversight network utilising risk criteria related to the transit of SCM in

Table 12.1 Role of Blockchain in Implementation Stages of Supply Chain Healthcare

S. No.	*Stages*	*Function*
1	Initiation stage	The organisation considers various aspects of innovation.
2	Adoption decision	The organisation decides whether and how to implement the innovation.
3	Implementation	The organisation deploys large-scale implementation and integrates the innovation into its structure.

pharmaceutical industry. The government and other players in this part of the supply chain could scrutinise them, view transaction data, and safeguard the integrity of these drugs. The initiation phase aids in the imagining of an efficient blockchain ecosystem for the SCM and further facilitates its user usability.[29]

Adoption Decision Stage

Organisations need to make strategic, financial, and technological assessments in order for them to move from the initiation up to the adoption decision stage. At this stage, inter-organisation resources are assessed and distributed to facilitate the adoption of technology. For example, in other implementations of technology such as RFID and IoT, there is a strategic level involvement that includes adoption decision stage commitment by top management because this kind of adoption may change the structure and resource needs of the organisation. It is good to use stakeholder support at this stage to follow the in-house development of culture related to Blockchain within organisations and obtain knowledge related to Blockchain. Stakeholders need the cost model to argue how Blockchain can be beneficial for the entire PSC financially. It has the potential to convince large enterprises to implement the pilot project due to the long-term benefits of Blockchain. Moreover, to solve the technological problems, we need blockchain platform companies. Blockchain allows interoperability with various other systems and drug flows rather than connecting different medical information systems and an ERP from a pharmaceutical manufacturer.[30]

Implementation Stage

The implementation stage is the actual usage of Blockchain at the organisational level or supply chain level. So, in such a case, a few supply chain participants can run a pilot project with BT to check its scalability in the SCM. Pilot projects on a smaller scale can yield a lot of meaningful and valuable lessons, too. The FDA's most prominent pilot initiative to date is MediLedger, which emphasises package-level surveillance and includes 25 major pharmaceutical companies and additional supply chain collaborators. A greater number of participants, particularly small enterprises within the blockchain-based pharmaceutical industry ecosystem, are expressing interest in this pilot initiative. However, after piloting efforts gain traction, the next level is scaling up with a supply chain. But as noted many times now, scalability (especially in terms of transaction speed and interoperability across multiple nodes) is a roadblock that must be cleared. Blockchain, if successful, may achieve widespread popularity among users and will require fewer technical issues and implementation costs.[31]

Implementation Factors of Supply Chains in Blockchain Healthcare

The unprecedented potential offered by BT makes it a promising candidate to resolve PSC issues, and various practitioners have taken a step towards illustrating technical proof of concept (PoC) for Blockchain-based applications in SC, initiating targeted pilot initiatives with pharmaceutical producers, distributors, and hospitals, such as IBM. With the help of internal and external regimes, this multi-participant cooperation in SC is galvanised to conduct a successful blockchain implementation.

Internal Factor

The thematic analysis identified three internal factors essential for the successful integration of BT in the supply chain. Figure 12.2 illustrates the relevance of enhanced data security, visibility, and transparency for augmenting the operational efficiency of SCM.[27]

Enhanced Transparency and Visibility

Patient medical records are generally maintained in hospitals, whereas manufacturers and distributors solely aggregate demand forecasts for pharmaceuticals. However, the provenance of drugs is not accessible to patients. Hence, gaining complete transparency and visibility in SCs is unprecedented compared to any supply chain, but it can help achieve higher collaboration, trust, and efficiency. Hence, the immutable nature of Blockchain, which is also Tamper-proof and interoperable, helps in mitigating the above challenges.[27]

These features make it very attractive to manage personal health records with Blockchain in compliance with data protection regulations. SC stakeholders will release their transactional data this way without exposing it to third parties. Moreover, it can assist with ensuring data accuracy while helping minimise information delays. Recently, the pharmaceutical ecosystem BlockRx collaborated with several pharmaceutical producers, merchants, and pharmacies to integrate their existing information systems, dismantle information silos, and enhance transparency in the supply chain.[27,33]

Enhanced Data Security

The centralised cloud storage of electronic medical records offers a processing benefit as the conventional approach for managing distributed data; however, this centralisation renders it highly susceptible to damage from cyber-attacks. Upon

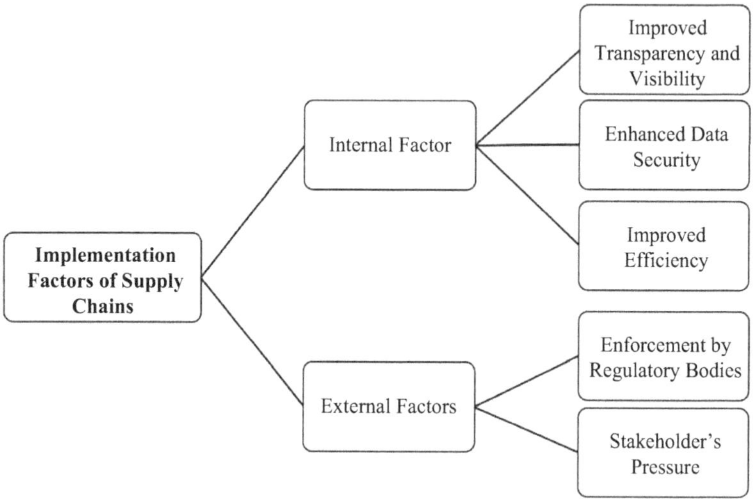

Figure 12.2 Implementation Factors of Supply Chains (SC) in Blockchain Healthcare.

implementation, Blockchain generates immutable blocks of time-stamped transaction records that can be disseminated via a decentralised distributed ledger. Hence, Blockchain safeguards healthcare and medicine/drug information against hacking threats or cyber criminals.

Blockchain in SC has attracted great attention, especially for medical data management. Certain pharmaceutical items, such as vaccinations, require meticulous temperature and humidity control during transportation. IoT devices (GPS, temperature sensors, etc.) can be used at the time of shipment to instantly record any unqualified environmental conditions for drugs and sound an alarm to authorised responsible entities on the Blockchain platform. They can also ensure transport conditions of vaccines throughout the supply chain for patients.[27,34]

During this process, smart contracts are useful in authenticating products and automated procedures and protocols as per preset guidelines, along with automatic contract termination and refunds. For instance, many Blockchain companies suggest Blockchain-based projects like 'SmartHub,' which helps to track and trace the properties of pharmaceutical goods such as location, product images, ingredients, and temperature settings during international business deals. The other use case, called 'LedgerDomain,' uses BRUINchain and barcoding for patients to trace the drugs and track them. In short, the SC-level implementation using BT is due to the need for Drug traceability and security.[35]

Improved Efficiency

This enhances the efficiency of the supply chain by adopting a chain. It is expected that smart responses to emergencies will be improved by blockchain, which can accelerate payments and accurate forecasting these days. Past studies have shown that the SC could take long periods to notify, recall, and suspend a drug due to cumbersome manual paperwork and inefficient, fragmented, complex systems, causing delayed response times and leaving healthcare services displeased. Blockchain acts as a catalyst in the processing time due to high levels of trust and data transparency between different parties within the supply chain, and it can quickly inform any supply chain party about drug recalls. In addition, smart contracts can eliminate other intermediates and reduce labour costs since, within the Blockchain network, the validation process is finalised. The agreement will be executed automatically when the predetermined conditions, rights, and obligations of each party are fulfilled. In addition to this, Blockchain expands the range of information exchanges, which represents an effective way for spotting bottlenecks, preventing overstock, and ultimately enabling more efficiency in the PSC.[36]

External Factors

The market environment comprises external factors, including legislation, competitive pressures, and macroeconomic conditions, all of which influence the adoption of new technology. Furthermore, external entities including governments, pharmaceutical regulatory bodies, suppliers, and patients affect external factors.

Enforcement by Regulatory Bodies

Government agencies such as the FDA and FMD (Falsified Medication Directive), along with non-profit organisations like the WHO, oversee the pharmaceutical sector. Organisations need to adhere to the regulations, and counterfeit products are fought against. Developed nations are doing much closer practical initiatives in countering fake medicines as compared to developing countries. The Blockchain pilot projects (MediLedger and PharmaLedger) aim to collaborate with multinational pharmaceutical manufacturers, distributors, hospitals, and pharmacies to document transactions on the distributed ledger. The European Federation of Pharmaceutical Industries and Associations is dedicated to identifying counterfeit products in the supply chain and is working to eliminate inferior medications.[27] FMD directives are followed by the National Health Service (United Kingdom), which assembles the pharmacies that supervise this movement of drugs. India, Brazil, etc., are underdeveloped countries that promote blockchain projects to raise the standard of their healthcare service layer.[37]

Stakeholder's Pressure

Patients are more concerned about where their medicines come from and what is inside, so they check for side effects/issues or simply follow sustainability and quality certificates.[38] Also, during the COVID-19 pandemic, local pharmacies had consumers to a limited extent follows from. There before then, it went up gradually upwards for buying drugs online. Therefore, rigorous regulation of online pharmacies was required from the governments, especially for their legitimacy and validity, in order to avoid purchasing counterfeited medicines. An example of the latter is My Net Doctor, a registered online pharmacy that recently subscribed to join UK-based MediConnect's Blockchain network. Such collaboration improves the SC traceability of online drugs, particularly prescription drugs. Confidential customer prescription data and provenance data for medicines will be tracked through the private, MediConnect's permissioned distributed ledger aims to mitigate the overuse and overprescription of pharmaceutical medications.[27,39]

Blocks to Blockchain Technology in Supply Chain Management

The obstacles to blockchain-based SCM in healthcare can be understood by discussing system adoption barriers, conception and regulations, and data security cyber risks, which are shown in Figure 12.3.

System Adoption

The predominant challenges faced during technology adoption are technical and operational in nature. Multidisciplinary research indicates that the primary barriers to blockchain adoption are the design of smart contracts, scalability issues, and elevated adoption costs.

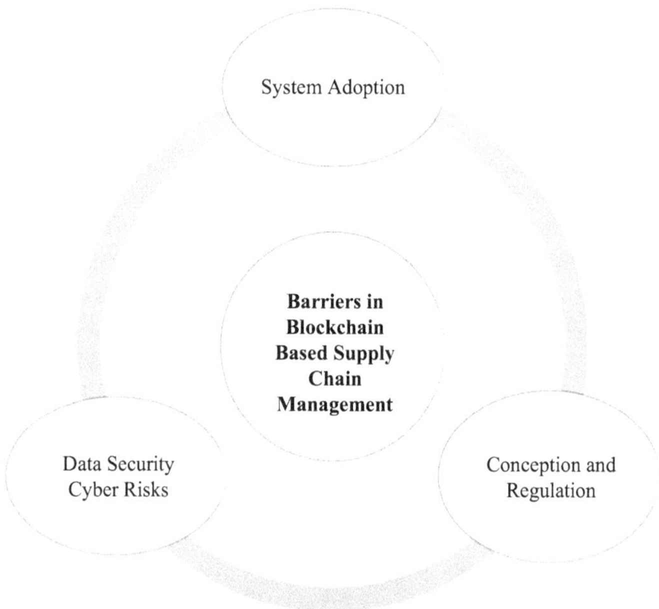

Figure 12.3 Barriers in Blockchain-Based Supply Chain Management.

Scalability

The plausibility and feasibility of new technology adoption have been market-tested hundreds of times. There have been very few successful pilot projects on blockchain applications in the healthcare sector so far, which means it is still early for such applications. As outlined by the previous studies, there is a need to scale the Blockchain on a supply chain network level and achieve scale in thousands of transactions per second while also handling very big data. The feasibility of 10 billion drugs driven by Taiwan's healthcare insurance was established through healthcare and pharmaceutical industry transactions. The current Gcoin Blockchain system, being a Blockchain-based drug governance solution, can fictively handle millions of transactions in a day; thus, sometime latency in confirming the transaction data will be apparent. In addition, the complexity and magnitude of medical supplies along with a decentralised distributed ledger implies that each transaction requires multiple nodes to process it; hence, generic scalability in the case of the supply chain is true for wider adoption of blockchain, too.[40,41]

Smart Contract Design

Moreover, if there were multiple permissionary parties, the self-executive smart contract design and verification between parties would also make mistakes. However, mapping the supply chain operations and regulations to smart contracts is challenging as the conflicts and interests of different stakeholders need to be balanced.[27] The clause that is generated in the interpretation may mislead you if you are not paying close attention and possibly result in failing a transaction or getting a bad transaction. Plus, these first smart contracts are only able to perform simple procedures such as executing payment transactions; there are no verification clauses for laws or regulations. Due to large transaction volumes and contracts, it may be impossible for smart contracts to verify counterfeit. In response, IBM created a mechanism called the 'crypto-anchor' platform to deliver correct products by letting users authenticate/certify the delivery receipt.[42]

Operational Cost

The high cost of system adoption and related expenses such as system maintenance and specialist consultant costs will likely delay blockchain adoption. As a result, practitioners from pharmaceutical companies are currently having difficulty perceiving whether efficiencies and cost savings associated with the adoption of Blockchain could offset the high cost of technology implementation. This can also translate into high adoption costs and technical issues during the adoption as a result of the current 'immature' BT market. Due to the financial risks of this technology, large enterprises might become 'early adopters,' but medium and small enterprises are expected to shun such a leap. Certain researchers also evident the combined approach of blockchain with other tech concepts such as Cloud, IoT, and

RFID for optimum operations. Hence the high expense of system-wide integration. Furthermore, there will be fairly high technical training costs for employees and the cost of implementing consultants for blockchain adoption in the entire supply chain.[43]

Conception and Regulation

Support from top management is a critical factor for successful implementation. The literature research indicates that leadership engagement and commitment are critical success factors for Blockchain deployment in the healthcare sector. However, due to a complex supply network, the interest of healthcare stakeholders in the order of blockchain projects is different from others. Consequently, the outcomes are few successful pilot projects, and consequently, it is challenging to rationalise an accord for substantial investment by the senior management. Nonetheless, an additional perceptual obstacle is the absence of an industry governance framework aligned with the blockchain network and the standardisation of information flow. Although certain government sectors have implemented measures to regulate counterfeit drugs, the laws and regulations pertaining to blockchain are currently under short-term strain, posing significant risks and pressures for managers in both healthcare and the pharmaceutical industry regarding the integration of blockchain into decision-making processes. Blockchain adoption in the supply chain is evidently influenced by industrial architecture and managerial support.[27,44]

Data Security Cyber Risks

In the coming years, digital supply chains will face a growing risk from all types of cyber threats. Similarly, cyber security problems involved with data control are yet another challenge inside the healthcare and even pharmaceutical industries. Its original cryptographic mechanism that protects a patient's medical records and medicine transaction information from cyber threats is still in the field test phase. So patients are worried their privacy may leak and do not want to provide useful information for the blockchain one. Past incidences like the AMCA (American Medical Collection Agency) data breach in 2018 are haunting examples of how privacy leakage questions the confidence of patient about their data safety.

But most importantly, the immutable aspect of blockchain could impede the accuracy of data. Even if wrong data in the blockchain can be fixed, the corrector transaction comes after the first transaction. Nevertheless, it complicates the search within a blockchain system and may be time-consuming. This is highly problematic for the blockchain if emergent cases like drug recalls occur, and yet we have wrong input data. Furthermore, in the blockchain, when codes are verified and interpreted into text, many errors may occur due to misinterpretation of these coding languages.[45]

Conclusion

BT has the potential to transform SCM in healthcare, and it can solve many issues with existing SCMs in healthcare. Many healthcare systems have been criticised for inefficiencies, opacity, and susceptibility to fake medicines in their traditional supply chains. The inherent characteristics of Blockchain, which is decentralised, immutable, and transparent, make it a challenging potential solution for such issues, providing enhanced traceability, accountability, and security across the supply chain.

Blockchain seems to show particular promise when used within the context of PSC as a solution for drug authenticity, reduction of counterfeiting risk, and enhanced visibility across the supply chain. By facilitating the sharing and verification of data between parties in near real-time, blockchain can help create end-to-end traceability from manufacture through the delivery of medicines to patients. This builds trust among different stakeholders, including manufacturers, distributors, regulators, and consumers, so that there are no counterfeit or unsafe products in the market.

The process for implementation of blockchain-based SCM in health care can be segmented into several stages, including the initiation stage (introduction of concept) and the adoption decision stage (evaluation/impact). In this last phase of implementation, the blockchain is actually integrated into supply chain processes, which would require collaboration across many different entities. Some of the important internal factors contributing to the adoption of BT are increased transparency, better data security, and operational efficiency, which can help businesses make supply chain operations effective and minimise costs. In addition to internal drives, external factors like regulatory mandates and stakeholder pressure also facilitate the swift adoption of BT in the healthcare sector.

However, big obstacles remain, such as the scalability of the blockchain systems, the complexity of smart contract designing, and the high operational costs to implement. Meanwhile, regulatory issues and data security, as well as cyber risk concerns, can both be threats that hinder state adoption. Blockchain possesses significant potential to transform healthcare SCM; however, these obstacles must be surmounted by a collaborative effort between industry stakeholders and regulators to actualise that potential.

References

1 Detmer, Don E., Elaine B. Steen, and Richard S. Dick, eds. "The computer-based patient record: An essential technology for health care." (1997). Washington, D.C.: National Academy Press.

2 Giannakis, Mihalis, Konstantina Spanaki, and Rameshwar Dubey. "A cloud-based supply chain management system: Effects on supply chain responsiveness." *Journal of Enterprise Information Management* 32, no. 4 (2019): 585–607.

3 Aditya, Dixit. "Synthesis & characterization of 4-hydroxyacetanilide starting from acetanilide." *Journal of Medical Pharmaceutical and Allied Sciences (June_2016)* 73, no. 077 (2016): 73.

4 Amiri, Mohammad Javad, Divyakant Agrawal, and Amr El Abbadi. "Permissioned blockchains: Properties, techniques, and applications." In *Proceedings of the 2021 International Conference on Management of Data*, pp. 2813–2820. 2021.

5 Sylim, Patrick, Fang Liu, Alvin Marcelo, and Paul Fontelo. "Blockchain technology for detecting falsified and substandard drugs in distribution: Pharmaceutical supply chain intervention." *JMIR Research Protocols* 7, no. 9 (2018): e10163.

6 McKone-Sweet, Kathleen E., Paul Hamilton, and Susan B. Willis. "The ailing healthcare supply chain: A prescription for change." *Journal of Supply Chain Management* 41, no. 1 (2005): 4–17.

7 Prokofieva, Maria, and Shah J. Miah. "Blockchain in healthcare." *Australasian Journal of Information Systems* 23 (2019), pp. 1–22.

8 Akhtar, Mohd Majid, and Danish Raza Rizvi. "Traceability and detection of counterfeit medicines in pharmaceutical supply chain using blockchain-based architectures." *Sustainable and Energy Efficient Computing Paradigms for Society* (2021): 1–31.

9 Srivastava, Shefali, and Rohit Kr Singh. "Exploring integrated supply chain performance in healthcare: A service provider perspective." *Benchmarking: An International Journal* 28, no. 1 (2021): 106–130.

10 Zheng, Jurong, Elmer Bakker, Louise Knight, Heather Gilhespy, Christine Harland, and Helen Walker. "A strategic case for e-adoption in healthcare supply chains." *International Journal of Information Management* 26, no. 4 (2006): 290–301.

11 Wahab, SitiNorida, Nusrat Ahmed, and Md UzirHossain Uzir. "Healthcare supply chain system challenges and mitigation measures: A systematic review of qualitative evidence." *Operations and Supply Chain Management: An International Journal* 16, no. 2 (2023): 164–176.

12 Mandal, Santanu. "Influence of human capital on healthcare agility and healthcare supply chain performance." *Journal of Business & Industrial Marketing* 33, no. 7 (2018): 1012–1026.

13 Jayaraman, Raja, Khaled Salah, and Nelson King. "Improving opportunities in healthcare supply chain processes via the internet of things and blockchain technology." *International Journal of Healthcare Information Systems and Informatics (IJHISI)* 14, no. 2 (2019): 49–65.

14 Jayaraman, Raja, Kamal Taha, and Angelica Burbano Collazos. "Integrating supply chain data standards in healthcare operations and Electronic Health Records." In *2015 International Conference on Industrial Engineering and Operations Management (IEOM)*, pp. 1–9. IEEE, 2015.

15 Tesfaye, Dessalegn. "The study of Ethiopia public health supply chain management: before and after pharmaceuticals fund and supply agency (PFSA)." PhD diss., St. Mary's University, 2015.

16 Wang, Luyao, and Yuqiao Hu. "Third party healthcare logistics: A study of third-party logistics providers in China." China: DiVA portal (2018).

17 Chen, Jessica Alice. "MedSupply network: An integrated logistical marketplace system for buyers and sellers in the medical supply industry." PhD diss., Purdue University Graduate School, 2024.

18 Betcheva, Lidia, Feryal Erhun, and Houyuan Jiang. "OM Forum—Supply chain thinking in healthcare: Lessons and outlooks." *Manufacturing & Service Operations Management* 23, no. 6 (2021): 1333–1353.

19 Falasca, Mauro, Scott Dellana, William J. Rowe, and John F. Kros. "The impact of counterfeit risk management on healthcare supply chain performance: An empirical analysis." *International Journal of Productivity and Performance Management* 71, no. 7 (2022): 3078–3099.

20 Urkude, Shubhangi V., Himanshu Sharma, Seethamsetty Uday Kumar, and Vijaykumar R. Urkude. "Anatomy of blockchain implementation in healthcare." Sandeep Kumar Panda, Ajay Kumar Jena, Santosh Kumar Swain, Suresh Chandra Satapathy (eds), In *Blockchain Technology: Applications and Challenges*, pp. 51–76. Cham: Springer International Publishing, 2021.
21 Abdallah, Salam, and Nishara Nizamuddin. "Blockchain-based solution for pharma supply chain industry." *Computers & Industrial Engineering* 177 (2023): 108997.
22 Raj, Praveen Vijaya Raj Pushpa, Sunil Kumar Jauhar, M. Ramkumar, and Saurabh Pratap. "Procurement, traceability and advance cash credit payment transactions in supply chain using blockchain smart contracts." *Computers & Industrial Engineering* 167 (2022): 108038.
23 Sunny, Justin, Naveen Undralla, and V. Madhusudanan Pillai. "Supply chain transparency through blockchain-based traceability: An overview with demonstration." *Computers & Industrial Engineering* 150 (2020): 106895.
24 Omar, Ilhaam A., Raja Jayaraman, Mazin S. Debe, Khaled Salah, Ibrar Yaqoob, and Mohammed Omar. "Automating procurement contracts in the healthcare supply chain using blockchain smart contracts." *IEEE Access* 9 (2021): 37397–37409.
25 Rejeb, Abderahman, John G. Keogh, Steven J. Simske, Thomas Stafford, and Horst Treiblmaier. "Potentials of blockchain technologies for supply chain collaboration: A conceptual framework." *The International Journal of Logistics Management* 32, no. 3 (2021): 973–994.
26 Rizzardi, Alessandra, Sabrina Sicari, and Alberto Coen-Porisini. "IoT-driven blockchain to manage the healthcare supply chain and protect medical records." *Future Generation Computer Systems* 161 (2024): 415–431.
27 Ghadge, Abhijeet, Michael Bourlakis, Sachin Kamble, and Stefan Seuring. "Blockchain implementation in pharmaceutical supply chains: A review and conceptual framework." *International Journal of Production Research* 61, no. 19 (2023): 6633–6651.
28 Paliwal, Vineet, Shalini Chandra, and Suneel Sharma. "Blockchain technology for sustainable supply chain management: A systematic literature review and a classification framework." *Sustainability* 12, no. 18 (2020): 7638.
29 Vishwakarma, Amit, G. S. Dangayach, M. L. Meena, Sumit Gupta, and Sunil Luthra. "Adoption of blockchain technology enabled healthcare sustainable supply chain to improve healthcare supply chain performance." *Management of Environmental Quality: An International Journal* 34, no. 4 (2023): 1111–1128.
30 Hartley, Janet L., William Sawaya, and David Dobrzykowski. "Exploring blockchain adoption intentions in the supply chain: Perspectives from innovation diffusion and institutional theory." *International Journal of Physical Distribution & Logistics Management* 52, no. 2 (2022): 190–211.
31 Chang, Shuchih Ernest, and YiChian Chen. "Blockchain in health care innovation: Literature review and case study from a business ecosystem perspective." *Journal of Medical Internet Research* 22, no. 8 (2020): e19480.
32 Suwanposri, Chavisa, Veera Bhatiasevi, and Thanarerk Thanakijsombat. "Drivers of blockchain adoption in financial and supply chain enterprises." *Global Business Review* (2021): 09721509211046170.
33 Bamakan, Seyed Mojtaba Hosseini, Shima Ghasemzadeh Moghaddam, and Sajedeh Dehghan Manshadi. "Blockchain-enabled pharmaceutical cold chain: Applications, key challenges, and future trends." *Journal of Cleaner Production* 302 (2021): 127021.
34 Bhatti, David Samuel, Muhammad Mueed Hussain, Beomkyu Suh, Zulfiqar Ali, Ismatov Akobir, and Ki-Il Kim. "IoT-enhanced transport and monitoring of medicine

using sensors, MQTT, and secure short message service." *IEEE Access* 12 (2024) 46690–44673.

35 Laturkar, Kasturi, and Kaustubh Laturkar. "Revolutionizing pharmaceutical supply chains-harnessing the power of blockchain technology." In *Achieving Secure and Transparent Supply Chains with Blockchain Technology*, pp. 92–112. IGI Global, 2024.

36 Wang, Shuai, Liwei Ouyang, Yong Yuan, Xiaochun Ni, Xuan Han, and Fei-Yue Wang. "Blockchain-enabled smart contracts: Architecture, applications, and future trends." *IEEE Transactions on Systems, Man, and Cybernetics: Systems* 49, no. 11 (2019): 2266–2277.

37 Banerjee, Arnab. "Blockchain in the pharmaceutical and healthcare ecosystem." In Malaya Dutta Borah, Roberto Moro Visconti, Ganesh Chandra Deka (eds), *Blockchain in Digital Healthcare*, pp. 209–230. New York: Chapman and Hall/CRC, 2021.

38 World Health Organization. "The safety of medicines in public health programmes: Pharmacovigilance, an essential tool." Switzerland: WHO Press (2006).

39 Saberi, Sara, Mahtab Kouhizadeh, Joseph Sarkis, and Lejia Shen. "Blockchain technology and its relationships to sustainable supply chain management." *International Journal of Production Research* 57, no. 7 (2019): 2117–2135.

40 Huang, Weng-Foung, and Hung-Chi Chiang. "Pharmaceutical benefit scheme and cost containment in Taiwan's National Health Insurance." In Albert l. Wertheimer (ed), *International Drug Regulatory Mechanisms*, pp. 132–149. Boca Raton: CRC Press, 2022.

41 Angeles, Rebecca. "Blockchain-based healthcare: Three successful proof-of-concept pilots worth considering." *Journal of International Technology and Information Management* 27, no. 3 (2019): 47–83.

42 Kumar, Tanesh, Vidhya Ramani, Ijaz Ahmad, An Braeken, Erkki Harjula, and Mika Ylianttila. "Blockchain utilization in healthcare: Key requirements and challenges." In *2018 IEEE 20th International Conference on e-Health Networking, Applications and Services (Healthcom)*, pp. 1–7. IEEE, 2018.

43 Yadlapalli, Aswini, Shams Rahman, and Pinapala Gopal. "Blockchain technology implementation challenges in supply chains–evidence from the case studies of multi-stakeholders." *The International Journal of Logistics Management* 33, no. 5 (2022): 278–305.

44 Hastig, Gabriella M., and ManMohan S. Sodhi. "Blockchain for supply chain traceability: Business requirements and critical success factors." *Production and Operations Management* 29, no. 4 (2020): 935–954.

45 Rai, Bipin Kumar. "BBTCD: Blockchain based traceability of counterfeited drugs." *Health Services and Outcomes Research Methodology* 23, no. 3 (2023): 337–353.

13 Emerging Trends NFTs and Healthcare Data Ownership

Akhil Sharma, Ashish Verma, Akanksha Sharma, Sunita, Shaweta Sharma, Shivkanya Fuloria

Introduction

Non-fungible tokens (NFTs) are one of the most important implementations of blockchain technology to date, as they are uniquely identifiable and non-interchangeable. In contrast, cryptocurrencies (i.e., bitcoin or ether) are fungible assets that can be traded on a one-to-one basis. In contrast, an NFT is a non-fungible digital asset that provides ownership of and exclusive rights to a unique item or piece of content. Every NFT contains a unique identifier that verifies ownership and authenticity, making it impossible for two tokens to be identical. The ability to take its knowledge outside a specific context is what facilitates such a diverse range of applications in art, music, gaming, and now more than ever healthcare as well. Essentially, NFTs can contain any digital file and offer a secure and verifiable way to verify ownership and provenance through decentralised ledgers.[1,2]

Overview of Healthcare Data Ownership

Healthcare data ownership refers to the entitlements and obligations concerning personal health information (PHI), personal health records, electronic health records (EHR), and other healthcare-related data created along the patient care continuum. Traditionally, ownership has stayed largely with healthcare providers and institutions, creating an uneven power dynamic in which most people have little control over their health data. Nonetheless, a paradigm shift has taken place towards patient-centric care that acknowledges individuals are becoming stakeholders in the management of their health data. This change embodies the concepts of autonomy and informed consent that empower patients with more insight into their data collection, use, and sharing.[3]

Ownership of healthcare data is also complicated by regulatory environments such as the United States Health Insurance Portability and Accountability Act (HIPAA), which mandates data protection involving PHI. However, if regulations protect the privacy of patients, they may also unintentionally make it harder for data ownership to evolve in ways that empower them. With healthcare systems backwards, there is an immediate need to take a look at forward ideas that can allow patients to wrest back control of their data.

DOI: 10.4324/9781003529910-13

Importance of Merging NFTs with Healthcare

NFTs in healthcare offer a window for switching up the ownership and access narrative around data. Healthcare stakeholders can build a more equitable and efficient system for managing health data by taking advantage of unique NFT features (like provenance, immutability, and trustless transactions).

NFTs are used within healthcare to improve data provenance and security. By issuing ownership of health data or medical records as an NFT, each NFT can be tied to a certain set of health data. This protects the data integrity and builds trust between patients, doctors, and researchers. With data breaches and unauthorised access to PHI still being some of the biggest threats our industry faces, the blockchain behind NFTs provides a decentralised, immutable shield against such attempted abuses.[4]

Patients can be custodians of their health data, and NFTs enable this. Utilising smart contracts, patients can set their terms, dictating access to data and guidelines for its use. This makes for a much more granular way to share information where individuals can permit their data to be used in other clinical trials, research studies, or commercial purposes. This control prevents them from being stripped of their autonomy but also opens monetisation channels, thus allowing the patient to get paid for their data.

NFTs also have a great potential to boost interoperability within the healthcare ecosystem. NFTs can provide a standard of exchange for health data, which is most relevant to stakeholders who both impact and benefit from it, such as providers, insurers, researchers, and patients. Such standardisation enables a more streamlined exchange of data between platforms and systems, solving one of the biggest challenges to the delivery of quality healthcare.[5]

Concept of NFTs

NFTs are a new kind of digital asset that cannot be exchanged for or replaced by an identifiable item or value, unlike fungible tokens like cryptocurrency. The underlying idea behind NFTs is that they can be used as verifiable proof of ownership for many different digital assets like healthcare data.[6]

Unique Digital Assets

At the core of NFTs is the notion of uniqueness. NFTs are non-fungible. One major difference between fungible assets such as Bitcoin or Ethereum, which can easily be exchanged for another with equal value and represent a traded commodity, is that NFTs are unique. The details on the asset, such as ownership history, provenance, and transaction, will be recorded within metadata and then stored on a blockchain when an NFT is created. This unique identification ensures authenticity and also allows the tracing of ownership through the unchangeable ledger of the blockchain.

NFTs are distinct and are, therefore, beneficial to industries needing proof of work and originality. For example, in the field of healthcare, patient records, medical images, and research data can be converted into NFTs with verifiable and immutable records of ownership and access permissions. This structure is powerful as it allows patients to take control over their health data, which enables the shift needed in care to be more patient-centred.[7]

Blockchain Technology in NFTs

The technology on which NFTs are built and stored, or recorded and tracked, is blockchain, the decentralised, distributed ledger that keeps track of transactions across many different computers. The decentralised approach strengthens security and eliminates the risk of data manipulation or loss. The protection offered by the invisible exchange of data involves employing cryptographic principles that uphold integrity and confidentiality, which are characteristic features of blockchain technology. This means that when an NFT is created, it goes through a process called minting, which registers the token on the blockchain and ties it to a specific digital asset. Anytime the NFT is transferred or sold, that information is recorded in the blockchain, which can be tracked and verified. In the healthcare domain, for example, having a verifiable record of who owns and accesses data is certainly useful in supporting compliance with regulatory frameworks such as HIPAA.[8]

Often, Smart contracts, which are self-executing contracts with the terms of the agreement directly written into code, are also used with NFTs. They can schedule processes such as access to health data or a transaction, thus increasing efficiency and agility while minimising intermediaries.

NFTs rely on blockchain for a solid foundation to secure ownership and authenticity of unique digital files. NFTs can be used in many sectors, with the greatest impact probably being realised in healthcare, as they challenge conventional notions of data control and ownership, providing security and transparency while restoring individual power. NFT technology is still fairly new, but its applicability goes far beyond digital art and collectables; it has the potential to push health data management and patient engagement forward in a significant way.[9]

Types of NFTs in Healthcare

NFTs provide a revolutionary alternative in terms of ownership, privacy, and access to your healthcare data. NFTs are digital assets with unique identification codes and metadata for specific instances of blockchain use; they provide new opportunities to manage different kinds of healthcare data. This may be patient records, medical images, or research data, as illustrated in Figure 13.1. This discussion is developed around these three types of NFTs that are specific to the healthcare domain.

Patient Records

NFTs can also change the way we manage patient records due to their ability to create a secure, immutable, and easy-to-access method of storing PHI. Traditionally, patient records are siloed in disparate healthcare systems, resulting in

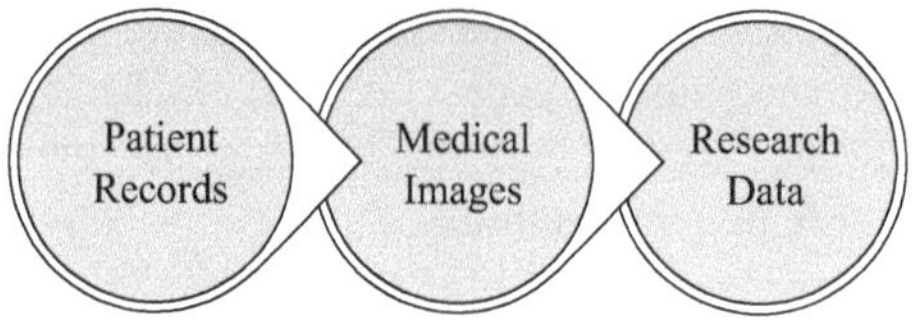

Figure 13.1 Types of NFTs in Healthcare.

inefficiencies, breaches of data as well and a lack of interoperability. Tokenising patient records into NFTs could help create a unified and searchable digital storehouse of verifiable information related to a person's health history.

Each NFT could represent a fundamental aspect of a patient's medical history, such as diagnosis, treatment, medication, and laboratory results. This increases data accuracy while giving patients more control over their information. By using smart contracts, patients can allow special healthcare providers and even researchers to access their records for general but personalised care. In addition, NFTs can enable secure data sharing between involved parties, such as stakeholders like insurers and specialists, while providing a comprehensive perspective on every aspect of the patient's health journey.[10]

Medical Images

Medical imaging includes MRI, CT scans, and X-rays, which are essential for diagnosis and treatment planning. Such images are now ubiquitous in the healthcare setting through digitisation, but questions about ownership, access, and reproducibility remain. Using NFTs, medical images can be attributed and stored in an immutable manner by having each NFT represent a single image with its metadata.

NFTs create a strong framework for validation and provenance of medical images. Each token may contain information such as imaging modality, acquisition date of the image, and clinical information about that particular image to provide more context about the image. NFTs also have a potential application beyond art by providing institutions with the means to license their images for research and educational usage while being able to monetise their imaging assets without losing control over how their images are used. This could enhance collaboration between researchers, radiologists, and institutions to drive innovation and progress in medical imaging technologies.[11]

Research Data

Healthcare research data covers everything from clinical trial results to genomic data. One major hurdle of research data is its management and sharing, where matters such as data privacy, reproducibility, and access are debated. With NFTs, researchers can still make verifiable and shareable representations of their datasets for collaboration while easily ensuring their data is not corrupted.[12]

With NFTs, researchers will have a clear and verifiable record of their data usage, enabling them to trace how their data is accessed and used by others. This is especially relevant, given the ethical discussions about data ownership and consent. When used in conjunction with NFTs, researchers can use smart contracts to ensure that their contributions are properly rewarded and used in clear terms. Additionally, the approach would allow for datasets to be tokenised and thus encourage people to participate in clinical research and share their data with other organisations as long as privacy is protected during that process.[13]

Current Trends in Healthcare Data Ownership

Shift towards Patient-Centred Care

The paradigm of health care delivery is rapidly changing with more focus on patient-centred and personal care, which includes moving the lens to see beyond reducing morbidity and mortality in acute settings and recognising nationally relevant priorities like heart failure. Instead, it emphasises the unique needs, preferences, and values of patients, who are seen as active participants in their health care. That means a very important change in terms of who owns the data. For most of the history of healthcare, data ownership will reside in the hands of providers and institutions. On the other hand, evidence-based practice encourages physicians to take into account patients' preferences when including them in their care plans; hence, patients need access to and control of their health data.

Patient engagement is essential to this trend, helping establish a collaborative relationship between patients and healthcare providers. By promoting patient involvement in health outcomes, this partnership empowers patients to be a part of their treatment decisions. An emerging component of practice called shared decision-making, where the providers share all relevant information and the patient's preferences and values about it to facilitate the decision, is gaining ground. Consequently, patients can comprehend their health information and, therefore, request access as well as ownership of this aspect.[14]

Digital health tools, including EHRs, patient portals, and mobile health applications, have revolutionised the manner in which patients engage with their existing health data. These technologies enable patients' immediate access to their medical records, lab results, and treatment trials. This allows patients to make more informed decisions about their care and reinforces the necessity of a reconceptualised framework for data ownership that identifies the patient as first among equal stakeholders.

A shift towards patient-centred care requires a rethinking of how patients are asked for permission to use their data. The unit of observation is even getting larger, and patients have started to realise how important their health data is in other domains, including research and population/public health, paving the way for calls for more transparent/interactive consent mechanisms. Such a demand for ownership necessitates that we move away from traditional models of consent, which are often based on one-time authorisation, into more granular types of acceptance for patients to declare what their data can and cannot be used for, reinforcing their rights as owners over their information.

Increasing Value of Personal Health Data

Personal health data is one of the most precious commodities of this decade in the new-age healthcare ecosystem. Advancements in technology, including artificial intelligence (AI) and machine learning, have increased the value of health data for facilitating individualised treatment and improving healthcare delivery. Wearable health devices and mobile health applications have proliferated; patients are now able to continuously monitor their health metrics, with vast amounts of data created that are ready for analysis.[15]

The growth of interest in personal health data is being fuelled partly by the recognition of its potential value to new healthcare payers and technology players. They are excited to use the knowledge from health data to improve clinical outcomes, design personalised medicines, and increase operational efficiencies. Consequently, the health data of patients is being turned into a commodity, and there are several deliberations on ownership of this data, privacy issues, and ethics around the usage of data.[16]

The term "data monetisation" is gaining popularity; individual payments for the use of health data in research or commercial applications may be a possibility in the future. It can also lead to wonders about the rights of patients as data owners and how they can preserve their ownership of such sensitive information. Also, ensure a regulating framework that provides enough information is delivered to the patient on how their data will be used and compensated.

Personal health data continues to become much more valuable; there is an increasing need for strong data governance frameworks that prioritise patient privacy and autonomy. With the rising value of health data comes an increased risk of data breaches and misuse. As a result, healthcare organisations face the challenge of protecting sensitive patient data against vulnerabilities as well as ensuring patients know they own that information.[17]

Regulations and Compliance

The regulatory frameworks are important in defining the ownership of healthcare data. HIPAA is one of only a few laws that enforce some aspects of health data privacy and security. HIPAA sets strict standards regarding the handling of protected health information (PHI) and requires healthcare providers and organisations to implement safeguards in order to guarantee the confidentiality and integrity of data.

Under HIPAA, patients have certain rights with respect to their health information, including access to their medical records and requests for corrections of inaccurate information. This is central to ensuring patient autonomy and empowering people to take control of their health data. But despite being a good start for protecting data, the evolving healthcare landscape means this no longer is fit for purpose, and change needs to occur in order to meet emerging challenges and trends.[18]

The increasing use of digital health technologies and the huge amount of health-related information created by mobile applications and monitored with wearable devices pose fresh challenges for regulation. The vast majority of these platforms should be seen as going beyond the regular healthcare system. Hence, there will always be ambivalence regarding whether existing regulatory frameworks will apply to data that has been collected under this interface. Such practice requires comprehensive regulatory guidance that covers these emerging data sources to ensure protections for patients remain strong.

With the rise of globalisation and the cross-border flow of health data, there is a greater recognition that international cooperation will be required to solve challenges related to the ownership of data. The European Union GDPR (General Data Protection Regulation) pioneered an individual rights and data ownership-centric approach to data protection law. In a world with healthcare systems that seem to grow increasingly interwoven, and need to harmonise regulatory frameworks across jurisdictions so as not to stifle the necessary sharing of data for research and innovation but also protect patients.[19]

Challenges in Data Ownership

However, many challenges remain that still prevent patient-centred data ownership from becoming a reality and continue to slow the movement towards citizen redefinition of healthcare data ownership. One of the biggest challenges is the complexity of health data ecosystems that often include various stakeholders. Decentralisation of data sources makes it difficult to delineate ownership rights and responsibilities.

The aspect of data interoperability presents high hurdles to data flow across stakeholders. Instead, multiple and scant standards exist for storing and exchanging healthcare data, with varying levels of technology sophistication among organisations that often lead to disparate systems that do a poor job utilising the overall dataset. Achieving interoperable health data cannot be achieved without the collaboration of industry players to set universal standards and protocols that allow for the secure transfer of ownership over such sensitive information.[20]

Another challenge lies in the fact that health data ownership involves legal and ethical issues. The exploitation risk and potential for misuse with these datasets are also increasing as health data continues to rise in value. Research with patients' data may become unethical without their consent. Such concern highlights the need for transparent data usage policies with an emphasis on seeking informed consent and ethical governance of the data.

Patients are not aware of their rights with respect to data ownership. The way most people do not know the control they have over their health information prevents them from being involved in data management systems. A lack of awareness further exacerbates this gap, and hence, educating the masses about this issue is a prerequisite to enabling patients with self-authorisation.[21]

Changes in cybersecurity threats set challenges for data ownership. A number of high-profile security breaches and leaks have highlighted the inherent weaknesses in systems that store health data, leading to serious questions about patient privacy and trust. Given that many organisations now use various digital solutions for managing data, it is crucial to adopt high-security systems so that sensitive health information is safe from unnecessary access and breaches.[22]

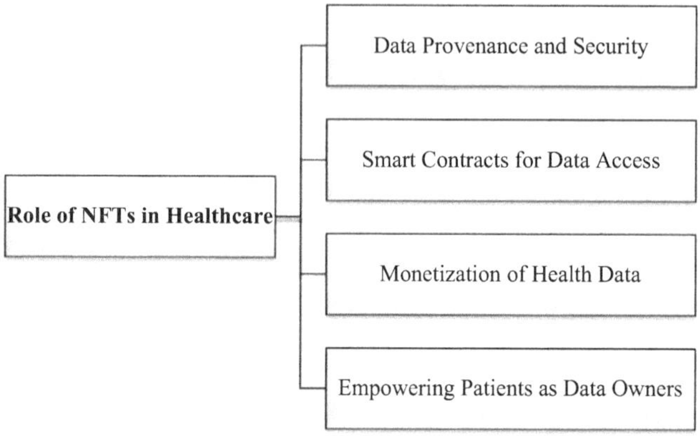

Figure 13.2 Role of NFTs in Healthcare.

Role of NFTs in Healthcare

As new technology, NFTs, enter the healthcare field, bringing a paradigm shift that includes new solutions to age-old issues of data provenance, security, and ownership. The functions that NFTs can perform in healthcare (data provenance and security, data access through smart contracts, monetisation of health data, and patients as data owners) are further discussed below and represented in Figure 13.2.

Data Provenance and Security

Data provenance in healthcare is nothing but the origin and lifecycle tracking of the data. It is essential for preserving the authenticity of medical records and making sure health information can be relied on. Through blockchain technology, NFTs can also support improved data provenance by creating a record (immutable, transparent) of who made the data/when, modified it/when, and accessed it.

Data provenance in the healthcare sector tracks where data comes from and what it passes through during its life cycle. This is essential to ensure that medical records are maintained and health data can be verified. Using blockchain technology, NFTs can allow for improved data provenance through an unalterable and transparent ledger of data creation, alteration, and access.

NFTs are, by design, unique and not replaceable. Hence, they can even ensure a strong mechanism for the authenticity of medical data. For example, if an NFT were minted based on a patient's medical record, every update to the record could be tracked in order on the blockchain. This creates a transparent audit chain, which is important for compliance with the HIPAA or simply maintaining trust with patients.[23]

NFTs improve data security by taking advantage of decentralised storage. Methods of data management in healthcare have a key feature; they are situated in one place, thus potential places where hackers could steal information or people who can access it illegally. On the other hand, NFTs can be distributed over a decentralised network of nodes, reducing single points of failure. Blockchain can support each NFT transaction and is therefore tamper-proof, which greatly reduces the risk of data corruption or unauthorised modification. NFTs can also enhance the overall integrity and trustworthiness of patient information by providing a secure, transparent mechanism for tracking healthcare data.[24]

Smart Contracts for Data Access

Smart contracts are computer programs (self-executing contracts) containing the terms of the agreement between buyer and seller. This is where smart contracts can ensure patient access to their patient data in a healthcare context. Employing NFTs with smart contracts can enable healthcare providers to automate data sharing in a way that respects and fulfils patient consent.

As an example, when the healthcare data of a patient is converted into an NFT, a smart contract can be implemented to define who has access to this data under what conditions and for how long. This special feature is especially helpful for queuing research scenarios in which patient data needs to be booked with third parties. Using a smart contract that complies with privacy regulations, only the necessary data can be accessed; it ensures that researchers use only data for its intended purposes.[25]

Moreover, smart contracts enable real-time data sharing that can be invaluable in an emergency healthcare context. As a simple example, if someone has been admitted into a hospital, their medical history may be saved on an NFT, and the smart contract can be read to identify any allergies or existing conditions quickly. Providing this timely access can enhance outcomes by informing the patient decision-making process.

Smart contracts enable automation, which also lowers the administrative overhead and cost of classic data-sharing agreements. Healthcare providers can remove large-scale reliance on third parties while keeping patient information tightly locked down within their networks.[26]

The Monetisation of Health Data

The emergence of NFTs in healthcare also creates new opportunities for the monetisation of health data. Historically, patients had minimal control over their data, at times being unaware of the commercial value associated with using patient data. NFTs are able to reshape the agency of patients, who can sell or license access to their data, and make them true participants in the data economy.

One example of this can be seen through NFT representations of a patient's health data, where the data collected from various wearable devices will be stored in an offshore database and tokenised as an NFT. That data can then be licensed to research institutions or drug companies studying trends or outcomes related to those conditions for a fee paid by the patient. That gives patients possible financial motivation, and it incentivises a more ethical practice of data usage.[27]

NFTs enable microtransactions and may allow for compensation based on data points or clinical trial participation directly to the patient. It is gradually fitting into an increasing paradigm of personalised medicine where information independent of an individual can be extremely beneficial for researchers and healthcare providers alike. NFTs and associated monetisation may open the way for a more equitable system in healthcare, where patients can be compensated for their data contribution to research with a transparent and efficient process.

This model also requires a broad framework when it comes to data privacy and consent. There should be clear guidelines to ensure that patients are aware of the implications of monetising their data and are in charge of the utilisation of their information.[28]

Empowering Patients as Data Owners

Perhaps one of the most revolutionary things about using NFTs in healthcare is that it allows patients to own their data. Historically, patient data was stored and managed within healthcare institutions, which kept patients disengaged from their health information. By enabling patients to take back control of their data, NFTs represent a way for individual patients to own and benefit from the value created by that data.

Healthcare data is tokenised as NFTs, allowing the patient to curate their health data by modifying who gets access to it. This could help increase the number of patients who play an active role in their health journeys. Easier access to health records, for example, can help patients actively engage in discussions with healthcare providers, which may facilitate better decision-making and health literacy.[29]

Moreover, since patients are the owners of these data, they can select and share their data according to their practices. Sharing data for research, getting paid, or simply letting health-care providers have the information they need. Enabling patients like this makes them more independent, and it creates the foundation for a new collaborative healthcare ecosystem to flourish because now, patients and providers are partners working towards the same goal of improving health outcomes.

The shift towards patient data ownership aligns with broader trends in healthcare, emphasising patient-centred care. By recognising patients as stakeholders in their health data, the healthcare system can move towards a more equitable and transparent model.

NFTs in healthcare offer many possibilities to improve the provenance, security, and ownership of data. With blockchain technology and smart contracts extracting, NFTs can provide more secure storage of health data and money for access to health records transfer from those who want to own such information. More importantly, NFTs can put patients in charge of their data, nurturing an approach to healthcare that puts the patient at the centre stage instead of being just a part of background noise. With an ever-changing landscape, the role of NFTs is only going to become more important for the future of healthcare data ownership and management.[30]

Benefits of Using NFTs in Healthcare

The four key benefits of NFTs in healthcare enhanced data privacy, improved interoperability, decentralised data management, and the potential for new revenue streams are discussed below and represented in Figure 13.3.

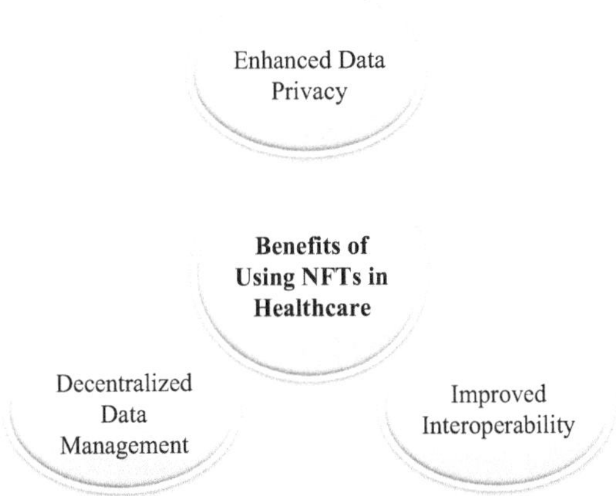

Figure 13.3 Benefits of Using NFTs in Healthcare.

Enhanced Data Privacy

Patient data is extremely sensitive and cannot be accessed by anyone outside of HIPAA guidelines. Databases in traditional data storage systems are often centralised, which allows them to be hacked, easily breached, and accessed unlawfully. In particular, NFTs can improve data privacy in a more transformative way because of the blockchain itself, which offers a secure and immutable ledger.[31]

NFTs are unique digital assets that can be tied to specific health data simply by nature. This linkage can be managed with cryptography, and patients can have total authority over who gets their data. NFTs can empower patients with the ability to control access to their data whenever they want, enabling something new for healthcare providers.

Improved Interoperability

Interoperability is a form of connective infrastructure that connects systems and organisations to remove friction from the flow of information. Interoperability in healthcare is key to enabling patient data to flow seamlessly between providers, payers, and other stakeholders. However, traditional systems often suffer from fragmented data silos, leading to inefficiencies and suboptimal patient care.

NFTs are essential for better interoperability as they provide a framework to represent medical data consistently. NFTs can encapsulate certain types of clinical patient information (e.g., EHRs, imaging data, and genome sequences) in a standardised format. Data normalisation enables different data sources to be blended so providers can see complete patient profiles.[32]

Decentralised Data Management

In the traditional model, healthcare data management relies heavily on centralised systems. The above can be solved using NFTs and other blockchain technologies, which provide a more decentralised way of managing data. This ensures that healthcare organisations do not have to depend on central authorities, thereby minimising the likelihood of data breaches.

On the other hand, in a decentralised model, patients own their health data as NFTs to represent ownership of information digitally. In such an ownership model, the control over data is moved from healthcare providers to patients, and they can now decide when their data is used, where it goes, and with whom it is shared. Patients share ownership and control of their data for different purposes, such as research, clinical trials, or delivery of care.

Decentralisation can make healthcare data systems more robust than centralised models, where data losses or service outages at a single point of failure can be catastrophic. On the other side, decentralised systems assign risk to many nodes, creating redundancy and availability. Such resiliency has become even more essential in health care, where access to data (e.g., patient records) can be a matter of life and death.[33]

Potential for New Revenue Streams

In addition, the adoption of NFTs in healthcare also opens the doors for new revenue streams to be created and distributed to both patients and healthcare providers. Earning from their data in return for sharing high-quality datasets with researchers, pharma companies, or other agents in the marketplace. More and more patients can own and control their health records.

For example, patients can use clinical trials or research studies to allow researchers to access their anonymous data history. NFTs can grant and automate consent and payment via smart contracts, allowing access to unique content. NFTs can give patients an economic incentive to part with their data by creating a marketplace for health data and enabling them to monetise their personal information in exchange for services like scientific discoveries.[34]

NFTs open up new business opportunities to healthcare providers. They could offer NFT-powered subscription services, which grant patients access to personalised data-driven health insights, customised treatment plans, or exclusive health resources. Such services improve patient engagement and generate continuous revenue for healthcare organisations.

NFTs can allow for the tokenisation of any asset within the healthcare ecosystem, such as medical devices, pharmaceuticals, or research findings. Such tokenisation can lead to fractional ownership and enable investors to invest in innovations in the healthcare spectrum while diversifying their portfolios. NFTs have the potential to open up liquidity in otherwise illiquid assets, which can help direct investment into healthcare innovation, which will ultimately lead to better outcomes for patients and society as a whole.[35]

Challenges in the Adoption of NFTs for Healthcare Data Ownership

Healthcare's transformative paradigm for NFTs also poses multiple interrelated challenges and concerns, and sequential solution pathways are needed to catalyse successful adoption. This segment explores the technological obstacles to adoption, ethical and legal aspects, data breach threats, and regulatory compliance challenges of NFTs in healthcare.

Technical Barriers to Adoption

However, some technical challenges must be overcome when making the switch from traditional healthcare data ownership to an NFT-based model. Most importantly, the compatibility of blockchain technologies with current healthcare information systems is a major obstacle. At the same time, most healthcare organisations house their data in numerous proprietary systems for archival and management purposes that are unlikely to be compatible with blockchain architecture. The absence of standardisation leads to multiple repositories for health data, making it difficult to tokenise the records.

One of the very first hurdles that many blockchain solutions are still facing is handling scales. Most blockchain networks, and especially the ones based on proof-of-work mechanisms, have limitations in the ability to process transactions (transaction speed/capacity). In healthcare, when timely information access and transfer are paramount for patient care, such constraints can delay the entire system.[36]

Managing and implementing NFT systems requires quite a good technical knowledge. Healthcare professionals may not have an adequate understanding of blockchain technology, which may cause operational inefficiency. Thus, thorough training and educational resources are required to give all healthcare stakeholders the necessary information to deal with this complicated technological environment.[37]

Legal and Ethical Considerations

The integration of NFTs into healthcare introduces complex legal and ethical challenges that need to be navigated carefully to protect patient rights and data integrity. The biggest question that is emerging is ownership of health data. Despite NFTs possibly enabling decentralised ownership, the legal frameworks behind them are opaque on data ownership. This relates specifically to patients transferring data for research or commercial purposes, which can influence the transferability of ownership. Clear legal precedents and guidelines should be established to prevent disputes over data ownership and usage rights.[38]

Consent and privacy have to be taken into consideration from an ethical perspective. Patients have to be well-notified about how their data will be tokenised and used, potentially even commercialised. Because NFTs can change hands with relative ease, acquiring informed consent becomes even more of a challenge. Trust in the system will require patients to retain ownership of their data while being allowed to consent to its use.

However, the commodification of health data for NFTs has its ethical considerations. Data shared for research purposes can be incentivised by monetisation, but this could also create opportunities for the exploitation of vulnerable populations. NFT ecosystem must tread between the need to provide incentives for data sharing and ensuring that patient welfare is protected, which is an ethical obligation.[39]

Data Security Risks

While blockchain technology is lauded for its built-in security attributes, NFT use in healthcare does not completely mitigate risk to the privacy or security of data. One of the greatest fears is those vulnerabilities existing in the blockchain network itself. Decentralisation improves security, but it also brings its threat: In 51% of attacks where one malicious actor controls the majority and can tamper with the integrity of whatever we are putting on-chain.

One of the challenges with the blockchain is that all transactions are permanent. It can become incredibly hard to remedy the situation if sensitive health data is tokenised and later hacked. In traditional data systems, when we make a mistake in database entries, such as pasting wrong patient data, it can be corrected, but in the case of blockchain, once information like personal health details has been entered into the system, it cannot be removed resulting in permanent disclosure of sensitive patient records.

When it comes to data security, the digital divide is a major issue. Data tokenisation could exacerbate inequitable access to healthcare among populations without high-tech resources. It is critical to ensure that security measures are not ignored and made accessible to all patients, else the ones who need it the most will be left out, and data exploitation and marginalisation may take place.[40]

Regulatory Compliance Issues

One of the major barriers to the adoption of NFTs for healthcare data ownership is regulatory compliance. We already have existing regulations like the HIPAA in the US that require us to treat patient data as sensitive information. Healthcare has its own set of regulations that any adoption of NFT use will have to comply with in order to protect patient rights by ensuring some anonymity.[41]

Blockchain comprises a range of decentralised systems and processes, which gives compliance professionals headaches. Since many regulatory frameworks are built around centralised actors, this makes it difficult to impose traditional regulations on decentralised systems such as the ones based on NFTs. This vagueness causes non-compliance, exposing healthcare organisations and entities to legal liabilities.

The NFT landscape is progressing at lightning speed, and regulators must keep pace with it by establishing NFT-guided policies that address the distinctiveness of both NFTs and blockchain technology in health care. This eventually establishes the benchmarks surrounding data privacy, informed consent, and rights regarding the usage of patient data. Policymakers need to work with stakeholders of the healthcare ecosystem in designing an environment that promotes innovation with respect for patient interest.[42]

Future Directions in NFTs and Healthcare Data Ownership

The infusion of NFTs into the healthcare landscape represents a radical change in data ownership, privacy, and interoperability. A number of emerging technologies, in tandem with NFTs and at various stages of acceptance, will support this growing field. Forecasts regarding the role of NFTs in healthcare will clarify how this segment may develop. Lastly, policymakers and various stakeholders would play a significant role in integrating these in an ethical and sustainable manner.

Emerging Technologies Complementing NFTs

Various developing technologies are ready to make NFTs more effective and useful in healthcare. The backbone that supports an NFT) is Blockchain technology, which provides unchangeable records and data provenance, leading to a trust-building process while managing patient data. Interoperability standards like Fast Healthcare Interoperability Resources will ensure data can be shared across platforms seamlessly, allowing the NFT to capture multiple different types of health records accurately.

Features of AI can be integrated into the analysis of NFT-oriented structures to enable real-time aggregation of healthcare data. The analysis process of AI algorithms on large hypotheses can identify patterns and insights, which NFTs can also impact to represent the novel paradigms of patient care and research. IoT devices can also facilitate the collection and validation of data. Real-time health data can be generated using Internet of Things devices, which can be minted as NFTs, allowing patients to take ownership of their health records.[43]

Predictions for the Integration of NFTs in Healthcare

In upcoming years, it expects a massive uptick in NFTs being used for patient empowerment and data monetisation. NFTs could well become a leading use case for personalised medicine, in which patients can retain ownership of their genomic data and share it anonymously. Such democratisation of data could catalyse research and drug development since, in anonymised datasets, pharmaceutical companies would be able to tap into such datasets while also being mindful of individual privacy.[44]

NFTs could unlock a new paradigm for clinical trials and research funding. Policymakers and researchers streamline recruitment, improve transparency, and compensate data contributors equally when tokenising patient consent. This will obviously support the incorporation of a wider and more diverse population in research designs, enhancing generalisability and applicability.

Role of Policymakers and Stakeholders

To make it work, NFT healthcare experts claim that policymakers and others must actively bring people together. Such regulatory frameworks must also be established to deal with the legal implications related to data ownership and patient privacy.

Regulators need to develop standards that balance patient safety and protection with innovation. Establishing standards for NFT interoperability, security, and ethical use will be critical to building trust among patients and providers for example.

Collaboration among stakeholders, including healthcare providers, technology developers, and patient advocacy groups, will be needed to develop best practices for the use of NFT. Such a multidisciplinary approach can mitigate the complexities related to NFT, especially data consent and privacy issues. Finally, education and awareness campaigns will be critical in giving patients the knowledge necessary to understand this changed landscape so that they can be informed participants in their healthcare journey.[45,46]

Conclusion

This combination of NFTs and healthcare data ownership opens up an exciting new paradigm in how our PHI is controlled, accessed, and used. As healthcare moves to a more patient-centric approach, having patients in control of their data has become more critical than ever. This transition reveals the necessity of emerging solutions such as NFT, which can be uniquely verified digital objects to securely represent various health-related data elements (physical or mental patient records, medical images, research data, and medicinal data).

NFTs leverage blockchain technology for greater security and provenance solutions to nearly perennial data integrity and privacy problems with digital information. The integrity of medical data ensured by NFTs would build better trust between patients and healthcare provider organisations. Furthermore, NFTs can theoretically be tied to smart contracts relevant to data access, which allows patients to both grant and revoke access to their information while enabling compliance with HIPAA.

There are multiple potential advantages of using NFTs in healthcare. This system not only supports data privacy and security but also improves interoperability among the diverse healthcare systems, allowing for a seamless exchange of information across various platforms. Additionally, NFTs can enable more patient control over health data; with decentralised data management, patients are in control of their health information, and they can choose when/how to use it. Such empowerment can help patients create new revenue streams by opting to sell or monetise their health data for research or other purposes.

The Challenges Ahead: However, there are many problems accompanying NFT adoption in healthcare. This means it can be implemented at scale, but various technical barriers need to be overcome. Legal and ethical considerations must also be taken into account, as well as data security risks and regulatory compliance issues. Establishing strong frameworks for stakeholder collaboration will be integral to surmounting those barriers.

The integration of emerging technologies will complement NFTs, enhancing their capabilities and utility within the healthcare ecosystem. Policymakers play a crucial role in establishing guidelines that protect patient rights while promoting innovation, ensuring that the benefits of NFTs can be realised without compromising ethical standards.

References

1 Xi, Ran. "Application-oriented: A polycentric framework for non-fungible tokens." *Rutgers Computer and Technology Law Journal* 50 (2023): 205.

2 Arjunwadkar, Maithili Vijay, and Bharati Mahadev Ramageri. "Metaverse and NFT." In Abdelkader Mohamed Sghaier Derbali (eds), *Blockchain Applications for Smart Contract Technologies*, pp. 72–99. New York: IGI Global, 2024.

3 Kalkman, Shona, Johannes Van Delden, Amitava Banerjee, Benoît Tyl, Menno Mostert, and Ghislaine Van Thiel. "Patients' and public views and attitudes towards the sharing of health data for research: A narrative review of the empirical evidence." *Journal of Medical Ethics* 48, no. 1 (2022): 3–13.

4 Esmaeilzadeh, Pouyan. "Evolution of health information sharing between health care organisations: Potential of nonfungible tokens." *Interactive Journal of Medical Research* 12, no. 1 (2023): e42685.

5 Kuznetsov, Oleksandr, Emanuele Frontoni, Kateryna Kuznetsova, Ruslan Shevchuk, and Mikolaj Karpinski. "NFT technology for enhanced global digital registers: A novel approach to tokenization." *Future Internet* 16, no. 7 (2024): 252.

6 Osterrieder, Joerg, Stephen Chan, Jeffrey Chu, and Yuanyuan Zhang. "Metaverse non-fungible tokens." Available at SSRN 4733153 (2024): 1–29.

7 Razi, Qaiser, Aryan Devrani, Harshal Abhyankar, G. Sai Sesha Chalapathi, Vikas Hassija, and Mohsen Guizani. "Non-fungible tokens (NFTs) a survey of current applications, evolution and future directions." *IEEE Open Journal of the Communications Society* (2023): 2765–2791.

8 Chen, Jim Q., and Allen Benusa. "HIPAA security compliance challenges: The case for small healthcare providers." *International Journal of Healthcare Management* 10, no. 2 (2017): 135–146.

9 Twinomurinzi, Hossana, Patrick Ndayizigamiye, and Khulekani Sibanda. "Non-fungible tokens (NFTs) in healthcare: A thematic analysis and research agenda." *Frontiers in Digital Health* 6 (2024): 1377531.

10 Bang, L. K., P. H. T. Trung, H. G. Khiem, N. T. K. Ngan, T. B. Nam, N. N. Hung, L. T. Nhi, and P. T. Nghiem. "Towards medical record keeping with blockchain, RSA-encrypted NFTs, and smart contracts." In *International Conference on Computer Information Systems and Industrial Management*, pp. 60–73. Cham: Springer Nature Switzerland, 2024.

11 Biesecker, Leslie G., James C. Mullikin, Flavia M. Facio, Clesson Turner, Praveen F. Cherukuri, Robert W. Blakesley, Gerard G. Bouffard, et al. "The ClinSeq Project: Piloting large-scale genome sequencing for research in genomic medicine." *Genome Research* 19, no. 9 (2009): 1665–1674.

12 Quy, T. L., Nguyen DP Trong, H. V. Khanh, H. L. Huong, T. D. Khoa, H. G. Khiem, N. T. Phuc et al. "Transforming child health records: Integrating blockchain, NFTs, and IPFS for enhanced medical data management." In *International Conference on Mobile, Secure, and Programmable Networking*, pp. 120–138. Cham: Springer Nature Switzerland, 2023.

13 Esmaeilzadeh, Pouyan, and Tala Mirzaei. "Role of incentives in the use of blockchain-based platforms for sharing sensitive health data: experimental study." *Journal of Medical Internet Research* 25 (2023): e41805.

14 Stiggelbout, Anne M., Arwen H. Pieterse, and Johanna CJM De Haes. "Shared decision making: Concepts, evidence, and practice." *Patient Education and Counseling* 98, no. 10 (2015): 1172–1179.

15 Williamson, Steven M., and Victor Prybutok. "Balancing privacy and progress: A review of privacy challenges, systemic oversight, and patient perceptions in AI-driven healthcare." *Applied Sciences* 14, no. 2 (2024): 675.

16 Diaz, Mabeth. "Data integration and analysis in healthcare: A pivot within the industry." PhD diss., University of Pittsburgh, 2022.

17 Abouelmehdi, Karim, Abderrahim Beni-Hessane, and Hayat Khaloufi. "Big healthcare data: Preserving security and privacy." *Journal of Big Data* 5, no. 1 (2018): 1–18.

18 Riad, ABM Kamrul Islam, Md Abdul Barek, Md Mostafizur Rahman, Mst Shapna Akter, Tahia Islam, Md Abdur Rahman, Md Raihan Mia, Hossain Shahriar, Fan Wu, and Sheikh Iqbal Ahamed. "Enhancing HIPAA compliance in AI-driven mHealth devices security and privacy." In *2024 IEEE 48th Annual Computers, Software, and Applications Conference (COMPSAC)*, pp. 2430–2435. IEEE, 2024.

19 Raut, Neha, Komal Bajaj, Prathmesh Matte, Muskan Vhora, Vinita Kale, Milind Umekar, and Suankit Harane. "Building bridges: Harmonization efforts for enhanced collaboration between developed and developing countries." *International Journal of Drug Regulatory Affairs* 11, no. 3 (2023): 68–79.

20 Kouroubali, Angelina, and Dimitrios G. Katehakis. "The new European interoperability framework as a facilitator of digital transformation for citizen empowerment." *Journal of Biomedical Informatics* 94 (2019): 103166.

21 Kutz, Daniel O., and Hamid R. Ekbia. "Designing for the invincible: Health engagement and information management." *In 2011 44th Hawaii International Conference on System Sciences*, pp. 1–10. IEEE, 2011.

22 Li, He, Sungjin Yoo, and William J. Kettinger. "The roles of IT strategies and security investments in reducing organizational security breaches." *Journal of Management Information Systems* 38, no. 1 (2021): 222–245.

23 Bandyopadhyay, Anjan, Jyotirmoy Karmakar, Kartikeya Raj, and Sujata Swain. "Fake medicine detection using blockchain in metaverse domain." In Saurav Mallik, Anjan Bandyopadhyay, Ruifeng Hu, Pawan Kumar Singh, Soumadip Ghosh, Sujata Swain (eds), *Healthcare Services in the Metaverse*, pp. 154–169. Boca Raton: CRC Press, 2024.

24 Poston III, Howard E. *Blockchain Security from the Bottom Up: Securing and Preventing Attacks on Cryptocurrencies, Decentralized Applications, NFTs, and Smart Contracts*. New Jersey: John Wiley & Sons, 2022.

25 Desai, Harsh, Kevin Liu, Murat Kantarcioglu, and Lalana Kagal. "Adjudicating violations in data sharing agreements using smart contracts." In *2018 IEEE International Conference on Internet of Things (iThings) and IEEE Green Computing and Communications (GreenCom) and IEEE Cyber, Physical and Social Computing (CPSCom) and IEEE Smart Data (SmartData)*, pp. 1553–1560. IEEE, 2018.

26 Li, Jennifer, and Mohamad Kassem. "Applications of distributed ledger technology (DLT) and Blockchain-enabled smart contracts in construction." *Automation in Construction* 132 (2021): 103955.

27 Chiruvella, Varsha, and Achuta Kumar Guddati. "Ethical issues in patient data ownership." *Interactive Journal of Medical Research* 10, no. 2 (2021): e22269.

28 Kaplan, Bonnie. "How should health data be used?: Privacy, secondary use, and big data sales." *Cambridge Quarterly of Healthcare Ethics* 25, no. 2 (2016): 312–329.

29 Smith, Sian K., Ann Dixon, Lyndal Trevena, Don Nutbeam, and Kirsten J. McCaffery. "Exploring patient involvement in healthcare decision making across different education and functional health literacy groups." *Social Science & Medicine* 69, no. 12 (2009): 1805–1812.

30 Lakshmi, D., Isha Kondurkar, Raj Kumar, and Roshni Banerjee. "Intelligent healthcare systems in the Metaverse: Architecture, applications, challenges, and opportunities." *The Metaverse for the Healthcare Industry* (2024): 17–32.

31 Bertino, Elisa, and Ravi Sandhu. "Database security-concepts, approaches, and challenges." *IEEE Transactions on Dependable and Secure Computing* 2, no. 1 (2005): 2–19.

32 Quy, T. L., Nguyen DP Trong, H. V. Khanh, H. L. Huong, T. D. Khoa, H. G. Khiem, N. T. Phuc et al. "Blockchain-driven animal healthcare: Leveraging NFTs, IPFS, and smart contracts for comprehensive animal medical record." In *International Conference on Mobile, Secure, and Programmable Networking*, pp. 100–119. Cham: Springer Nature Switzerland, 2023.
33 Avula, Ramya. "Addressing barriers in data collection, transmission, and security to optimize data availability in healthcare systems for improved clinical decision-making and analytics." *Applied Research in Artificial Intelligence and Cloud Computing* 4, no. 1 (2021): 78–93.
34 Spencer, Karen, Caroline Sanders, Edgar A. Whitley, David Lund, Jane Kaye, and William Gregory Dixon. "Patient perspectives on sharing anonymized personal health data using a digital system for dynamic consent and research feedback: A qualitative study." *Journal of Medical Internet Research* 18, no. 4 (2016): e5011.
35 Graham, Luke, and Andrew Baum. "A piece of the action: Innovations in fractional ownership and use of space." Available at SSRN (2023).
36 Zhou, Qiheng, Huawei Huang, Zibin Zheng, and Jing Bian. "Solutions to scalability of blockchain: A survey." *IEEE Access* 8 (2020): 16440–16455.
37 Krishnasamy, Sathya. "My holistic data share: A WEB3 data share application: Extending beyond finance to privacy-protected decentralized share of multi-dimensional data to enhance global healthcare." *Blockchain in Healthcare Today* 7, no. 2 (2024): 1–8.
38 Al Amin, Md, Amani Altarawneh, and Indrajit Ray. "Informed consent as patient driven policy for clinical diagnosis and treatment: A smart contract based approach." In *SECRYPT*, pp. 159–170. 2023.
39 Škoro, Ivana Emily. "Blockchain art activism: Examining four blockchain-based artworks for social, political, and environmental good." PhD diss., Aalborg University, 2024.
40 Jansky, Bianca, Tereza Hendl, and Azakhiwe Z. Nocanda. "Patient-led innovation and global health justice: Open-source digital health technology for type 1 diabetes care." *Bioethics* 38, no. 6 (2024): 511–528.
41 Edemekong, Peter F., Pavan Annamaraju, and Micelle J. Haydel. "Health insurance portability and accountability act." (2018).
42 Alshater, Muneer M., Nohade Nasrallah, Rim Khoury, and Mayank Joshipura. "Deciphering the world of NFTs: A scholarly review of trends, challenges, and opportunities." *Electronic Commerce Research* (2024): 1–57.
43 Sai, Siva, Aanchal Gaur, Vikas Hassija, and Vinay Chamola. "Artificial intelligence empowered digital twin and NFT-based patient monitoring and assisting framework for chronic disease patients." *IEEE Internet of Things Magazine* 7, no. 2 (2024): 101–106.
44 Abbott, Ryan. "Big data and pharmacovigilance: Using health information exchanges to revolutionize drug safety." *Iowa Law Review* 99 (2013): 225.
45 Liu, Zhen, Zulan Yang, Mingjie Liang, Yi Liu, Mohamed Osmani, and Peter Demian. "A conceptual framework for blockchain enhanced information modeling for healing and therapeutic design." *International Journal of Environmental Research and Public Health* 19, no. 13 (2022): 8218.
46 Henwood, Flis, Sally Wyatt, Angie Hart, and Julie Smith. "'Ignorance is bliss sometimes': Constraints on the emergence of the 'informed patient'in the changing landscapes of health information." *Sociology of Health & Illness* 25, no. 6 (2003): 589–607.

14 Global Perspectives

Implementing Blockchain in Healthcare Systems

Shaweta Sharma, Sunita, Ashish Verma, Akanksha Sharma, Neeraj Kumar Fuloria, Akhil Sharma

Introduction

Blockchain is a powerful technology that has the potential to revolutionise healthcare by putting patients at the centre of healthcare ecosystems and contributing to increased security, privacy, and interoperability of health data. This might create an alternative structure for health information exchanges (HIE), helping electronic health records become more efficient, direct-to-consumer, and secure. While not a panacea, this new and fast-moving area is well worth the investment for experimentation and proof of concept. Real interoperability is only possible with a blockchain-powered HIE. The ability of blockchain-based systems to shave off or eradicate the friction and costs currently charged by intermediaries.

The promise of blockchain makes a difference to every stakeholder in the healthcare ecosystem. Drawing on that technology could be a way to link isolated systems to create insights and, ultimately, more accurately measure care value. Over the years, a national blockchain system for electronic healthcare information could streamline efficiencies and enable wiser health results among patients.[1,2]

Importance of Understanding Global Perspectives

Blockchain can significantly change existing global healthcare systems, and therefore, it is important to view this in an international context. Blockchain gives more precise data security and protects the rights of people through sharing patient information without compromising privacy or integrity, which is extremely critical in a world where access to health records is flooded with data breaches or frauds. Moreover, its interoperability lays the groundwork for data exchange between fragmented healthcare systems and people such as patients, providers, and insurers. Such an ability is key to addressing what traditional models often struggle with care coordination and efficiency.

Blockchain can also help put patients in control of their health records so they can determine who will be able to access and use their data. As the costs for healthcare rise across continents, pure efficiencies of blockchain would lead to a drastic cut out on unwanted spending and bring quality healthcare closer to the masses. Global perspectives also give stakeholders the opportunity to identify best

DOI: 10.4324/9781003529910-14

practices and shape solutions that are considered in the context of specific regional challenges, which contributes to a more equitable healthcare landscape.[3,4]

The goal of this chapter is to explore the paradigm-shifting capability of blockchain in healthcare, in (i) strengthening data protection, (ii) confidentiality, and (iii) interoperability within and among health information systems. Starting with the basics of blockchain, it will delve into its uses in healthcare, such as electronic medical records, HIEs, and clinical trials. That chapter will look at regulatory considerations, different levels of adoption, and challenges around the world. Customisation will be followed by prominent test beds, where relevant case studies and examples from the real world that demonstrate effective implementations will be presented along with future directions for ongoing research and development in the field.

Regional Insights of Blockchain in Healthcare

The various regional insights of blockchain in healthcare are described in Figure 14.1.

Trends in U.S. Healthcare Blockchain Technology Market

The United States held the most market share for blockchain technology in the healthcare industry in 2023. The proactive actions of the major U.S. players exposed the rapidly expanding market for blockchain technology in the healthcare industry.[5] As an example, Avaneer Health, a U.S. healthcare blockchain technology leader, announced a significant push from major healthcare payers in Jan 2022. This network is backed by USD 50 million of seed funding from these organisations combined.[5,6]

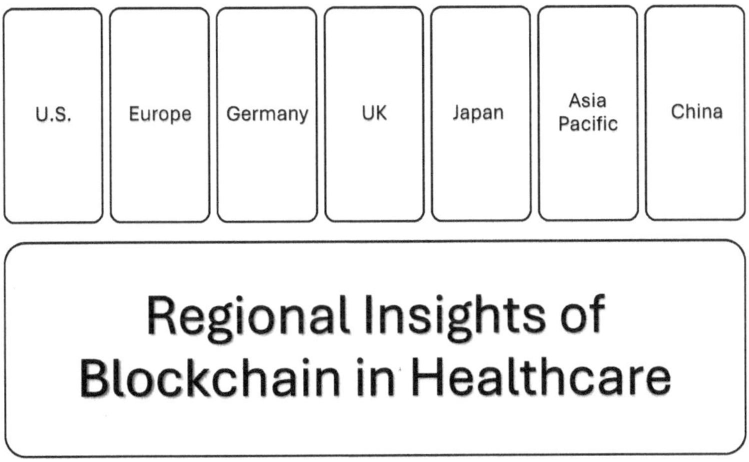

Figure 14.1 Regional Insights of Blockchain in Healthcare.

European Trends Blockchain Technology Market for Healthcare

Europe is the largest market for blockchain technology in healthcare, accounting for 34.8% of the global market in 2023. One of the primary factors propelling market expansion is the increasing adoption of blockchain technology in countries such as Germany, France, and the UK. For example, IBM, Accenture, and others are actively developing blockchain solutions for the healthcare sector. In February 2022, the European digital healthcare business Epillo Health Systems unveiled INTRx, a blockchain-based digital pharmaceutical solution. A Bangalore-based digital health pioneer with reasonably priced goods that combines blockchain, artificial intelligence, and machine learning for use in digital healthcare applications. Since blockchain technology enhances operational efficacy, security, and transparency for all parties involved in managing prescription medication programs and other services via the electronic health record system, Epillo Health Systems' adoption of it in the healthcare industry is a major factor driving the market's expansion.[5,7–9]

Blockchain Technology in Healthcare in Germany

Due to the widespread use of new healthcare technologies and expanding government spending, which also accounts for the largest portion of the industry, blockchain technology in healthcare is expected to develop at the fastest rate in Germany in 2023. The nation's dedication to embracing technology for the sake of healthcare is further demonstrated by the numerous initiatives and collaborations that have been formed to evaluate its use case in healthcare applications. The German Camelot Consulting Group, for instance, implemented blockchain administration for private medical data in April 2018. The business provided a digital platform to encourage safe patient data interchange in the healthcare industry with their Hypertrust X-Chain data management solution.[5,10]

Blockchain Technology in the UK's Healthcare Field

Over the anticipated period, the UK market for blockchain technology in healthcare is anticipated to grow rapidly. The National Health Service (NHS) is currently looking into integrated architecture for administrative duties, drug traceability, and data security. NHS looks into how blockchain technology might be used to manage drug traceability, health data security, and administrative work process operational continuity. The UK government's interest in and ongoing work in the field to improve data security, interoperability, and general efficiency of healthcare sectors demonstrated the significance of blockchain in this decentralised paradigm.[5] For instance, 30 million UK patients now have immediate smartphone access to their primary care information thanks to the UK NHS's introduction of the MyPCR blockchain platform through the software company Guardtime. This portal, which was created in partnership with Instant Access Medical and Healthcare Gateway, connects to all three of the major NHS GP platforms in the UK. These are the variables that are expected to drive growth in the UK market.[11,12]

Trends in the Asia-Pacific Healthcare Blockchain Market

Over the course of the projection period, blockchain technology's application in the Asia Pacific healthcare market is anticipated to expand dramatically. The promise of blockchain technology is attracting the attention of governments throughout the area, who actively encourage its advancement through strategic initiatives and policy changes.[5,13]

Blockchain Technology in the Healthcare Sector in Japan

In 2023, the top market for blockchain technology in healthcare was Japan. Japanese businesses are increasingly attempting to leverage blockchain technology's potential by creating solutions for the pharmaceutical and healthcare industries. For instance, in April 2019, the startup Susmed Inc. started a certified pilot project to monitor clinical data securely using mobile health apps and blockchain technology. In a similar vein, pharmaceutical behemoth Takeda co-led an international initiative utilising blockchain technology to create robust registries and patient passports for rare diseases.[5] This comes as part of initiatives against incidences of falsified data.[5]

Blockchain Technology in the Healthcare Sector in China

In the upcoming years, blockchain technology in the healthcare market in China is expected to increase significantly. Blockchain is being swiftly adopted by Chinese healthcare institutions to improve patient-centered care as well as the transparency and quality of data. There are also ongoing government pilot projects for inter-institution medical record exchange and drug traceability. Businesses throughout the country launched their own solutions in response to blockchain technology's capacity to securely store prescription medications, medical records, and insurance claims.[5] In May 2021, Tencent, the Chinese tech giant, collaborated with Waterdrop, a health insurance provider focused on crowdfunding of medical costs, the world's first commercialised blockchain-based medical & insurance solution. It also included deploying this solution into Tencent's most popular WeChat messenger, which already has over a billion active Chinese users a month. The partnership was focused on providing users with the ability to access their medical bills efficiently and securely using blockchain technology.[5,14,15]

Global Challenges in Blockchain Adoption

Global challenges in blockchain adoption in healthcare encompass a variety of technical, organisational, and regulatory hurdles that impede widespread implementation. Some challenges are shown in Figure 14.2.

Lack of Trust and Awareness

Despite its widespread potential interest, a lack of familiarity and knowledge of blockchain technology leads to many stakeholders being sceptical about the capabilities it offers. Such scepticism creates resistance to change at all levels across healthcare organisations, complicating buy-in.[16]

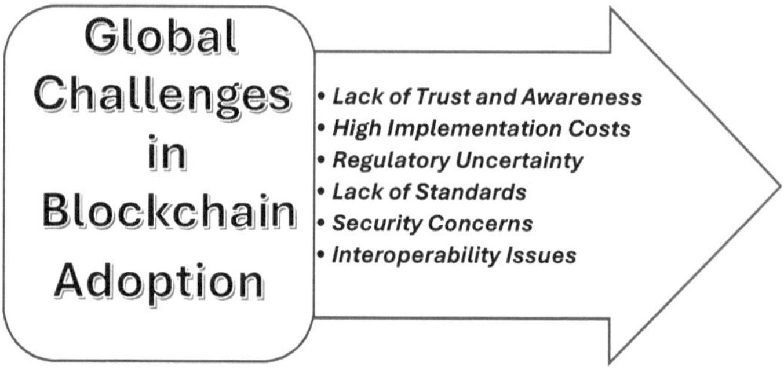

Figure 14.2 Global Challenges in Blockchain Adoption.

High Implementation Costs

There is a heavy financial burden when it comes to building the blockchain infrastructure. The high costs associated with acquiring, training on, and maintaining technology can prevent healthcare organisations from investing in blockchain solutions due to opportunity costs.[17]

Regulatory Uncertainty

Organisations looking to use a blockchain in healthcare are left wondering whether the existing legislation on data privacy applies to their specific circumstance. Adding to this challenge, organisations need to show that blockchain solutions do not clash with existing data protection laws like the very stringent HIPAA regulation in the United States.

Interoperability Issues

Interoperability issues in blockchain need to be integrated with other existing healthcare systems. These systems are not built to accommodate decentralisation, and this means that data can be hard to share between health-tech companies or even different organisations within one company.[18]

Security Concerns

Despite being praised for its security features, the technology does not remain unscathed from cyber warfare. Data breaches and the risk of unauthorised access continue to be major adoption concerns.

Lack of Standards

Available standards and regulatory guidelines are generally not sufficient to guide blockchain implementation in a way that allows interoperable solutions to be developed. Different organisations may follow different protocols, resulting in fragmentation of the ecosystem.[19]

Opportunities for Improvement of These Challenges

Despite these challenges, they could act as a hindrance to the adoption of blockchain in healthcare while there still exists an opportunity to improve on the limitations mentioned above. To tackle financial barriers and to stimulate research into best practices, government support, and investment have a significant role to play. Moreover, educational programs to enhance the knowledge and comprehension of blockchain technology among franchise leadership within health systems can build confidence and willingness for rapid adoption of new solutions.

In summary, while the path to widespread blockchain adoption in healthcare is fraught with challenges, addressing these issues through collaboration, education, and regulatory clarity could unlock significant benefits for the industry.[20,21]

Blockchain Use Cases in Global Healthcare

This section examines seven blockchain application cases that address different healthcare issues, as outlined below:

Opioid Prescription Tracking

The opioid epidemic has proven a challenge in the United States, which is forcing systems that track prescriptions to do their job. Today's systems incentivise data hoarding, doctor shopping, provider ignorance, and over-prescription. Blockchain presents an especially attractive solution for prescription monitoring. It can improve the security of prescriptions and reduce their volume. Such as healthcare providers, pharmacies, and patients are rewarded for pumping the opioid pipeline because they provide immediate comfort but also lead to a chronic illness of addiction. It is plausible that a technological solution can re-incentivise this and make headway in the opioid epidemic.[22]

A solution for securely storing opioid-linked transactions is the blockchain-based system, which would connect hospitals and pharmacies into a trusted network. It enables providers to access their silos even in the absence of an explicit trust relationship, thus reducing the opioid epidemic. The stakeholders are motivated to onboard more members, resulting in the formation of a more comprehensive dataset. This ecosystem brings value as it could solve a number of problems in the current opioid system. Specifically, it provides a more thorough prescription history, reveals patterns of overprescription and doctor shopping, and improves the quality of care. Such functionality of tracking opioid prescription history might lead to less addictive and longer-acting treatment.[23,24]

Data Exchange between Traditional Care and Telemedicine

Telemedicine is a substantial trend among remote patients who want to have easier access when it comes to medical care. As the new smart mobile device is becoming smarter, organisations have started to give you 24/7 access to care. Technological applications such as Apple Health make it easy for patients to track and report their health. However, most telemedicine services need providers to be in different regions or networks, which means poor continuity of care and a lack of access to health information.[25]

Blockchain has the potential to eliminate third-party authority and can allow healthcare providers to communicate directly with each other. However, it cannot tackle the intricate data-sharing problem on its own. It needs to fit within the confines of current health systems and standards for clinical data. Data transactions are governed by a smart contract, which creates the transaction of an immutable history.[26]

Patient-Controlled Exchange of Cancer Data

Cases of cancer are often not straightforward, meaning many considerations go into diagnosis and treatment plans due to the complexities surrounding tumour cases and the treatment options available. If the peers are specialists in their field, then it can help narrow down and potentially shorten the time from (suspected) diagnosis to treatment for a cancer patient. Today, tumour boards (which include all medical, surgical, and radiation oncologists participating in the care of individual cancer patients who meet to review details of each patient's condition and treatment with a team-focused interdisciplinary approach) have been incorporated into most U.S. hospitals. Patients and their families continue to be passive participants in the decision-making process, despite increased efforts to encourage doctor participation in cancer care. Specialists from a variety of specialisations may be participating in a large enterprise hospital, but budget limitations may make it challenging to expand the scope of tumour boards in a smaller care facility. Cancer patients' quality of life is important, and thus patient detachment may disregard it.[27,28]

Cancer Registry Sharing

Data exchange is crucial in cancer care because the situation is usually complex and there are rarely one-size-fits-all treatments.[29] The ability to share cancer data promotes the integrity (even if only individual affirmation and validation) of results gained from clinical trials, and it can also aggregate intelligence collected together to limit unnecessary duplication at the level of conducting clinical trials. This helps the distributed clinical trials reach a large enough cohort, enabling better cancer treatments. Nowadays, around 3% of cancer patients in the United States are being treated in clinical trials. Consequently, the vast majority of cancer patients are treated based on observations made upon the small cohort of a highly selective group of patients with varying demographics, family history, secondary diagnoses, etc., as population-based cancer registries attempt to record at least some rough data from incidences of cancer in geographical regions and for keeping track for planning an arbitrary population-wide attack against cancer.

Like EHRs, cancer registries are frequently fragmented and siloed. Blockchain technology can help speed up information sharing. Furthermore, prognostic and predictive models were created to help care practitioners make decisions as more reliable data was gathered from the broader patient population through artificial intelligence. A learning environment that facilitates the exchange of prediction models and the collaborative enhancement of the accuracy of learnt medical insights might be established using blockchain technology.[29–31]

Patient Digital Identity

Patient identification matching, which finds a patient from a healthcare database using specific information, is one of the most important aspects of sharing health information. To manage patient identities within a trusted network or healthcare organisation, technologies like the Enterprise Patient Master Index and Master Patient Index were created.[32] Even with the extra development effort, getting good, consistent, and accurate matching of patient data is difficult. Errors in patient identity have led to repeated entries of patients and also incomplete or wrong medical data. One study estimated that 195,000 deaths occur each year due to medical errors, with 10 of 17 errors being identified. This duplication wastes resources and burdens healthcare organisations that keep duplicate records and acquire mistakes from the wrong merge of patients with repeated tests or delays in treatment. Apart from that, it translates into a loss in reimbursement bills due to the denial of claims because of false information, as well as security threats when patients give out their confidential data.[33]

PHR (Personal Health Records)

EHRs are now frequently used by doctors to store and manage patient data, even though PHRs are apps that people, who are the true owners of their health data, use to see and manage personal healthcare information. PHRs' ultimate objective is to make it safe and simple for patients to collect, track, and manage all of their medical records from a range of sources, such as information on provider visits, prescriptions, vaccinations, physical activity data collected by smartphones, and much more. Patients can utilise PHRs to ensure that their medical records are accurate, manage who can access them, and correct any mistakes. Businesses and IT companies like Apple and Microsoft have started to express interest in so-called centralised solutions in recent years because of their products, Apple Health and Microsoft HealthVault. However, centralised approaches do not address the data sharing issue at its source and might hit the same hurdles faced by current fragmented EHR systems.[29,32–35]

Adjudication of Health Insurance Claims

In addition to protecting all personal assets from the financial burden of a major accident, acute illness, or chronic disease, health insurance aims to guarantee that the appropriate care will be available when needed. Depending on the type of coverage, health insurance can pay for surgeries, hospital stays, doctor visits, preventative care, and long-term care.[29] At the point of care, patients could pay a share of out-of-pocket costs, if applicable, but the rest ask for allowable claims from their health insurance companies. Through the claim adjudication process, insurers determine how much they'll pay, if anything at all, to healthcare providers. The insurer will either approve the payment of claims, reject the claim, or settle for less to be paid. When the insurance company believes that the service was inappropriate or medically unnecessary for a diagnosis (or procedure) code, payment to the provider will usually be down-coded. So, proper coding of all claims submitted for payment is essential. The moment a claim for medical treatment is made to the insurance company, it launches an in-depth investigation into the details of the alleged conduct. Even simple mistakes like a typographical error in the patient's name can lead to the rejection of a claim at times. While most of the claims today are processed automatically with no manual involvement, claim adjudication is a difficult task as they become complex and error-prone and face challenges such as fraud detection.[36,37]

Security and Ethical Considerations

As organisations explore the use of blockchain technology for data privacy, security considerations become top of mind. Although blockchain is a novel approach to data privacy in principle, it also leaves many security threats and ethical issues for organisations to address.

What will be key in ensuring that blockchain can deliver on its promise, but not at the cost of security and ethical standards, is the holistic approach for combining adequate cybersecurity efforts with moral principles.[38]

Security Concerns

The security of blockchain is based on cryptographic concepts and consensus algorithms. These features protect data integrity but are not without their vulnerabilities. The risk of a 51% attack is when somebody controls most of the network computing power. Moreover, if not coded securely, smart contracts, self-executing pieces of code on the blockchain, are also subject to exploitations. This means that organisations need to implement strong security measures in order to minimise these risks, preventing the data on the blockchain from being changed and requiring it to be kept private.[39]

Ethical Considerations

Using blockchain technology for data privacy poses ethical issues, unlike other data management techniques. While this is one of the strengths of any blockchain, it can also lead to unwanted visibility into data. Finding the right point between transparency and privacy is important to avoid blockchain being one more surveillance or data access tool. Furthermore, the application of blockchain in sectors such as healthcare, finance, and identity management calls for an ethical review process. For the ethical adoption of blockchain solutions, privacy, consent, and control over user data must be prioritised.[40]

Responsible Implementation

A responsible approach to blockchain and data privacy includes treating security vulnerabilities seriously while addressing ethical issues with the technology. They have the right to transparency regarding how their data is handled and shared and should be made aware of any potential consequences arising from it being kept on a blockchain.[41]

Interoperability and Technological Integration

Compatibility with Existing Systems

Integration with EHRs and Legacy Health IT System: Interaction with EHR and legacy health IT systems: The true promise of Blockchain within healthcare will be maximised only if it can work in integration with current Electronic Health Records (EHR) and other legacy health IT systems. This ultimately allows for a smoother transition, minimises disruption, and leverages the benefit of blockchain for data sharing, security, and efficiency.[42]

Adopting Standards (e.g., FHIR which stands for fast healthcare interoperability resources) for Data Exchange: Utilising established standards like FHIR facilitates data exchange across diverse systems. This standardisation helps create a unified framework for sharing patient information securely and efficiently across different platforms.[43]

Combining Blockchain with Emerging Technologies

AI, IoT, and Big Data for Real-time Health Monitoring

Real-time monitoring of identified health issues is made possible by the combination of blockchain technology, artificial intelligence (AI), the Internet of Things (IoT), and big data analytics. These technologies are well-aligned with the continuous data collection and analysis needs of patients; blockchain can provide a foundation for encrypted, integrity-secured sources of patient data and consent to utilise their care records or other processes.

Leveraging Wearable Devices for Data Collection

Integration of blockchain networks with wearable devices to collect health-related indicators such as heart rate, glucose level, and physical activity. The data can then be encrypted and saved on a blockchain to offer accuracy, privacy, traceability, and other valuable data necessary for precise personalised healthcare.[44]

Future Trends and Opportunities

Table 14.1 shows future trends and opportunities in healthcare blockchain technology, indicating key areas where significant advancements could occur.

Table 14.1 Future Trends and Opportunities in Healthcare Blockchain Technology

Future Trends and Opportunities	*Description*
Decentralised Healthcare Models	
Empowering patients with self-sovereign health data	Enables patients to own and control their health information, granting access as needed.[45]
Tokenised data markets for research collaboration	Creates marketplaces where patients can share de-identified health data for research.
Global Standardisation and Collaboration	
Establishing international blockchain standards	Developing unified guidelines to ensure interoperability across different blockchain networks.
Multinational partnerships and regulatory alignment	Encouraging countries to collaborate on regulations to facilitate cross-border data exchange.[46]
Research and Development Priorities	
Blockchain performance and scalability improvements	Focus on enhancing transaction speeds and reducing energy consumption for broader adoption.
Exploring new use cases for healthcare innovation	Investigating novel applications, such as supply chain management and personalised medicine.[47]

Strategic Recommendations for Implementing Blockchain Globally

These strategic recommendations provide a roadmap for successfully implementing blockchain technology in the global healthcare sector:

Implementation Guidelines

Steps for Successful Blockchain Adoption in Healthcare

Evaluating current infrastructure by choosing the right blockchain technology enables data interoperability and integrates easily with legacy systems. Pilot programs work really well as a first step in getting your strategies fine-tuned and figuring out where the biggest challenges might lie.[48]

Best Practices from Successful Global Initiatives

Learn from existing projects worldwide that have successfully integrated blockchain into healthcare, such as Estonia's e-health system or the use of blockchain for supply chain management in pharmaceutical industries. Adapt and apply these lessons to other regions, considering local regulations and infrastructure.[49]

Partnerships and Collaboration

Stakeholders across conversions to create an adequate ecosystem. Engaged key stakeholders like blockchain firms, regulators, and healthcare providers to co-create blockchain solutions. It creates an event of governmental intervention in providing a regulatory framework leading to data security and compliance to promote innovation.[50]

Education and Training Programs

Develop specialised training modules to improve blockchain literacy among healthcare practitioners, IT staff & clinicians. These programs could teach the basics of blockchain and its use cases in healthcare, as well as practical training on deploying blockchain-based solutions.[51]

Setting Benchmarks for Blockchain Adoption

Identifying Key Performance Indicators (KPIs)

Define KPIs to assess the effectiveness of blockchain projects in healthcare, such as greater data security, lower administrative cost, improved patient outcomes, and higher patient involvement.[52]

Tracking Progress and Outcomes Globally

Track blockchain progress and performance in different countries and regions using standardised metrics to measure progress. Encourage information sharing and collaboration within the industry to develop solutions for overcoming challenges, leading towards a cohesive approach to blockchain in healthcare across the globe.[53]

Conclusion

Blockchain technology has the potential to remake health data storage, transmission, and usage across the globe. Blockchain has the potential to create an improved healthcare landscape that is more transparent, efficient, and patient-centred by tackling larger challenges such as data security, interoperability, and empowering patients. The chapter, with examples of human experiences around the world using blockchain technology, has highlighted developments that pave the way for strategy enhancement, regulatory support, and the facade landscape that oversees this adoption implementation process.

Decentralised healthcare models, self-sovereign health data, and tokenised data markets are encouraging signs for the future of healthcare. Yet, for blockchain to reach its potential, international standards will need to be developed, scalability issues will be worked through, and world governments will have to cooperate. As with any nascent technology, partnerships between governments, healthcare organisations, and technology providers will be key for tackling the complex world of regulatory compliance while assisting in widespread utilisation.

Going forward, broad strategic efforts, such as more detailed guidance on incorporating blockchain technology, education and training of the labour force, and established benchmarks to guide adoption, will be essential. Such steps can assist in ensuring that blockchain not only furthers improving data security and efficiency but also promotes positive patient empowerment options along with a more inclusive and collaborative approach to overall healthcare.

Blockchain has the potential to revolutionise healthcare delivery around the world. To fully harness this transformative potential, the healthcare industry needs to learn from successful case studies and embrace innovative practices to establish a future that is secure, interoperable, and patient-centric.

References

1 Gordon, William J., and Christian Catalini. "Blockchain technology for healthcare: Facilitating the transition to patient-driven interoperability." *Computational and Structural Biotechnology Journal* 16 (2018): 224–230.
2 Esmaeilzadeh, Pouyan. "Benefits and concerns associated with blockchain-based health information exchange (HIE): A qualitative study from physicians' perspectives." *BMC Medical Informatics and Decision Making* 22, no. 1 (2022): 80.
3 Burnouf, Laura. "Global awareness and perspectives in global education." *Canadian Social Studies* 38, no. 3 (2004): n3.
4 Wells, Karen. *Childhood in a Global Perspective*. John Wiley & Sons, 2021.
5 Blockchain Technology in Healthcare Market Size, Share & Trends Analysis Report by Network Type (Private, Public), by End-Use (Providers, Payers), by Application, by Region, and Segment Forecasts, 2024–2030. https://www.grandviewresearch.com/industry-analysis/blockchain-technology-healthcare-market
6 Sabbagh, Parisa. "Developing an innovative blockchain-based model to contribute to the implementation of the 2030 agenda in Italy." (2022).
7 Bittins, Soeren, Gerhard Kober, Andrea Margheri, Massimiliano Masi, Abdallah Miladi, and Vladimiro Sassone. "Healthcare data management by using blockchain technology." *Applications of Blockchain in Healthcare* (2021): 1–27.
8 Radanović, Igor, and Robert Likić. "Opportunities for use of blockchain technology in medicine." *Applied Health Economics and Health Policy* 16 (2018): 583–590.
9 Pane, Josep, Katia M. C. Verhamme, Lacey Shrum, Irene Rebollo, and Miriam C. J. M. Sturkenboom. "Blockchain technology applications to postmarket surveillance of medical devices." *Expert Review of Medical Devices* 17, no. 10 (2020): 1123–1132.
10 Namasudra, Suyel, and Ganesh Chandra Deka, eds. *Applications of Blockchain in Healthcare*. Vol. 83. Singapore: Springer, 2021.
11 Leeming, Gary, James Cunningham, and John Ainsworth. "A ledger of me: Personalising healthcare using blockchain technology." *Frontiers in Medicine* 6 (2019): 171.
12 Massaro, Maurizio. "Digital transformation in the healthcare sector through blockchain technology. Insights from academic research and business developments." *Technovation* 120 (2023): 102386.
13 Kshetri, Nir, and Elena Loukoianova. "Blockchain adoption in supply chain networks in Asia." *IT Professional* 21, no. 1 (2019): 11–15.

14 Schinckus, Christophe. "A Nuanced perspective on blockchain technology and healthcare." *Technology in Society* 71 (2022): 102082.
15 Hou, Heng. "The application of blockchain technology in E-government in China." In *2017 26th International Conference on Computer Communication and Networks (ICN)*, pp. 1–4. IEEE, 2017.
16 Momoh, Muyideen Omuya, P. U. Chinedu, W. Nwankwo, D. Aliu, and M. S. Shaba. "Blockchain adoption: Applications and challenges." *International Journal of Software Engineering and Computer Systems* 7, no. 2 (2021): 19–25.
17 Kumar, Rakesh, Muhammad Faizan Tahir, Surendra Kumar, Ahmed Zia, Hallar Memon, and Waqas Mahmood. "Challenges in the adoption of blockchain in developing countries." In *2019 4th International Conference on Emerging Trends in Engineering, Sciences and Technology (ICEEST)*, pp. 1–8. IEEE, 2019.
18 Carlos Ferreira, João, Luís B. Elvas, Ricardo Correia, and Miguel Mascarenhas. "Enhancing EHR interoperability and security through distributed ledger technology: A review." In *Healthcare*, vol. 12, no. 19, p. 1967. MDPI, 2024.
19 Saxena, A., and Bang Han Chiu. "BOFUS and CLARITY: Streamlining blockchain architecture and assessment for advanced standardization and interoperability in distributed ledger technologies." *Frontiers in Blockchain* 6 (2023): 1235088.
20 Joshi, Sudhanshu, and Manu Sharma. "Assessment of implementation barriers of blockchain technology in public healthcare: Evidences from developing countries." *Health Systems* 12, no. 2 (2023): 223–242.
21 Riedel, Tino. "Addressing challenges: Adopting blockchain technology in the pharmaceutical industry for enhanced sustainability." *Sustainability* 16, no. 8 (2024): 3102.
22 Buchmueller, Thomas C., and Colleen Carey. "The effect of prescription drug monitoring programs on opioid utilization in Medicare." *American Economic Journal: Economic Policy* 10, no. 1 (2018): 77–112.
23 Zhang, Peng, Breck Stodghill, Cory Pitt, Cavin Briody, Douglas C. Schmidt, Jules White, Alan Pitt, and Kelly Aldrich. "Optrak: Tracking opioid prescriptions via distributed ledger technology." In *Alternative Pain Management: Solutions for Avoiding Prescription Drug Overuse*, Information Resources Management Association (IRMA), pp. 103–123. IGI Global, 2020.
24 Angraal, Suveen, Harlan M. Krumholz, and Wade L. Schulz. "Blockchain technology: Applications in health care." *Circulation: Cardiovascular Quality and Outcomes* 10, no. 9 (2017): e003800.
25 Asim Kichloo, Michael Albosta, Kirk Dettloff, Farah Wani, Zain El-Amir, Jagmeet Singh, Michael Aljadah, Raja Chandra Chakinala, Ashok Kumar Kanugula, Shantanu Solanki, Savneek Chugh. "Telemedicine, the current COVID-19 pandemic and the future: A narrative review and perspectives moving forward in the USA." *Family Medicine and Community Health* 8, no. 3 (2020): 1–9.
26 Aashima, Mehak Nanda, and Rajesh Sharma. "A review of patient satisfaction and experience with telemedicine: A virtual solution during and beyond COVID-19 pandemic." *Telemedicine and e-Health* 27, no. 12 (2021): 1325–1331.
27 Perocchia, Rosemarie Slevin, Julie Keany Hodorowski, Laurie A. Williams, Julie Kornfeld, Nydia Lassalle Davis, MaryAnn Monroe, and Mary Anne Bright. "Patient-centered communication in cancer care: The role of the NCI's Cancer Information Service." *Journal of Cancer Education* 26 (2011): 36–43.
28 Treiman, Katherine, Lauren McCormack, Murrey Olmsted, Nancy Roach, Bryce B. Reeve, Christa E. Martens, Rebecca R. Moultrie, and Hanna Sanoff. "Engaging patient advocates and other stakeholders to design measures of patient-centered

communication in cancer care." *The Patient-Patient-Centered Outcomes Research* 10 (2017): 93–103.

29 Zhang, Peng, Douglas C. Schmidt, Jules White, and Gunther Lenz. "Blockchain technology use cases in healthcare." In Pethuru Raj, Ganesh Chandra Deka (eds), *Advances in Computers*, vol. 111, pp. 1–41. Elsevier, 2018.

30 Bando, H., N. Okita, Y. Sakamoto, H. Sokuoka, Y. Nakamura, T. Hashimoto, T. Misumi et al. "Cancer registry as external control data for regulatory submission in Japan." *ESMO Real World Data and Digital Oncology* 6 (2024): 100072.

31 Chambers, David A., Eitan Amir, Ramy R. Saleh, Danielle Rodin, Nancy L. Keating, Travis J. Osterman, and James L. Chen. "The impact of big data research on practice, policy, and cancer care." *American Society of Clinical Oncology Educational Book* 39 (2019): e167–e175.

32 Morris, Genevieve, Greg Farnum, Scott Afzal, Carol Robinson, Jan Greene, and Chris Coughlin. "Patient identification and matching final report." *Office of the National Coordinator for Health Information Technology* (2014): 1–93.

33 Alsahafi, Yaser A., and Valerie Gay. "An overview of electronic personal health records." *Health Policy and Technology* 7, no. 4 (2018): 427–432.

34 https://dokumen.pub/blockchain-technology-platforms-tools-and-use-cases-111-0128138521-9780128138526.html

35 Roehrs, Alex, Cristiano André Da Costa, Rodrigo da Rosa Righi, and Kleinner Silva Farias De Oliveira. "Personal health records: A systematic literature review." *Journal of Medical Internet Research* 19, no. 1 (2017): e5876.

36 Genitsaridi, Irini, Haridimos Kondylakis, Lefteris Koumakis, Kostas Marias, and Manolis Tsiknakis. "Towards intelligent personal health record systems: Review, criteria and extensions." *Procedia Computer Science* 21 (2013): 327–334.

37 Harish, Ravindran, Ranjana S. Suresh, S. Rameesa, P. M. Laiveishiwo, Prosper Singh Loktongbam, K. C. Prajitha, and Mathew J. Valamparampil. "Health insurance coverage and its impact on out-of-pocket expenditures at a public sector hospital in Kerala, India." *Journal of Family Medicine and Primary Care* 9, no. 9 (2020): 4956–4961.

38 Poelman, Michelle, and Sarfraz Iqbal. "Investigating the compliance of the GDPR: Processing personal data on a blockchain." In *2021 IEEE 5th International Conference on Cryptography, Security and Privacy (CSP)*, pp. 38–44. IEEE, 2021.

39 Arabsorkhi, Abouzar, and Elham Khazaei. "Blockchain technology and GDPR compliance: A comprehensive applicability model." *International Journal of Web Research* 7, no. 2 (2024): 49–63.

40 Sharif, Monica M., and Farshad Ghodoosi. "The ethics of blockchain in organizations." *Journal of Business Ethics* 178, no. 4 (2022): 1009–1025.

41 Lee, Wanbil W., Wolfgang Zankl, and Henry Chang. "An ethical approach to data privacy protection." (2016).

42 Chen, Catherine, Terhilda Garrido, Don Chock, Grant Okawa, and Louise Liang. "The Kaiser Permanente electronic health record: Transforming and streamlining modalities of care." *Health Affairs* 28, no. 2 (2009): 323–333.

43 Merhej, Joseph, Hassan Harb, Abdelhafid Abouaissa, and Lhassane Idoumghar. "Toward a new era of smart and secure healthcare information exchange systems: Combining blockchain and artificial intelligence." *Applied Sciences* 14, no. 19 (2024): 8808.

44 Idrissi, Zineb Kamal, Mohamed Lachgar, and Hamid Hrimech. "Blockchain, IoT and AI in logistics and transportation: A systematic review." *Transport Economics and Management* 2 (2024): 275–285.

45 Narayan, Aditya, Kydo Weng, and Nirav Shah. "Decentralizing health care: History and opportunities of Web3." *JMIR Formative Research* 8, no. 1 (2024): e52740.
46 Khorsandroo, Sajad, Adrián Gallego Sánchez, Ali Saman Tosun, José M. Arco, and Roberto Doriguzzi-Corin. "Hybrid SDN evolution: A comprehensive survey of the state-of-the-art." *Computer Networks* 192 (2021): 107981.
47 MohammedAbdul, ShezonSaleem. "Navigatingblockchain'stwinchallenges: Scalability and regulatory compliance." *Blockchains* 2, no. 3 (2024): 265–298.
48 Haleem, Abid, Mohd Javaid, Ravi Pratap Singh, Rajiv Suman, and Shanay Rab. "Blockchain technology applications in healthcare: An overview." *International Journal of Intelligent Networks* 2 (2021): 130–139.
49 Akbar, Muhammad Azeem, Víctor Leiva, Saima Rafi, Syed Furqan Qadri, Sajjad Mahmood, and Ahmed Alsanad. "Towards roadmap to implement blockchain in healthcare systems based on a maturity model." *Journal of Software: Evolution and Process* 34, no. 12 (2022): e2500.
50 Singh, Yuvraj, M. A. Jabbar, Shishir Kumar Shandilya, Olena Vovk, and Yaroslav Hnatiuk. "Exploring applications of blockchain in healthcare: Road map and future directions." *Frontiers in Public Health* 11 (2023): 1229386.
51 Bali, Shivani, Vikram Bali, Rajendra Prasad Mohanty, and Dev Gaur. "Analysis of critical success factors for blockchain technology implementation in healthcare sector." *Benchmarking: An International Journal* 30, no. 4 (2023): 1367–1399.
52 Biswas, Baidyanath, and Rohit Gupta. "Analysis of barriers to implement blockchain in industry and service sectors." *Computers & Industrial Engineering* 136 (2019): 225–241.
53 Kassab, Mohamad, Joanna DeFranco, Tarek Malas, Phillip Laplante, Giuseppe Destefanis, and Valdemar Vicente Graciano Neto. "Exploring research in blockchain for healthcare and a roadmap for the future." *IEEE Transactions on Emerging Topics in Computing* 9, no. 4 (2019): 1835–1852.

15 The Future of Healthcare Industry

A Blockchain-Centric Landscape

Shaweta Sharma, Akanksha Sharma, Ashish Verma, Sunita, Shilpa Thukral, Akhil Sharma

Introduction

Many industries, including the healthcare sector, benefit from digital transformation, which is a vital advantage. Better patient care is sparked by it, and it also develops durable, effective operational procedures that meet the demands of patients, healthcare institutions, and carers. The healthcare sector is embarking on an exciting path away from fee-for-service and towards the value-based paradigm thanks to new generations of technologies like artificial intelligence, big data analytics, cloud computing, consumerism, customer relationship management, and the Internet of Things (IoT). The healthcare sector is benefiting from digital transformation by offering secure, high-quality patient care as well as more profitable incentives through more effective business processes.[1]

Such progress provides Healthcare providers with easier access to vast sets of patient data than ever before. It may involve data that is personally identifiable information about other people or business data. Healthtech cybersecurity solutions are particularly difficult to find. Cyber threats are now a huge concern for healthcare organisations to prevent it. In 2018, the healthcare sector experienced three times more patient records compromised in 503 breaches, totalling over 15 million records lost or stolen than had occurred during all of 2017.

By the middle of 2019, these figures had grown to over 25 million patient records. Another significant breach was revealed to the public in early May 2019 in an 8-K filing with the US Securities and Exchange Commission. The vendor for the American Medical Collection Agency (AMCA) was hacked for around eight months, compromising patient data worth up to 25 million. Phishing attacks and third-party providers were responsible for the majority of these security problems.[1,2]

The healthcare sector should be heavily regulated in terms of privacy and transparency, even though it is data-driven. Since sensitive and strictly regulated data, such as medical records, insurance claims, or private payment information, goes through each healthcare provider's system, they should also have first-rate data governance systems in place.[1] In addition to addressing growing IT architectural complexity and the expansion of data relative to the healthcare systems, network security and protection of health data from unauthorised access present a significant challenge.[1]

DOI: 10.4324/9781003529910-15

A low degree of interoperability and excessive patient medical costs might result from the loss of patient medical data when it moves between various healthcare facilities with different data standards. In 2009, the government pushed for the digitisation of all patient records through the electronic health information exchange (HIE). Over $35 billion in incentives have been made available as part of this law, which is known as the Health Information Technology for Economic and Clinical Health Act, to promote and assist the broad adoption and meaningful use of EHRs among qualified healthcare providers and hospitals.[1,3]

However, 96% of EHR programs are adopted in the healthcare sector, and there is still a long way to go before they become interoperable across all care settings. In 2015, just 6% of healthcare providers were able to send patient data to other clinicians using a different EHR system. That lack of interoperability is not moving the needle on improving healthcare from an administrative standpoint, and the shift to patient-centred care still seems very much out of reach.

Blockchain technology can also provide healthcare care with a strong decentralised data platform with the basic characteristics of transparency, traceability, and security to switch from volume-based care to value-based care, which is compliant with all health standards.[4] A survey report by the World Economic Forum says that blockchain will store 10% of the world's gross domestic product by 2027. When considering the healthcare system and its ecosystem, blockchain can offer a much-needed decentralised platform for the recording, tracking, and management of clinical history records, provider directory credentials evaluation records, drug supply chain information, insurance, and claim information. The cornerstone for enforcing strict medical regulations and providing flawless medical services, followed by efficient medication supply chain management care, is the automated protection of ledger, accuracy, and immutability. The healthcare sector has historically viewed data as a commodity and a source of competitiveness rather than as a source of care. In the healthcare sector, decentralisation of data, security, and transparency enhance interoperability and collaboration, which lowers overall administrative expenses.[1,5]

Evolution of Blockchain

Satoshi Nakamoto originally proposed blockchain as a distributed ledger technology and architecture platform for the financial industry back in 2008. Still, its evolution now has reached a point that can be regarded as a basic component technology to build diverse, decentralised applications on top of. Blockchain has come a long way now over the years. The five different versions of blockchain are blockchain technology 1.0–5.0.

The version of blockchain 1.0 is the simplest form of a decentralised transaction ledger to store information across many computers created by Nakamoto. The data stored on the first blockchains was only limited to an object (digital currency) whose ownership changes over time.

Blockchain 2.0 is the era of the emergence of Ethereum for an improved cryptocurrency experience. Ethereum was the first blockchain with built-in smart contract functionality. In simple terms, smart contracts are a set of scripts that execute themselves when the conditions are met. These contracts permit individuals or legal entities to perform more complex operations than just simple exchanges in cryptocurrency. Ideal for decentralised applications and autonomous organisations.[6]

Blockchain technology 3.0 is more widely applicable to distributed applications such as enterprise blockchain. The best of the blockchain 3.0 use cases are healthcare, cyber security, supply chain management, and manufacturing.

In order to support Industry 4.0 and Healthcare 4.0, blockchain technology has once again experienced a development known as Blockchain 4.0. It aims to enhance the user experience in the sector. There are two examples of blockchain 4.0: Rchain and Metaverse.

Blockchain 5.0 is the current or upcoming iteration of the blockchain technology. This is an effort to lessen the security concerns and other disadvantages of blockchain. Blockchain 5.0 apps include Hedra, Relictum Pro, and Hashgraph.[7]

Characteristics of Blockchain in the Healthcare Industry

Most of the traditional network applications have client-server architecture, whereby a central server controls and authorises all operations. With this centralisation, data cannot be shared, and there is less transparency. Blockchain operates on a classification of peer-to-peer distributed systems, where one copy of the same data is provided to all nodes, and all work according to the same set of rules. A blockchain is a set of blocks to which data is added in a distributed ledger. It continuously grows as new data keeps getting appended to it. User security and ledger consistency are protected by asymmetric cryptography and consensus algorithms,

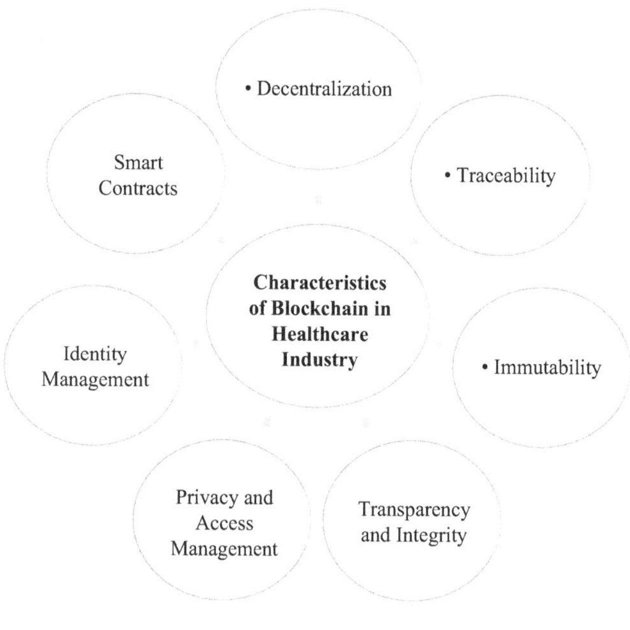

Figure 15.1 Characteristics of Blockchain in Healthcare Industry.

both distributed solutions.[8] The inherent nature of blockchain design provides multiple benefits, which are discussed in Figure 15.1.

Decentralisation

Blockchain maintains data in each network node at all times. Every node examines the block and adds it to the board as the data size grows. At any one time, every participant has identical data because they all have the same chain of blocks. It achieves standardisation by enabling live data querying, adding redundancy while avoiding central authority, and using a standardised data structure.[1]

High availability and network fault tolerance are facilitated by the data's partitioned form among all participating nodes. Cloud-based apps, however, are susceptible to Denial of Service attacks, in which a single malicious node can bring down the entire network. In contrast, the blockchain network's decentralisation and computational consensus techniques prevent fraudulent nodes from updating.[1]

That decentralised aspect of blockchain assures us that there is no singular governing body. This helps to keep the system secure and nice with matching transactions. Instead, it uses consensus mechanisms across the network of peers to transact with other users while relying on a single authority for vindication transactions and recording data in an intractable way. As a result, any recorded ledger information is truthful and precise.[9] It offers unchangeable transaction records and a high-quality service supply. Due to the distribution of its computing power, it is easy to manage and operate the network. Effectively, these transactions use blockchain mechanisms owing to the quality of service. The quality of service (QoS) parameters cover features such as data integrity with end-end traceability, availability, accountability, etc., a very high degree of reliability, and an increase in customers can be expected. Delivery of trusted quality is highly dependent on what data you decide to put into distributed ledgers. Instead of sending all data coming from the system into the blockchain network, some of the data are stored in local databases. If not, only applications that require immutability will be included in the blocks. This lowers the costs of replication, storage, and search for applications built on it. This network is easy to manage and run as its computing power is decentralised.[10]

Traceability

To peers, everything is clear; Finding out when something happened and who approved the transaction's execution is easy. Because of this characteristic, each person takes accountability and is forthright and truthful about all interactions.[7] After a few years of blockchain hype, a number of firms are offering solutions with the promise to trace. Still, almost all that has been delivered is merely on the block and chain level, and more importantly, nothing has improved in the quantity or quality of data that is being collected and shared.[11] This has created a lot of uncertainty about whether blockchain can truly be used in supply chain cases. Once a new transaction is added to a block, it will be irreversible and instantaneously timestamped. This allows for easy tracking of data and forces the information in the block to be unchangeable. All businesses must be trustworthy in order for any specific data or transaction that is stored on the blockchain to be authentic and traceable. Pharmacies, wholesalers, hospitals, manufacturers, raw material suppliers, and patients are all part of the complex network that is the healthcare supply chain.[7] Tracking supply through this network is challenging due to a number of factors, such as the lack of information or incentives within and across local networks, stripping ownership from stakeholders when supply chains become vertically integrated, and behaviours that create conflicts between stakeholders. Drug traceability has gained a lot of importance in recent times, with some countries also mandating it. As a result, the traceability of drugs has emerged to be one of the most important components of the pharmaceutical supply chain since it not only provides the authenticity of the product but also endeavours to track and even trace the entire chain of custody traversed by the product across the supply chain.[12]

Immutability

Another key property of blockchain is immutability. A blockchain ledger cannot be tampered with, and hence, there would be no changes in terms of hash on the blockchain added or persistent. Similarly, blockchain nodes are decentralised and distributed platforms that use the consensus until all the data is stored. This guarantees that the uniqueness of the data is maintained. There is no end to hacking and security breaches from centralised databases, which depend upon third-party trust to ensure they are safe. Blockchain keeps ledgers for all the transactions. Valuable ledgers are among blockchain participants. Once transactions are recorded in blocks using hash keys and stored in the blockchain, the data becomes unchangeable. The transactions in the subsequent block are validated using the same technique on each block, and these hash keys are linked to the preceding block. Because of this, when a transaction is altered, a new hash key is created, which also makes it possible for other blocks in the network to recognise it. In blockchain technology, ledgers are always open. All of the nodes share ledgers with it, and they are in real-time sync with one another.[13]

Transparency and Integrity

Blockchain: once the system records data in the blockchain, it cannot be changed. To place a block of data on the chain, blockchain leverages hashing and consensus (also known as proof of work). Once a transaction is prompted, it goes to a pool of transactions to be validated. The nodes in the blockchain are made aware of these transactions. Miner nodes select unconfirmed transactions from the memory pool; a block is created, and validated transactions are stored in it as data (a collection of transactions), along with a hash of the current state of the chain and previous hash that will link this block to the chain. Subsequent valid blocks are then validated by the rest of the node, adding it to their chain and continuing with the pending transactions. The rules determined as part of the network, and proof of work help solve the Byzantine General problem and achieve consensus among nodes so that transactions can be validated. As soon as some node tries to change any committed transaction, it will generate a new hash and break the link.[14]

Management of Privacy and Access

Traditionally, a central authority (i.e., a sharing institute) controls access and privacy management in cloud-based repositories. Attacks that have infiltrated the system over time are always present in such systems. The system's fundamental problems include the fact that users have no control over their data outside of institutions they share and that anonymised data sets are nonetheless vulnerable to user re-identification.

The first issue with current data-sharing techniques is that they can share data but have poor control over it. As a result, an organisation or user loses ownership of data once it is shared. The fact that there is no technical barrier to re-identification even in cases where a data set has been anonymised further exacerbates these problems. The latter still maintains strict control over the data, but this will make sharing it ineffective, negating the whole point.[15]

Blockchain provides access control and privacy through the use of sophisticated cryptographic techniques like hashing. Blockchain users can use both public and private cryptographic keys to develop their identities. These keys enable you to take advantage of access control and can be utilised in scalable, distributed, and safe ways for identification, authentication, and other purposes. The private key is used to encrypt the data, while the public key is used to identify the user. The fact that a public key's identification may or may not be directly linked to the user's true identity is another significant characteristic that highlights pseudo-identity; as a result, this behaviour supports privacy-preserving identity in a public ledger. In a private or permissioned blockchain, the same mechanism can also be helpful in converting public keys into actual identities.[16]

Management of Identity

The growing requirement to unify a single source of truth and share data makes the necessity for decentralised identification already quite clear. There are currently several identity systems that are divided into the following categories: user-central network anonymity scheme, where identity is owned and controlled by the user; federated identity management scheme, where identity is established in one system and can be trusted to be used in another system, such as single sign-on systems; and central identity management scheme, where identity is controlled by a central authority.[1]

Identity management and the decentralised nature of the blockchain itself can be combined to create and write a digital ID into the blockchain network. An encrypted digital ID serves as its public-private key. While private keys serve as security controls by encrypting data, the public key aids in identification. A digital ID is similar to a digital fingerprint that may be used to confirm identification; once it is saved to the blockchain, it cannot be altered or tampered with. Digital ID is unique in that it can identify the correct patient information, which is necessary to deliver better care. Finally, in the case of blockchain, the distinctive behaviour can be used.[17]

Smart Contracts

The term "smart contracts" was first used by Nick Szabo, who also provided the following definition: A computerised transaction protocol that carries out a contract's conditions is called a smart contract. Smart contracts are executable scripts that reside on the blockchain and allow for the processing of distributed, highly automated workflows.[1] Every smart contract is associated with an address and can be called by making a transaction at that address. Unlike these constructs, a smart contract is not dependent on anything else. Smart contracts allow the use of a multi-step transactional process without the need to trust third parties. Smart contracts can eliminate the middle player and, consequently, speed up the process timeline, ensuring a more efficient transaction cost. Such behaviour of smart contracts creates a new paradigm where, besides distributing data in a secure and verifiable way among non-trusting stakeholders, there is also the possibility to execute an action on that data at runtime.[18]

Smart contracts can transparently and securely support healthcare marketplace services like medical billing and claim processing. By keeping this out of the healthcare industry, administrative costs are avoided, and fraud involving important processes like billing and insurance is successfully challenged.

Role of Blockchain in Addressing Key Healthcare

Technology issues, privacy concerns, and the lack of a system governing the usage or sharing of data are the main causes of the lack of cooperation among medical organisations. There are situations when real-time access to patient health data and other healthcare facilities is not possible. These are the shared and fundamental characteristics of blockchain-based healthcare systems that can address potential issues.[19]

Personalised Healthcare Records

The medical records contain confidential information on surgical procedures, medications, and recovery. In traditional health systems, these documents are still archived on paper manually. While healthcare supply chains are becoming increasingly digital, and electronic health records will only grow in number moving forward, no full-funnel ecosystem exists for the immediate updating and distribution of these records across organisations and geographic regions. This scenario may turn out to be far more troublesome, owing to patient data confidentiality and privacy issues. Medical data can be generated instantly through IoT-enabled devices. The latest advancements in blockchain technology, also known as distributed ledger technology, can help address some of the problems with data access and transfer. Patients may be able to take control of their care if they have safe, personalised, and thorough access to their medical data through digital health records.[20]

Personalised health records allow us to create a platform that combines smart contracts, digital medicines, and medical data collection and retrieval. In addition to encouraging patients to use their data to promote their therapy, their strategy offers strong consent capabilities for sharing with other institutions and applications. The integration of smart contracts, patient monitoring and control systems, and event-driven health record data requires the use of blockchain-based solutions for customised healthcare records.[7,21]

Security

At every stage of a hospital's operation, the healthcare system is in charge of creating, transmitting, storing, and analysing vast amounts of data. It uses various contemporary digital technologies to help safeguard the system against data loss or misuse and offers thorough, layered security for all cloud destination data transfers. The platform will often operate in accordance with the strictest privacy and data security regulations in a nation. The risk of data breaches is decreased by this hospital system's hosted cloud-based servers, which are situated outside the buildings.

Blockchain-based solutions for healthcare frequently promote transparency, ensure privacy, prevent data breaches, and create a safe and secure environment for medical facilities to operate in. Using a Hyperledger blockchain network, two healthcare organisations can share data across a distributed database without needing to trust each other. Additionally, it makes healthcare transactions swift, safe, and transparent.[7,22]

Performance

Blockchain-based healthcare systems greatly boost the system's speed, agility, and efficiency as many processes get streamlined and integrated seamlessly. Due to its intra-operability and flexibility, it enhances the performance and patient treatment scopes of a healthcare facility. Ability to customise its features specifically for outpatient department (OPDs), IPDs (inpatient department), diagnostics management, emergency care response invoicing and payments, operations, etc. It allows users to provide role-based control and access for single or multiple functions, helping in monitoring all activities needed to track operations related to the provision of healthcare.

Reliability

The healthcare system based on blockchain technology is very resistant to any disruption, downtime, or breakdown of other technological systems. It is really safe in terms of data safety and has an easy-to-use and professional-looking user interface, which makes it easier to navigate. The maintenance functions can be grouped into pre-planned periods whenever there is a minimum demanding atmosphere, and upgrading takes very little time. It brings in remote updates and upgrades to the medical records without affecting the regular functionality.[23]

Interoperability

Patient participation, security, privacy, governance, and consent are among the issues raised by the paradigm change to patient-centered interoperability. By offering a foundation for the safe movement of data, blockchain technology presents an alluring answer to these problems. In conclusion, blockchain provides a theoretical illustration of how a patient can safely communicate with several parties, authenticate themselves at multiple institutions, and compile their medical records in a format compatible with blockchain technology.

Access Control

Patients should be asked for consent from a doctor before they are allowed to access them. If the doctor has not acted otherwise, the system will refuse access. Similarly, if the patient wants a regular access privilege, then a doctor must ask that personally. For the patient, this means that he has first to grant permission before anyone sees his medical records. It also allows the patient to, temporarily, if needed, provide access and grant or revoke any access for others using the system.[24]

Advanced Blockchain Applications in the Healthcare Sector

Blockchain is poised to revolutionise the healthcare system; by virtue of its decentralised principles, blockchain can enhance the accessibility and security of patient information, therefore changing the hierarchy of healthcare (wherein doctors prescribe, but patients call others to their treatment). The privacy of sensitive medical records has become a very serious data breach, as there is no safe framework to store them in a traditional healthcare system. Another problem, which is becoming increasingly prevalent as wearable technology and customised therapy proliferate, is that people do not yet have complete control over their medical data. Both of these situations have important moral implications that require consideration.[25] The application of blockchain technology in the healthcare industry is shown in Figure 15.2.[7]

Patient Data Management

Blockchain emerged as a tool for the management of patient data, with applications focused primarily on enhancing security and cost-effectiveness. Electronic storage of medical data, patient scheduling, billing/accounts management, and lab tests are among the numerous EHR systems used in the healthcare system. The focus is on providing a secure, immutable, and cross-platform sharing of medical records. With multiple levels of management by the patient, physicians, regulators, hospitals, insurers, and others, blockchain stores every single medical record of each patient in a manner that allows such data to be securely recorded and retain an extremely detailed history profile for every person.[26]

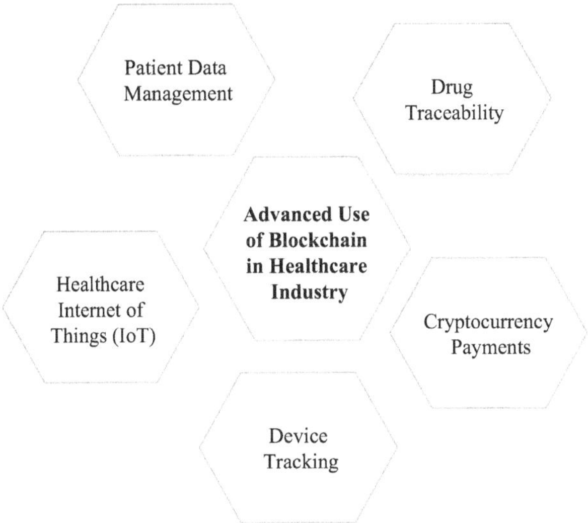

Figure 15.2 Advanced Use of Blockchain in Healthcare Industry.

Drug Traceability

Counterfeit medicines are the cause of harm and even death in millions of people every single year. Medicine counterfeiting costs pharmaceutical companies immensely, both financially and reputationally. Blockchain-based drug traceability makes it possible to eliminate a significant amount of the supply chain management process by removing fraud and counterfeit pharmaceuticals. In a study including stakeholders and their interactions with the smart contract and medication monitoring system, a medicine traceability system was developed. The front-end layer, represented by a dApp that interacts with the smart contract, decentralised storage system, and on-chain resources through an API, provides software devices to stakeholders that rely on them. A G-coin blockchain was developed to protect public health data and enable transparent medical transactions.[7,27]

Cryptocurrency Payments

Using blockchain technology, a ledger keeps track of all transaction kinds. All of the coin's owner information is contained in the saved data. That ensures the transactions being conducted are legitimate. Decentralised currency is digital cash that does not control the bank or the government. The person or company that created the digital cash owns it. Patients can make exchanges through blockchain. In this manner, the absence of contacts like merchants, agents, and banks does not necessitate a focal body sanction to execute the exchanges. This makes the entire charging process easier. This identification style does not just hold for tests conducted on patients, notwithstanding the fact that the ones that take a break at clinical exercises are straightforwardly distinguished on the framework. It validates the legitimacy of the particulars presented by them and the credibility of trades.[28]

Device Tracking

The tracking of medical devices from the moment they are manufactured until they get decommissioned is yet another critical process that would need to be revolutionised in terms of how healthcare functions. Any hospital faces challenges when it comes to its inventory of certain medical equipment that is shared between departments and patients. Finding the right supplies in a medical emergency requires quick thinking. Medical device tracking and monitoring are therefore essential to enable timely device recovery (preventing needless repurchases) and fraud analytics from the supply chain to decommissioning. There are several advantages to using a blockchain-based approach over conventional location monitoring solutions. Immutability and resistance to tampering are two of the most prevalent and significant characteristics of blockchain technology. In addition to a device's creator, reseller, and serial number, blockchain technology may create an immutable record that shows not just the device's current location but also its history of travel, which aids in regulatory compliance. A hostile individual cannot alter or remove the location history of any device contained in the database by using this method with blockchain. We can better understand how medical equipment is used, ensure that it stays in approved locations, and make sure that end users use it thanks to blockchain technology. Keeping an inventory process log, automating the utilisation process, and conveniently locating equipment in an emergency are a few advantages.[29]

Healthcare IoT

The IoT envisions a completely networked world where objects may communicate with one another via data. There are numerous smart applications across a wide range of industries, including wearables, smart cities, smart grids, smart homes, and the automobile sector. An enormous amount of data is produced by the continuous growth of the IoT. One major issue that needs to be resolved is preserving the reliability of its data. Using blockchain technology to give creditability in IoT data includes elements like distributed services that are authorised by each participant and making the data write access irreversible.[30]

Blockchain, however, in the future not only provides security and transparency to the IoT data but also gives IoT efficiency, scalability as well as standardisation for the healthcare industrymaking this technology is a critical solution for those who want to grow with smart devices. Blockchain-enabled IoT devices used in healthcare will allow the patients themselves to choose who can access the data so that these devices cannot be hacked and they are monitored who accessed them. In fact, it is even possible that supply chain payments will become automated through the use of blockchain-based systems implemented with smart contracts based on conditions monitored by IoT sensors.

The healthcare sector is generating huge interest in the IoT to help patients and physicians due to sensors that can be embedded into small devices for monitoring the health condition of the patient and transmitting data for analysis. The IoT can convert hospitals into intelligent hospitalsin which different procedures are made easy for medical professionals.[31]

Future Scope of Blockchain in Healthcare Sectors

A decentralised, public, unchanging, and corruption-proof databank that includes every individual whose history is used through complex, protected codes that can secure the privacy of medical data can be maintained with the aid of blockchain technology. Patients, doctors, and other healthcare workers can all simply and securely access the same information thanks to this collaborative design. Some of the specific future applications of blockchain technology in the healthcare sector are covered in the section that follows.

Blockchain in Authentication Aspects and Security

Blockchain can permanently secure medical records at every level. Any type of blockchain-based ledger storage model used in the healthcare industry typically creates a decentralised network of nodes using cryptographic computations made by the participants in different sections using hash chains, digital signatures, and consensus mechanisms. These models offer a number of service qualities, including traceability, integrity, security, and non-repudiation, in addition to extremely dependable storage capabilities. Usually, these records are kept in a decentralised, public, yet private way.[32,33]

Patient files and medical information related to the gathering, use, and other resources during and after hospital care make up medical records. These are obtained from several automated applications, patient body sensors, and various departmental units. Because medical records are computerised, they require even more security and a role-based level of privileges for health information. Access controls, authentication, confidentiality, nonreproduction (i.e., guaranteeing the integrity of information or documents that have not been altered), and availability (for authorised users at the appropriate time) are all used in healthcare records security.[34]

Blockchain in Precision Medicine and Clinical Trials

In the medical field, clinical trials are essential preconditions for analysing the drug results for each designated condition and the associated adverse effects. It has been acknowledged that patient recruitment is a difficult aspect of the clinical trial designer's work. If timely goals are not met, money and time are wasted, statistical results are incomprehensible, or the study's duration is extended, which will probably lengthen the planned patient recruitment timeline. 86% of clinical studies are found to fall short of their recruitment goals on time, and 19% of registered clinical trials were closed or abandoned due to the inability to reach the anticipated enrolment. In order to avoid outcome failure, which could result in the early termination of the experiment, systematic and valid patient recruitment is essential in clinical trials. A novel approach to stakeholder participation in clinical trial recruitment is supported by data security and patient privacy as well as the features of a peer-to-peer external audited transaction system.[33,35]

Additionally, the blockchain paradigm offers fundamental features including public auditability, immutability guaranteeing data provenance, and data decentralisation. Every transaction in a blockchain-based network model is dispersed and saved in every node of any operational electronic device, negating the need for any hardware. Entering information into the system: Before being recorded in the blockchain, every transaction must be validated by the user. The system is infallible since it is decentralised and all transactions may be utilised and audited by anybody for anybody. A smart contract is a self-executing protocol that establishes protocols between various parties on the blockchain; it builds a system over the blockchain based on the needs for task prioritisation.[33] Nick Szabo originally proposed a smart contract system in 1996 as an agreement or coded protocol between the two parties (sender and receiver) that govern all transactions on the distributed ledger system.[36]

Smart contract features have been incorporated into the protocols of most of the blockchain systems that have been presented in clinical trials (e.g., Ethereum and Hyperledger). Any computable problem, like matching patients for recruitment or verifying the validity of a clinical trial, can be expressed as an execution of a Turing machine, which is why smart contracts are written on the Ethereum blockchain, a distributed computing platform with an integrated Turing complete programming language. Conventional recruiting technology and its dependence on patient interaction, automated subject matching, patient recruitment, and trial-based contract administration present a new set of difficulties that blockchain-based smart contract systems can address.[37]

Blockchain in Customising Medical Services

Implementing secured data sharing and interoperability of applications, data sources, and other external systems is one of the biggest challenges for digital healthcare systems. To enable personalised care delivery, the digital healthcare system creates personal healthcare records that are inter-operative and give patients limited access and control over their data. However, government guidelines highlight privacy and private data protection in the areas of consent, anonymisation, and data ownership, which need to be maintained as well as security and transparency. Patients can be permitted to make use of the data by token-based permission on a platform based on blockchain technology. Patients can, at the same time, give consent in order for doctors and researchers to check their health history and well-being and get medical services from the global market in an unalterable way so as to promote their health.[38]

Blockchain in the Management of Healthcare Data

By design, a blockchain is a particular kind of database that may be thought of as an immutable read-once-and-read-only database. No one, either internal or external, is permitted to alter or remove data from blockchain databases since they are built and constructed once. Until the private keys are owned by the real owner, no one may access the data in a blockchain decentralised ledger, which functions similarly to a transaction-type database. Compared to centralised databases, these database file systems offer superior security, speed, and cost advantages by storing data locally. The use of blockchain technology in the healthcare industry has created new dimensions in the data management space by reducing data duplication through the use of cloud components with cryptographic algorithms and data encryption logics, which enable user sharing. EMR data management for blockchain, healthcare data protection, PHR data management with blockchain, point-of-care genomics, and EHR data management blockchain are examples of potential healthcare data management systems.[33,39]

Using Blockchain to Improve Public Health Monitoring

Blockchain technology offers the chance to restructure the healthcare system and enhance the calibre of its offerings through the exchange of health-related data across numerous stakeholders, including patients, physicians, hospitals, and the government, while guaranteeing information security and selective privacy. It additionally offers a way to facilitate genuine patient-centered data sharing by other stakeholders, which can assist with remote management and monitoring of general health status, thus reinforcing disease surveillance systems in any nation for imminent chances of outbreak leading to local and global health emergencies. An optimal system for implementing public health surveillance in the context of such enhanced scalability, security, interoperability, and authenticity is, therefore, a blockchain-based real-time surveillance system. The features of blockchain technology are a good candidate to improve Global health security and networking capabilities, as it provides privacy for the health information of an individual patient, which can facilitate healthcare research.[40]

A blockchain-based decentralised care records network records all data and transaction changes with real-time updates at every network node involved. This manages the data records so that any information is kept and cannot be changed or removed at one node without the other nodes' knowledge. As a result, this feature of blockchain technology, as seen in healthcare surveillance, fosters independence and transparency within the network (WN) system. It also likely has the potential to improve the quality of healthcare services for shared data interflow between all stakeholders by offering interoperable, immutable, highly secure, affordable, and rapid delivery access. Additionally, the speed at which health record passages are occurring makes blockchain technology even more prominent. Blockchain-based surveillance solutions guarantee the methodical gathering and evaluation of data as well as the prompt distribution of information to all relevant parties so that appropriate action can be taken. In order to promote disease surveillance, infectious disease control, and the prevention of epidemic spread, it enhances the quality of public epidemiologic monitoring pertaining to infectious and noncommunicable illnesses in national health systems.[33,41]

Blockchain in e-Healthcare to Customers

The current systems for electronic medical records are built to serve only one hospital. Whenever a patient tries to get medical facilities at other hospitals, the majority of the time, electronic medical records cannot be integrated from different hospitals, which means that another hospital is not able to access the patient's emerging medical profile. As such, minimum benefits can be rendered to such patients. Additionally, the hospitals are unable to handle more from other hospitals for e-healthcare facilities and patients do not trust data security and privacy due to the inferiority of the software used. These problems are sourced from three main issues that include completeness of data, sources, and status of information, and data security in sharing.

Therefore, the e-healthcare system requires patient records with accuracy and completeness of data. Unlike many e-healthcare systems, which require multiple authenticated individuals to access or authenticate patient information, data from the blockchain is available to anyone else who has permission to use the blockchain architecture. The networked features of the healthcare industry will be solved using this system whereby these elements are visible and transparent to patients as well as all stakeholders via data usage.[42]

Blockchain in Medicine Management and Healthcare Administration

Using its intrinsic properties, blockchain can enable participants in the healthcare ecosystem to exchange patient, clinical information, and treatment while maintaining confidentiality by providing information provenance and suitability. An immutable log combined with availability across providers and treatment sites completes the administration use case for patients without sacrificing accessibility. Blockchain possesses characteristics that enable healthcare systems administrators to enhance the degree of authentication, confidentiality, accountability, and data exchange – all key factors when dealing with sensitive information. The incorporation of localised databases to enable the design of a modularity-based healthcare system enables interoperability, system convenience, and flexibility.[43] The medicine management system with blockchain enables medical stakeholders to access the network as executives or scientists. Implementation of medical records as blockchain also enables competent and sufficient risk analysis to detect blockchains from different relevant domains, develop new therapies and medicines, or enable precision medicine.

Blockchain in Telemedicine and Telehealth

The legitimacy of telemedicine and telehealth services can be enhanced with the use of blockchain technology. By using a decentralised management strategy with blockchain backing, telehealth, and telemedicine become more decentralised, safe, transparent, traceable, trustworthy, and foolproof. It encourages telehealth and telemedicine services to assist remote healthcare services in order to systematically avoid and manage the spread of pandemics and chronic diseases while making the best use of limited resources in hospitals.[44]

This system allows confident care monitoring, diagnosis, and treatment of remote patients as a cost-effective service by reducing patient reach in addition to workforce limitation, enhancing technology capabilities, and minimising physician, staff, or patient exposure to pandemic disease. Through the use of information communication and computation technology (ICCT), telehealth and telemedicine enhance the quality of medical services by giving patients access to preventive education, support networks, and health awareness. Many authenticity-based improvements, such as the infallible establishment and provenance of clinical data, the legitimacy of agent users requesting patient data, working-based device identification for remote patient monitoring, firewalls to protect patient anonymity, and payment settlement, can be enforced by integrating the current telehealth and telemedicine ecosystem with standard blockchain technology.[45]

Blockchain in Managing Medical Imaging

Blockchain technology gives us a unique ability to create an anonymous ledger with optional proof-of-presence to the participants, if necessary. That is, this characteristic enables blockchain technology to facilitate the decentralised and interoperable health system sharing of medical images multi-organisationally, under patient control, without central authority consent. Before digital imaging was made possible by high-speed network connectivity and blockchain-based image storage and sharing, medical image copies were physically stored on CDs or DVDs and sent between consumers and providers. Since this is an intrinsically wasteful and inefficient system, the solution is to encrypt a digital asset on the optical medium, which is frequently only read once during importation at the receiving location. Each stage of the procedure might be isolated. Furthermore, the fact that these photographs cannot be misplaced, destroyed, or intercepted during transit puts an undue burden on the patient. Research, teleradiology, implanted medical device tracking, picture sharing of direct patient ownership of images, and artificial intelligence are a few examples of particular medical imaging-related possible uses for blockchain technology.[46]

Blockchain in Developing Smart Healthcare Systems

In order to address the issues with traditional smart healthcare and continue expanding applications of user-centred smart healthcare systems, such as a multi-party medical alliance chain made up of the government, businesses, and society, blockchain and smart healthcare conduct cross-disciplinary research and leverage the benefits of blockchain in information sharing, data security, and privacy conservation. This system demonstrates how blockchain technology can be used in healthcare in an automated and intelligent manner.[33]

Smart healthcare systems exploit the underlying technologies of ICCT, such as Artificial Intelligence & Machine learning, big data and business Intelligence, Cloud computing, IoT, Wireless sensor networks, Robotic surgery, wearable and mobile technology, information storage, etc. Blockchain technology and smart healthcare systems enhance security features such as data availability and authorisation to stakeholders in a distributed, decentralised, and centralised setting as well as confidentiality and integrity.[33] ICCT underlying technologies and blockchain further underscore the need for secured electronic health records, with ICCT enabling easier sharing and access, coupled with a secured but quicker method of medical information exchange in the current scenario.[47]

Blockchain in Information Systems for Healthcare

The role of blockchain information systems in the hospital industry would be to integrate subsystems horizontally and vertically so that they bring reliable management information, efficient patterns of delivery, and effective integrated and inter-organisational information management for healthcare organisations as well as the healthcare systems of the country. The blockchain technology, in this instance, can be used as a bridge that enables different healthcare information systems to share records for information transactions. It allows team members and other stakeholders to transfer data securely and transparently between each other while ensuring you log the history of what they traded and when. Instead of a lone, hackable computer, records are kept on multiple computers. Because this information is extremely difficult to tamper with or erase, it provides the other part of that code: the immutability feature. Another way in which the information management process offers value is because it guarantees that all the information entered into the blockchain-based healthcare solution is immutable, and thus creates a landscape of trust between team members.[48]

Limitations of Blockchain in Healthcare Industry

Using blockchain technology in the healthcare industry comes with limitations, which are discussed below.

The data must be accessible at any time and from any location while still adhering to the patient's desired access-control policies. In the meanwhile, different locations and types of data may require different expressions for access-control policies. As a result, establishing universal guidelines for data accessibility is difficult. Permissioned blockchains have the drawback of being consortium-oriented, which means that once established, they cannot be made globally (i.e., a single consortium with common governance).

Although it is crucial from a medical standpoint that healthcare data be unchangeable, due to their extremely sensitive nature, such data cannot be completely unchangeable on a chain (unless encrypted). In fact, many of the current cryptographic infrastructures around the world face an existential threat from quantum computing. Some specific implications of data availability may come as a surprise, such as the impact on the patient's relatives of storing genomic data on the blockchain. In this sense, a lot of focus should be placed on creatively designing on- and off-chain data structures, interoperability methods between ledger and off-chain data storages, and privacy-preserving protocols.[1,49]

It does not guarantee that the right (majority Share) State is held by every peer in a network. Malicious attacks or malfunctions in hardware or software can render a peer invalid. Nevertheless, the peer may still be linked to the network in the event of a partial or complete failure. In this manner, even if some nodes are rogue, the user or client must still receive accurate information from the blockchain. Policy and other procedures for querying the blockchain nodes are essential for obtaining and reading reliable responses from the blockchain.[1]

Using off-chain data storage (for data storage or for performing calculations over the healthcare data) and membership services in the case of a permissioned blockchain increases the risk of a single point of failure. Cryptography (symmetric/asymmetric encryption, digital signatures, threshold encryption/homomorphic encryption), decentralising the data-storage computer/membership service, or trusted third parties are some ways to mitigate this limitation of the solution.[1,50]

It may not be that easy to satisfy healthcare requirements by using the technology. So, this means filling the gap between practical needs and technology capabilities may be needed. Even though distributed ledger technology is emerging as a great field of study within the research community, many shortcomings have already been identified, such as scalability, bounded data storage capacity, immutability issues related to the distributed ledger itself, the legal obligation for opting out from data, and standardisation.

The business logic in the form of a contract cannot be designed and verified fully automatically, so human intervention is needed here. The assigned individual should possess domain knowledge and be skilled (which means that the rules need to be created based on the use-case scenario). Also, the implementation of smart contracts must be verified to ensure compliance with all required principles.[51]

Conclusion

Abstract blockchain technology can solve long-standing issues by transforming data management, security, transparency, and efficiency in healthcare. Decentralisation, traceability, immutability, transparency, and improved privacy (the core characteristics of blockchain) can build a strong digital healthcare ecosystem. Blockchain removes the middleman, allowing health data to be exchanged freely and securely, all while maintaining patient privacy with identity access management tools that keep their information secure.

The framework provided by blockchain can help transform the transport of personalised healthcare records and strengthen security within the system while also improving its functionality and interoperability based on technology for innovations in future healthcare. At a more advanced level, some applications of blockchain are already disrupting patient data management, drug traceability, and medical device tracking while also enabling cryptocurrency payments and complimenting or supporting the healthcare IoT for real-time monitoring and care.

The future scope of blockchain in healthcare is vast. Blockchain can considerably improve healthcare delivery, from security and authentication to clinical trials, precision medicine, and personalised healthcare services. It offers the potential to enhance public health surveillance and transform administrative processes like telehealth, medical imaging, and the administration of health data. Blockchain technology can further help create a more intelligent and connected healthcare system by providing e-health services and telemedicine to patients in the quickest way possible.

If we may say so, some of the limitations are scalability, complicated implementation processes, regulatory issues, and stakeholder adoption. Even with these limitations, the outlook of blockchain in healthcare is bright since groundbreaking innovations are constantly pushing the envelope and transforming digital health to new dimensions. Blockchain can serve as one of the cornerstones in the transition to a more efficient, transparent, patient-centered healthcare system that opens up a new era for secure, interoperable, and tailored healthcare solutions if integrated effectively.

References

1 Narikimilli, Naga Ramya Sravanthi, Anup Kumar, Antara Debnath Antu, and Bin Xie. "Blockchain applications in healthcare–a review and future perspective." In *Blockchain–ICBC 2020: Third International Conference, Held as Part of the Services Conference Federation, SCF 2020*, Honolulu, HI, USA, September 18–20, 2020, Proceedings 3, pp. 198–218. Springer International Publishing, 2020.

2 Diaz Araque, Evelyne. "Active cyber defense in the healthcare sector." (2023). https://commons.clarku.edu/graduate_school_professional_studies/17

3 Holmgren, A. Jay, Moritz Esdar, Jens Hüsers, and João Coutinho-Almeida. "Health information exchange: Understanding the policy landscape and future of data interoperability." *Yearbook of Medical Informatics* 32, no. 01 (2023): 184–194.

4 Zhang, Rongen, Amrita George, Jongwoo Kim, Veneetia Johnson, and Balasubramaniam Ramesh. "Benefits of blockchain initiatives for value-based care: A proposed framework." *Journal of Medical Internet Research* 21, no. 9 (2019): e13595.

5 Yaqoob, Ibrar, Khaled Salah, Raja Jayaraman, and Yousof Al-Hammadi. "Blockchain for healthcare data management: Opportunities, challenges, and future recommendations." *Neural Computing and Applications* (2022): 1–16.

6 Anwar, Sidra, Sadia Anayat, Sheeza Butt, Saher Butt, and Muhammad Saad. "Generation analysis of blockchain technology: Bitcoin and Ethereum." *International Journal of Information Engineering and Electronic Business (IJIEEB)* 12, no. 4 (2020): 30–39.

7 Andrew, J., Deva Priya Isravel, K. Martin Sagayam, Bharat Bhushan, Yuichi Sei, and Jennifer Eunice. "Blockchain for healthcare systems: Architecture, security challenges, trends, and future directions." *Journal of Network and Computer Applications* 215 (2023): 103633.

8 Acharjamayum, Irani, Ripon Patgiri, and Dhruwajita Devi. "Blockchain: A tale of peer to peer security." In *2018 IEEE Symposium Series on Computational Intelligence (SSCI)*, pp. 609–617. IEEE, 2018.

9 Lashkari, Bahareh, and Petr Musilek. "A comprehensive review of blockchain consensus mechanisms." *IEEE Access* 9 (2021): 43620–43652.

10 Srivastava, Saijshree, Surya Vikram Singh, Rudrendra Bahadur Singh, and Himanshu Kumar Shukla. "Digital transformation of healthcare: A blockchain study." *International Journal of Innovative Science, Engineering & Technology* 8, no. 5 (2021): 414–425.

11 Mackey, Tim K., Tsung-Ting Kuo, Basker Gummadi, Kevin A. Clauson, George Church, Dennis Grishin, Kamal Obbad, Robert Barkovich, and Maria Palombini. "'Fit-for-purpose?'–challenges and opportunities for applications of blockchain technology in the future of healthcare." *BMC Medicine* 17 (2019): 1–17.

12 Musamih, Ahmad, Khaled Salah, Raja Jayaraman, Junaid Arshad, Mazin Debe, Yousof Al-Hammadi, and Samer Ellahham. "A blockchain-based approach for drug traceability in the healthcare supply chain." *IEEE Access* 9 (2021): 9728–9743.

13 Sahu, Dipansu, Namita Tiwari, and Meenu Chawla. "Blockchain as a solution for electronic health record management: A comprehensive review." In *2024 IEEE International Students' Conference on Electrical, Electronics and Computer Science (SCEECS)*, pp. 1–6. IEEE, 2024.

14 Sankar, Lakshmi Siva, M. Sindhu, and M. Sethumadhavan. "Survey of consensus protocols on blockchain applications." In *2017 4th International Conference on Advanced Computing and Communication Systems (ICACCS)*, pp. 1–5. IEEE, 2017.

15 Shen, Bingqing, Jingzhi Guo, and Yilong Yang. "MedChain: Efficient healthcare data sharing via blockchain." *Applied Sciences* 9, no. 6 (2019): 1207.

16 Thwin, Thein Than, and Sangsuree Vasupongayya. "Blockchain-based access control model to preserve privacy for personal health record systems." *Security and Communication Networks* 2019, no. 1 (2019): 8315614.

17 Lim, Shu Yun, Pascal Tankam Fotsing, Abdullah Almasri, Omar Musa, Miss Laiha Mat Kiah, Tan Fong Ang, and Reza Ismail. "Blockchain technology the identity management and authentication service disruptor: A survey." *International Journal on Advanced Science, Engineering and Information Technology* 8, no. 4-2 (2018): 1735–1745.

18 Sharma, Ashutosh, Sarishma, Ravi Tomar, Naveen Chilamkurti, and Byung-Gyu Kim. "Blockchain-based smart contracts for internet of medical things in e-healthcare." *Electronics* 9, no. 10 (2020): 1609.

19 Kumar, Tanesh, Vidhya Ramani, Ijaz Ahmad, An Braeken, Erkki Harjula, and Mika Ylianttila. "Blockchain utilization in healthcare: Key requirements and challenges." In *2018 IEEE 20th International Conference on e-Health Networking, Applications and Services (Healthcom)*, pp. 1–7. IEEE, 2018.

20 Leeming, Gary, James Cunningham, and John Ainsworth. "A ledger of me: Personalizing healthcare using blockchain technology." *Frontiers in Medicine* 6 (2019): 171.

21 Cernian, Alexandra, Bogdan Tiganoaia, Ioan Sacala, Adrian Pavel, and Alin Iftemi. "PatientDataChain: A blockchain-based approach to integrate personal health records." *Sensors* 20, no. 22 (2020): 6538.

22 Kumar, Naveen, and M. Dakshayini. "Secure sharing of health data using hyperledger fabric based on blockchain technology." In *2020 International Conference on Mainstreaming Block Chain Implementation (ICOMBI)*, pp. 1–5. IEEE, 2020.

23 Gupta, Sunil, Hitesh Kumar Sharma, and Monit Kapoor. *Blockchain for secure healthcare using the Internet of Medical Things (IoMT)*. Springer, 2023.

24 Tith, Dara, Joong-Sun Lee, Hiroyuki Suzuki, W. M. A. B. Wijesundara, Naoko Taira, Takashi Obi, and Nagaaki Ohyama. "Patient consent management by a purpose-based consent model for electronic health record based on blockchain technology." *Healthcare Informatics Research* 26, no. 4 (2020): 265–273.

25 Mondal, Susmita, Mehak Shafi, Sumeet Gupta, and Sachin Kumar Gupta. "Blockchain-based secure architecture for electronic healthcare record management." *GMSARN International Journal* 16, no. 4 (2022): 413–426.

26 Jabbar, Rateb, Noora Fetais, Moez Krichen, and Kamel Barkaoui. "Blockchain technology for healthcare: Enhancing shared electronic health record interoperability and integrity." In *2020 IEEE International Conference on Informatics, IoT, and Enabling Technologies (ICIoT)*, pp. 310–317. IEEE, 2020.

27 Agrawal, Divyansh, Sachin Minocha, Suyel Namasudra, and Amir H. Gandomi. "A robust drug recall supply chain management system using hyper ledger blockchain ecosystem." *Computers in Biology and Medicine* 140 (2022): 105100.

28 Katuwal, Gajendra J., Sandip Pandey, Mark Hennessey, and Bishal Lamichhane. "Applications of blockchain in healthcare: Current landscape & challenges." *arXiv preprint arXiv:1812.02776* (2018).

29 Alkhader, Walaa, Khaled Salah, Andrei Sleptchenko, Raja Jayaraman, Ibrar Yaqoob, and Mohammed Omar. "Blockchain-based decentralized digital manufacturing and supply for COVID-19 medical devices and supplies." *IEEE Access* 9 (2021): 137923–137940.

30 Azzawi, Mustafa Abdullah, Rosilah Hassan, and Khairul Azmi Abu Bakar. "A review on Internet of Things (IoT) in healthcare." *International Journal of Applied Engineering Research* 11, no. 20 (2016): 10216–10221.

31 Majumder, Sumit, Tapas Mondal, and M. Jamal Deen. "Wearable sensors for remote health monitoring." *Sensors* 17, no. 1 (2017): 130.

32 Ratta, Pranav, Amanpreet Kaur, Sparsh Sharma, Mohammad Shabaz, and Gaurav Dhiman. "Application of blockchain and internet of things in healthcare and medical sector: Applications, challenges, and future perspectives." *Journal of Food Quality* 2021, no. 1 (2021): 7608296.

33 Aithal, P. S., and Edwin Dias. "Innovations in the healthcare industry using blockchain technology: Concept, application areas, and research agendas." In Borah, Malaya Dutta, Zhang, Peng, Deka, Ganesh Chandra (eds), *Prospects of Blockchain Technology for Accelerating Scientific Advancement in Healthcare,* IGI Global, pp. 48–83, 2022.

34 Cerchione, Roberto, Piera Centobelli, Emanuela Riccio, Stefano Abbate, and Eugenio Oropallo. "Blockchain's coming to hospital to digitalize healthcare services: Designing a distributed electronic health record ecosystem." *Technovation* 120 (2023): 102480.

35 Shae, Zonyin, and Jeffrey J.P. Tsai. "On the design of a blockchain platform for clinical trial and precision medicine." In *2017 IEEE 37th International Conference on Distributed Computing Systems (ICDCS)*, pp. 1972–1980. IEEE, 2017.

36 Singh, Bhupinder, and Christian Kaunert. "Blockchain framework for precision medicine, clinical trials, and genomic biomarkers discovery: Focuses on monitoring and managing data in health dimensions." In Kittisak Wongmahesak, Roy Rillera Marzo (eds), *AI Technologies and Advancements for Psychological Well-Being and Healthcare*, pp. 255–288. New York: IGI Global, 2025.

37 Shae, Zonyin, and Jeffrey Tsai. "Transform blockchain into distributed parallel computing architecture for precision medicine." In *2018 IEEE 38th International Conference on Distributed Computing Systems (ICDCS)*, pp. 1290–1299. IEEE, 2018.

38 Aithal, P. S., and Architha Aithal. "Blockchain technology status and future research opportunities in various areas of the healthcare industry." *International Journal of Health Sciences and Pharmacy (IJHSP)* 5, no. 1 (2021): 130–150.

39 Zaabar, Bessem, Omar Cheikhrouhou, Faisal Jamil, Meryem Ammi, and Mohamed Abid. "HealthBlock: A secure blockchain-based healthcare data management system." *Computer Networks* 200 (2021): 108500.

40 Bhattacharya, Sudip, Amarjeet Singh, and Md Mahbub Hossain. "Strengthening public health surveillance through blockchain technology." *AIMS Public Health* 6, no. 3 (2019): 326.

41 Gul, M. Junaid, Barathi Subramanian, Anand Paul, and Jeonghong Kim. "Blockchain for public health care in smart society." *Microprocessors and Microsystems* 80 (2021): 103524.

42 Singla, Deepak, and Sanjeev Kumar Rana. "A systematic review on blockchain-based e-healthcare for collaborative environment." In *International Conference on Emergent Converging Technologies and Biomedical Systems*, pp. 361–376. Singapore: Springer Nature Singapore, 2022.

43 Dash, Sachikanta, Pradosh Kumar Gantayat, and Rajendra Kumar Das. "Blockchain technology in healthcare: Opportunities and challenges." *Blockchain Technology: Applications and Challenges* (2021): 97–111.

44 Ahmad, Raja Wasim, Khaled Salah, Raja Jayaraman, Ibrar Yaqoob, Samer Ellahham, and Mohammed Omar. "The role of blockchain technology in telehealth and telemedicine." *International Journal of Medical Informatics* 148 (2021): 104399.

45 Koshechkin, Konstantin, Georgy Lebedev, George Radzievsky, Ralf Seepold, and Natividad Madrid Martinez. "Blockchain technology projects to provide telemedical services: Systematic review." *Journal of Medical Internet Research* 23, no. 8 (2021): e17475.

46 De Aguiar, Erikson J., Alyson J. Dos Santos, Rodolfo I. Meneguette, E. Robson, and Jó Ueyama. "A blockchain-based protocol for tracking user access to shared medical imaging." *Future Generation Computer Systems* 134 (2022): 348–360.

47 Shukla, Rashmi G., Anuja Agarwal, and Shekhar Shukla. "Blockchain-powered smart healthcare system." In *Handbook of Research on Blockchain Technology*, pp. 245–270. Academic Press, 2020.

48 Prybutok, Victor R., and Brian Sauser. "Theoretical and practical applications of blockchain in healthcare information management." *Information & Management* 59, no. 6 (2022): 103649.

49 Alzahrani, Ahmed G., Ahmed Alhomoud, and Gary Wills. "A framework of the critical factors for healthcare providers to share data securely using blockchain." *IEEE Access* 10 (2022): 41064–41077.

50 Zhang, Peng, Jules White, Douglas C. Schmidt, Gunther Lenz, and S. Trent Rosenbloom. "FHIRChain: Applying blockchain to securely and scalably share clinical data." *Computational and Structural Biotechnology Journal* 16 (2018): 267–278.

51 Tern, Somboun. "Survey of smart contract technology and application based on blockchain." *Open Journal of Applied Sciences* 11, no. 10 (2021): 1135–1148.

Index